Positive Psychology as Social Change

Robert Biswas-Diener
Editor

Positive Psychology as Social Change

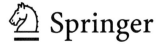 Springer

Editor
Robert Biswas-Diener
SE. Aldercrest Rd. 4625
97222 Milwuakie Oregon
USA
jayajedi@comcast.net

ISBN 978-90-481-9937-2   e-ISBN 978-90-481-9938-9
DOI 10.1007/978-90-481-9938-9
Springer Dordrecht Heidelberg London New York

Printed on acid-free paper

Springer is part of Springer Science+Business Media (www.springer.com)

Editor's Foreword

If you were to bring all of the authors who contributed to this volume and put them in a single room they would argue. In part it is because some of them are, by nature, argumentative. The other reason is that there is not universal agreement about the science of positive psychology. There is no agreement about the best methods for defining and measuring elusive concepts such as happiness or empathy. There is not even total agreement about how to interpret the results of solid peer-reviewed studies. As Scollon and King point out in the opening chapter, psychologists once interpreted the modest correlations between income and subjective well-being to mean that "money does not matter all that much to happiness." In more recent times, according to Scollon and King, scientists have looked at those same correlations and offered an interpretation of this relationship as being "always positive and robust." And so it should come as no surprise that a wide range of academics, hailing from different disciplines and various cultures, might argue about how to best approach the science and application of positive psychology. What is more surprising and—to me at least—more inspiring, is the fact that, despite all the obvious differences, the scholars represented between the pages of this book share in common a desire to engage in a productive dialogue on the topic of the good life. In this way the authors are a reflection of positive psychology itself: Although we have differences and disagreements, we can band together for a higher purpose and work toward the greater good.

For many years this dialogue on the good life focused heavily on personal well-being. This individualistic focus may be the result of the fact that positive psychology is deeply anchored in Western culture. The influence of classical Greek philosophy, the humanistic movement, and the predominance of North American scholars in the early days of modern positive psychology may have set the stage for a discipline that was primarily concerned with researching and intervening at the individual level. To some degree I think we can point to the influence of Ed Diener—my father—to explain the emphasis on individual well-being. He was part of the highly influential positive psychology steering committee in the early days of the field and his area of expertise—subjective well-being—was a natural place to look for a useful positive psychology outcome measure. Optimism, courage, and curiosity might all lead to growth and higher functioning but these, in turn, can be weighed against the gold standard of increases in personal happiness. I suggest no Machiavellian intent on behalf of my father; rather, happiness became a widely used outcome measure precisely because it was useful, sensible, and there were good assessments available. To his credit, my father has turned his attention toward the ways in which well-being intersects public policy and group level flourishing, as illustrated by his chapter in this volume.

Happiness-related measures tend to narrow our attention to the individual level of psychological experience, sometimes at the expense of other legitimate foci for positive psychologists, especially those that are specifically pro-social. Take the case of empathy. Despite the fact that a PsycInfo search reveals that there are more than twice the number of scholarly publications on "empathy" than on "happiness," papers on the latter topic are 33 times more likely to be paired with "positive psychology" as a keyword. In fact, empathy is rarely included in conferences or edited volumes specifically related to positive psychology. By way of illustration, the flagship journal of the field—*Journal of Positive Psychology*—has only two publications on empathy as opposed to 26 on happiness. Similarly, a PsycInfo search on the word "altruism" yields more than 2,300 results of which only five are explicitly coupled with the search term "positive psychology." Compare this to the term "strengths" which is paired with "positive psychology" in nearly 300 cases.

In all fairness, in their 2000 introductory article on positive psychology, Seligman and Csikzsentmihalyi discussed the emerging field as being concerned with both individual well-being and group-level concepts such as civic virtues and positive institutions. This sentiment was echoed again in Seligman's 2009 address to attendees of the conference of the International Positive Psychology Association. In this speech Seligman issued a challenge to measurably increase flourishing around the world. Although, on some level, this may be interpreted to mean the flourishing of individuals the mechanisms by which this goal is achieved must necessarily include group-level interventions, policies, and social change broadly. It is in this spirit that this volume is being published. I feel that positive psychology is at an important turning point: The idea that positive psychology is not a western pursuit alone, that it is not solely about the individual, and that it is not only about happiness are ideas that are gaining purchase. My editorial mission for this volume was to create a platform for scholars to weigh in on various aspects of the idea that positive psychology is about positive social change. As a basic science it is about promoting research and public policy that can be leveraged to enhance social welfare. As an applied science positive psychology is about creating tools and interventions by which we might advance both individual and group-level flourishing. It is my ultimate hope that this volume will become a seminal work for a new generation of positive psychologists who are interested in less individualistic and culturally constrained science.

By the same token I would hope this book offers a hushing counterpoint to those critics who charge positive psychology as being elitist, selfish, western, or individualistic. I took care when assembling contributors to bring on board a truly international cast of scholars. Their voices hail from Singapore, England, Scotland, Australia, Iceland, Germany, Canada, Italy, Norway, India, South Africa, Germany, and the Netherlands, as well as from the United States. Certainly they don't represent every corner of the globe but I am proud of the fact that American contributors are outnumbered by non-Americans in this book. What's more, I wanted to avoid the natural professional trap of believing that psychologists own the monopoly on positive psychology. Although we certainly play an overwhelmingly large role in the field, it is a mistake to overlook the many insights offered by people from other professions. As a result, the contributors to this volume include an anthropologist, a sociologist, coaches and consultants, educators, entrepreneurs, and a computer scientist in addition to research and practice related psychologists. In this way the authors also reflect positive psychology itself: What once was a principally American concern has become a truly global endeavor.

Despite the fact that my editorial mission was to shift the emphasis of positive psychology from individual to group-level well-being, I tasked the authors with a different set of instructions. I believe that if something is worth doing it is also worth having fun while doing. In this vein I asked the authors to take risks. I offered them a platform by which they might present arguments or theory that they might not otherwise get to voice. Gandhi famously introduced his own idea of "7 deadly sins" which included "science without humanity." With this in mind I wanted to offer the contributors a chance to bring some of their humanity to the table in a way that is often drained from more traditional academic works. I encouraged them to take linguistic risks, play with conventional style, and sprinkle humor in their chapters. In some cases, such as the chapters by Nic Marks and George Burns, the authors write in the first person. In others, such as the one by Antonella Delle Fave and Giovanni Fava, the authors present a more formal academic tone but their deep passion for their topic shines through. More than anything else, I wanted to avoid creating a collection that included authors' "staple chapters," the type of fare they can churn out in mildly modified form to reprint in volume after volume. I wanted fresh ideas and presentation and am pleased to report that, without exception, this is exactly what I received as you will soon discover.

What will you find sandwiched between the covers of this book? *Positive Psychology as Social Change* begins with Christie Napa Scollon and Laura King's chapter on folk theories of the good life. The authors do a wonderful job of democratizing science by amplifying the voices of everyday people on the fascinating topic of the good life. Importantly, they ask the question "Do scientists make proper assumptions about people when creating programs of research?" Their chapter is a nice launching point for the rest of the book. After this chapter the book is divided into seven parts. The first is what I think of as cautionary voices. Here Nic Marks and Neil Thin offer two chapters that encourage readers to connect to others. Marks outlines the pressing social issues of the day and offers both interesting ways to think about solving these problems and some actual solutions. Thin weighs in with a sobering critique of the ethnocentric elements of positive psychology and of the prospect of social engineering programs in general. Fortunately, he offers alternative frameworks related to cultural inclusiveness and the importance of looking at individuals within the social context of relationships and societies. He ends with thoughts on public policy, which dovetail nicely with the next part of the book, addressing exactly that topic.

Part II begins with Ed and Carol Diener's chapter on "monitoring psychosocial prosperity." In it the authors extend the recent professional conversation on creating well-being indicators to a more specific policy suggestion that includes candidate variables. George Burns follows with an interesting account of the Gross National Happiness policy of Bhutan, including some good examples of how that government balances competing factors such as environmental development with the well-being of its citizenry. This leads nicely into the following chapter by Tim Kasser on ecological and materialistic values. Kasser argues that a fundamental shift in values needs to occur that will promote both ecological sustainability and personal well-being. Far from being an environmental alarmist, Kasser offers practical examples of change strategies ranging from *time affluence* to restrictions on advertising. Rounding out the section on policy is a chapter on health promotion by Dora Guðrún Guðmundsdóttir. I am particularly intrigued by Guðmundsdóttir's chapter because it is far too seldom that we attend to physical health concerns within positive psychology and far too seldom that health policy looks at positive functioning.

The third part of this book is devoted to the intersection of poverty and positive psychology. This area is one of my personal passions and, indeed, I co-authored the first of two chapters in this part. It is my belief that the study of the emotional quality of life of people living in poverty represents the type of approach that Neil Thin would approve, and helps us gain greater knowledge about where and how social change needs to happen from a bottom-up approach. In this chapter, Lindsey Patterson and I explore the psychological dimensions intervention techniques related to poverty alleviation programs. In particular, we focus heavily on microfinance and the ways it can increase psychological empowerment. Our chapter is, in essence, a companion to that written by Alex Linley and his colleagues. Linley champions the idea of a strengths-based approach to community development and offers a variety of compelling case studies to illustrate how this might be accomplished. One of the unusual elements of this chapter is that Linley's co-authors are personally involved in one of the programs they describe. Rather than raising red flags related to bias and objective science I believe that this is a good example of what Gandhi meant when he advocated "science with humanity." This portion of the book is intended, in part, to remind readers of our obligation to offer both our science and intervention strategies to less privileged groups.

For good or ill, work constitutes an enormous part of how we spend our time. Work, at its best, provides a sense of purpose, economic security, and opportunities for growth. The office is a natural venue for the attention of positive psychologists, not least because much of applied positive psychology happens in the workplace in the form of coaching, consultation, and training. Part IV of this book is focused on positive psychology and organizations. It opens with Nicky Garcea and Alex Linley's chapter on building positive organizations. The strengths-based framework, the emphasis on bottom-up development strategies such as strengths recruitment, and individual strengths development all represent years of actual consulting experience with a wide range of businesses and governmental organizations. This chapter is one of those instances in which no one can criticize the content for being "academic" or otherwise divorced from real-world application. The same is true of the chapter by Traci Fention, the founder of WorldBlu, which certifies businesses as being "democratic." After providing a rationale for creating democratic workplaces Fenton offers extraordinarily clear theoretical guidelines for creating democratic organizations and illustrates these with a real world example of Da Vita, a Fortune 500 company. This part of the book should be a go-to source for any coach or consultant aspiring to use positive psychology in his or her practice.

Part V includes two chapters that introduce two topics that I feel have been somewhat overlooked by positive psychology: empathy and altruism. Both of these topics are inherently positive and their absence from conferences and volumes on positive psychology is conspicuous. Both of these topics are, by their very definition, "other focused" and are, therefore, a conceptual fit for the mission of this book. The first chapter in this portion is by Lara Aknin and her colleagues and concerns pro-social spending. The authors report on a new but growing research on the psychological effects of spending money on others. Importantly, they describe elements of giving that have rarely been explored in research such as factors that predict recipient happiness, how pro-social spending affects team performance, and how spending on others can create a positive feedback loop. The other chapter in this part is on an aspect of empathy known as perspective taking, and is written by Sara Hodges and her colleagues. Together, these authors tackle a complex research literature that spans empathic concern, accuracy, helping behaviors, and developmental psychology, to name just a few portions. They do an excellent job of making a case for the natural development of perspective-taking ability and tie this together with concern for others. Particularly interesting is their discussion of how perspective taking reduces prejudice, making it among the most powerful psychological mechanisms available for widespread social change.

I often find edited academic volumes frustrating. They are, by definition, written by academics. As a researcher I tend to love learning and enjoy asking endless questions but as an interventionist I tend to want more in the way of usable advice for translating research findings into practical tools. I think this is especially important in the case of positive psychology because it is both a basic and applied science. To better address the applied side I invited a number of contributors to weigh in on various intervention strategies for promoting social change. Part VI, which tackles interventions, begins with a chapter on coaching by Sunny Stout Rostron. Rostron offers a departure from the usual fare by presenting a series of interviews with a number of highly respected and influential coaches. For readers interested in how executive coaching can be integrated with positive psychology, and how this professional mode of work can affect positive social change, Rostron's chapter is heaven-sent. It is rare to have access to such a diverse range of professionals working at this high a level, and the interviews are as inspiring as they are informative. The next chapter, by Antonella Della Fave and Giovanni Fava, on positive psychology applications to psychotherapy, provides another exploration of a specific intervention methodology. Della Fave and Fava are world thought leaders in positive psychotherapy. In their chapter, they discuss vital aspects of mental health including

personal agency, responsibility, and a sense of meaning and offer important discussion of cultural caveats. I find their description of their short-term Well-being
Therapy (WBT) and its effectiveness to be particularly useful.

The next chapter in the "intervention" part of the book is on recreation, written
by my doctoral advisor and friend, Joar Vittersø. To pull back the curtain on the editorial process, this was the chapter I had the hardest time placing. Should a chapter
on leisure find a place next to a chapter on folk theories of the good life, or might
it sensibly be included with chapters on intervention techniques? Ultimately, I felt
Vittersø's discussion of recreation was framed as an intervention. At the heart of this
chapter is a provocative and elegant theory of pleasant emotion counter-balanced
against unpleasant engagement states. Vittersø argues that we must move between
these two psychological states for optimal mental health and discusses the role of
leisure pursuits in this context.

The final chapter in the intervention part of the book is on Positive Computing, by
Tomas Sander. I believe this is the seminal article on positive computing and brings
a fundamental part of daily life—the use of technology—into the wider positive
psychology discussion. This, in my opinion, is long overdue. Although Sander envisions far-reaching implications of affective and persuasive computing technologies
he is not a fantasist. He restrains his commentary to the ways in which computers
can potentially help individuals and groups function better. Notably, he brings his
expertise as a computer scientist to the table, discussing ethical issues related to
privacy and other concerns that might not immediately be on the minds of many
positive psychologists. Ultimately, Sander offers a challenge to positive psychology
in that he suggests that there may be ways that technology is actually better than
human intervention in delivering certain positive psychology services. There will,
undoubtedly, be those who are uncomfortable with the idea of a hand-held Personal
Happiness Assistant, but Sander makes an excellent case that it is *when*, not *if*, such
devices will appear in our lives.

The book closes—in my opinion—with a bang. Master storyteller and change
agent Scott Sherman invokes a rallying cry in his chapter, *Change the World*!
Sherman tells two stories, his own, and that of the most dangerous place in the
United States. I will leave it for him to tell the tale, for he does so better than I, but I
still feel compelled to mention the effect of his writing. Sherman is not a rosy-eyed
cheermonger, of the type that Neil Thin warns us against. Instead, Sherman is interested in proof that one person can make a positive impact, and he delivers nicely on
this point.

I would also like to take a moment and point out that although the chapters in
this book cover a huge range of topics by a diverse group of authors in various narrative styles there are two common themes that creep into this volume again and
again. The first is money. Humans are physical creatures shackled to this life by our
bodies. As such, we need a modicum of material comfort to enjoy life. How much
we need, how we use it, and the value we place on getting more of it are all topics
that contributors to this book address. Whether it is the way that wealth factors into
definitions of the good life or how spending money on others impacts happiness,
there is a sense that material concerns are relevant to social change. Social change

may be about increasing material wealth for those in need, or in sharing wealth, or in avoiding the trap of valuation wealth to toxic levels. There is no one correct answer about this sticky issue and so I leave it to the intelligence of the reader to tease your own conclusions out of the chapters that follow. The other theme implicit (and sometimes explicit) in this volume is that science—and positive psychological science in particular—possesses many of the answers to pressing social ills. The contributors in this volume, without exception, believe that a better world is possible. But it is not their instinctual optimism displayed in the pages of this book, it is their expert knowledge of cutting-edge science. In some cases it is anecdotal evidence drawn from years of working with clients while in other instances it is a showcase of careful laboratory research. In each chapter the contributors offer at least one tangible, useable tool by which we can affect positive social change. The only thing not on offer here is an excuse not to use them.

Coventry, UK   Robert Biswas-Diener

Contents

Contributors

Lara B. Aknin University of British Columbia, Vancouver, BC, Canada, laknin@psych.ubc.ca

Avirupa Bhaduri Centre of Applied Positive Psychology, Coventry, UK

Robert Biswas-Diener Centre for Applied Positive Psychology, Coventry, UK; Portland State University, Portland, OR, USA, jayajedi@comcast.net

George W. Burns Hypnotherapy Centre, Milton H. Erickson Institute, Western Australia, Australia, georgeburns@iinet.net.au

Brian A. M. Clark University of Oregon, Eugene, OR, USA, clark13@uoregon.edu

Antonella Delle Fave Università degli Studi di Milano, Milan, Italy, Antonella.dellefave@unimi.it

Ed Diener University of Illinois, Urbana-Champaign, IL, USA; The Gallup Organization, Washington, DC, USA, ediener@uiuc.edu

Carol Diener University of Illinois, Urbana-Champaign, IL, USA

Elizabeth W. Dunn University of British Columbia, Vancouver, BC, Canada, edunn@psych.ubc.ca

Giovanni A. Fava Università degli Studi di Bologna, Bologna, Italy, giovanniandrea.fava@unibo.it

Traci L. Fenton WorldBlu, Inc., Cedar Rapids, Iowa, USA, traci@worldblu.com

Nicky Garcea Centre of Applied Positive Psychology, Coventry, UK, Nicky.garcea@cappeu.com

Reena Govindji Centre of Applied Positive Psychology, Coventry, UK

Dora Guðrún Guðmundsdóttir Public Health Institute of Iceland, Reykjavík, Iceland, dora@publichealth.is

Sara D. Hodges University of Oregon, Eugene, OR 97403, USA,
sdhodges@uoregon.edu

Tim Kasser Knox College, Galesburg, IL, USA, tkasser@know.edu

Laura A. King University of Missouri at Columbia, Columbia, MO, USA,
kingla@missouri.edu

P. Alex Linley Centre of Applied Positive Psychology, Coventry, UK,
Alex.linley@cappeu.com

Nic Marks New Economics Foundation, London, UK,
nic.marks@neweconomics.org

Michael I. Norton Harvard Business School, Boston, MA, USA,
mnorton@hbs.edu

Lindsey Patterson Portland State University, Portland, OR, USA, lbp@pdx.edu

Sunny Stout Rostron Manthano Institute of Learning (Pty) Ltd, Cape Town,
South Africa, express@iafrica.com

Tomas Sander HP Labs, Princeton, NJ 08540, USA, tomas.sander@hp.com

Gillian M. Sandstrom University of British Columbia, Vancouver, BC, Canada,
gsandstrom@psych.ubc.ca

Christie Napa Scollon Singapore Management University, Bras Basah, Singapore,
cscollon@smu.edu.sg

Debasish Sen Sharma Centre of Applied Positive Psychology, Coventry, UK

Scott Sherman Transformative Action Institute, Los Angeles, CA, USA,
ssherman@transformativeaction.org

Neil Thin University of Edinburgh, Edinburgh, Scotland, n.thin@ed.ac.uk

Joar Vittersø University of Tromsø, Tromsø, Norway, joar.vitterso@uit.no

Michael W. Myers University of Tokyo, Tokyo, Japan, myers636@l.u-tokyo.ac.jp

Chapter 1
What People Really Want in Life and Why It Matters: Contributions from Research on Folk Theories of the Good Life

Christie Napa Scollon and Laura A. King

At the heart of social progress is the human capacity to notice a discrepancy between how things are and how they might be. Certainly, such progress requires more than simply this realization. It requires the belief that change is possible and right. It requires social cooperation and work by groups for the common good. But these activities would never occur without someone at some point noticing that things could be better: that profoundly difficult lives could be good and good lives could be better. Thus, the human capacity to imagine and envision a better or ideal life is linked to the emergence of social progress. Of course, this human capacity to imagine a future that is different from current circumstances can also be a force for social change in the opposite direction. When accompanied by greed, hatred for difference, or concern for power and dominance, we can see this capacity reflected in various historical and social atrocities and catastrophes.

In a sense, naïve notions of what constitutes the good life represent the ideals toward which individuals might aspire or actively strive. These naïve conceptions of optimal human functioning reveal the content of common human longings and can tell us against what standards current circumstances are judged.

Certainly, not-so-naïve conceptions of what makes a life good have had enormous impact on human intellectual thought, ethics, and the psychology of well-being. Since Aristotle (and certainly even before), philosophers, religious leaders, and humans more generally have puzzled over what it is that qualifies as a good life. Many thinkers have provided strong statements about how life ought to be lived and what aspects of life qualify it as a good one. Psychology, perhaps especially positive psychology, also provides guidelines in this regard, suggesting, for instance, ways to insure optimal happiness, thriving, or resilience or optimal psychological development, maturity, moral reasoning, etc. Knowledge of these prescriptions for the good life tells us about the values of psychologists, but may miss the ideals that lurk inside each person – the good life as defined by everyday people for themselves. The research we review here takes up just this question: What makes a life good for everyday people and what do these conceptions of the good life tell us about the

L.A. King (✉)
University of Missouri at Columbia, Columbia, MO, USA
e-mail: kingla@missouri.edu

R. Biswas-Diener (ed.), *Positive Psychology as Social Change*,
DOI 10.1007/978-90-481-9938-9_1, © Springer Science+Business Media B.V. 2011

values that everyday people wish to see realized in their own lives? Do everyday people think that money buys happiness? Do they privilege happiness over other values such as, the experience of meaning? Do they believe that career success is more important than relationships? In what ways does the naïve notion of the good life converge with psychological research and in what ways does it diverge? Notions of the good life are certainly contextualized in culture. How does culture influence naïve notion of the good life? Before describing the results of a number of studies on these provocative questions, we briefly discuss the value of studying folk theories of the good life.

situational desires   ~situational ethics

Why Study Folk Theories of the Good Life?

The prudential argument. There are at least three reasons to study folk theories of the good life. The first is prudential. As the title of this volume suggests, one of the goals of positive psychology is to improve lives. However, before we can begin to understand how people strive to achieve the good life or the resources that they draw upon in their pursuit of the good life, it is important to understand how people answer the question of "What makes a life good?" As positive psychology articulates its view of the good life, lay persons may well have a different, and possibly opposing, vision of the world (Kasser, 2004).

Folk theories and scientific theories complement each other. Fletcher (1995) has argued that scientific theories that take into account folk theories have the potential to produce insights beyond common sense. Moreover, the divergence of folk and scientific theories is more than an aha! opportunity to show that lay thinking is fallible. In fact, the divergence between folk and scientific theories is often where the action is. For example, part of the excitement about the early scientific finding that money and happiness are only weakly correlated was that, at the time, there was widespread belief that this finding ran counter to people's intuitions. For example, Myers and Diener (1995) included the belief that wealthy people are happier as one of the myths of happiness (see also Myers, 2000). Our research was the first to show how folk theories of the good life were actually far closer to scientific theories than researchers realized, although newer research has begun to show money does matter more than we (both scientists and laypersons) think.

On a more practical level, an understanding of the convergence and divergence among folk and scientific theories may further the aims of subjective well-being research by highlighting what everyday people already know or don't know. Even if a folk theory happens to be factually incorrect, it can serve as a good starting point for helping people to understand the scientific theory. Examining folk theories explicitly allows us to identify how and when psychologists have gotten human beings wrong. That is, folk theories are an excellent place to uncover the subtle misanthropic bias that sometimes creeps into psychological research (itself a central goal of positive psychology, Sheldon & King, 2001).

Folk theories as opportunity. If folk theories are "instruments of culture" as Bruner (1990) noted, then they seem particularly suited for examining the good life, both within and across cultures. After all, folk theories of the good life are probably more strongly shaped by culture than, say, folk theories about electricity and illness (although there are a wide range of beliefs on these topics as well). Rather than treat folk theories as error-ridden sources of information, we view them as a rich source of meaning – an intersection of individual values, local meaning systems, and shared cultural beliefs (Fletcher, 1995). As such, folk theories exert an enormous amount of influence on behavior and judgment (Bruner, 1990; Fletcher, 1995; Harkness & Super, 1996). For example, differences in the beliefs about the malleability of personality influence attributions for behavior, desire for revenge, views toward punishment (Chiu, Dweck, Tong, & Fu, 1997; Chui, Hong, & Dweck, 1997).

In terms of SWB research, a culture that defines the good life in terms of wealth has different priorities and therefore behaviors and judgments than a culture that defines the good life in terms of happiness. Thus, understanding how different cultures define the good life might lead us to clues as to why some societies are more conducive to happiness than others. Clearly, different societies have different values, so why shouldn't there be cultural differences in folk theories of the good life? At the same time, there may be some good which is so desirable that people around the world agree on the virtue of that good. Happiness may be one of these.

Our Research Paradigm

In all of our studies of the good life, we asked participants to judge the desirability and moral goodness of another person's life based on circumscribed attributes which we manipulated. Specifically, participants viewed a "Career Survey" ostensibly completed by another individual rating aspects of his or her job. In King and Napa (1998), the target survey was manipulated to reflect a life of high or low happiness, high or low wealth, and high or low meaning. All other target information was held constant across experimental conditions. In subsequent studies, we altered the various attributes included in the target survey, but the basic design of the study remained the same. After viewing the survey, participants made judgments about the target's life.

Independent variables. At this point some consideration of our independent variables is warranted. As noted above, in our research, we have generally manipulated three key variables, happiness, meaning, and money. These characteristics were chosen because they reflected the interests of psychologists and assumptions that psychologists had made about people. Clearly, a great deal of research within positive psychology has focused on happiness and ways to make people happier. From a psychological perspective, it is difficult to argue against the importance of happiness. Who doesn't want to be happy? Yet, the empirical question remained to be addressed: Do everyday people view happiness as an important aspect of the good life?

Furthermore, crossing happiness with differing levels of the experience of meaning in life allowed us to examine what was then (and continues to be) a burgeoning debate in the well-being literature, the contrast between hedonic and eudaimonic conceptions of well-being (e.g., Biswas-Diener, Kashdan, & King, 2009; Kashdan, Biswas-Diener, & King, 2008; Ryff & Singer, 2008). Hedonic well-being is essentially how an individual feels about his or her life; in a very general way this construct maps on to personal happiness. Following Aristotle's contrast between hedonistic happiness and eudaimonic happiness (for Aristotle, happiness that emerges out of living in accord with one's daimon), some psychologists had asserted that well-being ought to be understood not simply as hedonic feelings, but as the positive affect that emerges out of living in accord with one's authentic self (Waterman, 2008), actualizing one's potential (Ryff & Singer, 2008) or from the pursuit of organismic needs (Ryan & Deci, 2001). From the eudaimonic perspective, a life devoted to hedonic happiness runs the danger of a pleasant but meaningless existence. Would everyday people prefer a life of hedonic enjoyment, even if it were devoid of meaning?

Finally, we included income as an independent variable in the design. If there was a lesson in research on SWB prior to 1998 it was that money does not buy happiness. Research had shown that those who value extrinsic goods such as monetary success over more intrinsic values such as relatedness, autonomy, and competence were more likely to suffer both psychologically and physically (Kasser & Ryan, 1993). Other researchers noted with some surprise the lack of strong relationship between income and happiness. Such results were often described as having important relevance for everyday people who might think that money buys happiness. Thus, it was of interest to explore the question "Do everyday people think money does buy happiness?" In sum, then, in response to the issues that were relatively hot at the time, we manipulated levels of these three variables in the lives of the targets to be judged. Rather impersonal target lives were then evaluated by participants in terms of their "goodness." We defined goodness in two ways, the desirability of a life and its moral character. These dependent measures themselves now warrant some discussion.

Dependent measures. Faced with a very limited amount of information about a target life (see King & Napa, 1998 for a sample target form), participants were asked to rate the life on a variety of evaluative dimensions. First, they rated how "good" they thought the life was, how desirable it was, and how much they would like to live the life in question. Second, they rated the moral goodness of the life in two ways, by rating it on the descriptor "moral" and by rating the likelihood that the target *was to go to heaven.* This last evaluation provided a rather revealing glimpse of naïve notions of moral goodness. Individuals might balk at judging a life that was presented in so limited a way. They might feel especially uncomfortable casting moral judgments on an anonymous target. Yet, this question of whether the target was likely to go to heaven allowed us to sidestep some of these qualms, allowing participants to, in effect, note that although the participant might not find the life particularly objectionable, God wouldn't like it. Interestingly, the vast majority of participants answered this question. Across all of our studies and thousands of participants, only about 3% of respondents returned the survey without answering this question. The mean on the ratings, which ranged from 1 (likely to go to hell) to 10 (likely to go to heaven), typically hovered around 6.50. In a sense, just as the Protestant work ethic considers earthly success as a mysterious sign of God's good graces, this rating allowed participants to render their own similarly mysterious evaluation.

Putting the folk into folk theories: The participants. Before sharing the results of these investigations, it makes sense to give a bit of information about the participants who have taken part in these studies. The goal of studying folk concepts of the good life is to uncover the ways that everyday people think of the optimal human life. Thus, one might wonder who the everyday people were who participated in these studies. First, of course, some of the participants were college students. Although the use of students in psychological research is often criticized, it is worth noting that, contrary to popular belief, college students are, in fact, people. Second, we recruited participants from a wide variety of venues – in the waiting rooms of jury duty selections in Dallas County, TX (King & Napa, 1998; Twenge & King, 2005), in the waiting areas of major US airports (Scollon & King, 2004), and around downtown areas, near public transportation stations, and around local neighborhoods (Scollon & Wirtz, 2010). Participation in these studies takes approximately 5 min, which provided participants time to look over the target life and judge it accordingly.

What We Know: A Review of Research on Folk Theories of the Good Life

What makes a life good? In 1998, we noted that researchers often assumed, without empirical knowledge, that people think money is an important component of the good life. We set out to investigate how people weigh the characteristics of happiness, meaningfulness, and wealth in determining the overall value of a life. Using our Career Survey paradigm, we found that Americans overwhelmingly defined the good life in terms of happiness and meaning. Not only was happiness considered desirable, but happy people were judged as more likely to go to heaven in our studies. Further, the very best, most desirable, and morally good life was a life of happiness and meaning. Wealth, on the other hand, was relatively unimportant to people's notions of the good life.

Some intriguing generational differences also emerged in that older community adults gave more weight to wealth than college students, reflecting a less naïve and romantic world view. An interesting interaction also emerged among our independent variables of happiness, meaning, and wealth in judging the moral goodness, but not desirability, of a life. Respondents considered the happy, meaningful, and rich life, someone who "had it all," as most likely bound for heaven. Meanwhile, the poor, unhappy, person whose life had little meaning was judged harshly. The results were consistent with a Protestant view of morality. According to Weber's (1930/1976) analysis of the Protestant work ethic, a happy life with earthly economic success was a sign that the person was looked upon favorably by God. Such findings highlight how shared cultural beliefs and local meanings converge in folk theories, and that these can be captured using our paradigm.

More generally, King and Napa (1998) showed some convergence among folk concepts of the good life and the scientific research on subjective well-being. Early SWB research found the correlation between income and happiness to be modest (typically about 0.17–0.21 according to Lucas & Dyrenforth, 2006 meta-analysis). In addition, the very rich are somewhat happier than middle-class folks, but not hugely (Diener, Horwitz, & Emmons, 1985). Thus, it seemed that people, Americans at least, were not prioritizing wealth over happiness and meaning, as some early SWB researchers had feared. Furthermore, everyday folk were not hedonists who eschewed meaning for pleasure. Rather, for the everyday person in our study meaning and happiness were each robust predictors of lives being judged as good.

Since then, the research on wealth and happiness has taken an interesting twist. Whereas early researchers interpreted correlations of 0.20 between income and well-being as small and inconsequential, more recently, the pendulum has swung back somewhat. For example, in 1995 Myers and Diener included in their "myths about happiness" the belief that money could buy happiness. By 2008 Lucas, Dyrenforth, and Diener's myths of happiness included "small correlations between income and happiness [mean] that the rich are barely happier than the poor" (p. 2004). Researchers now recognize that the relation between wealth and well-being is, in fact, always positive and robust. Lucas and Schimmack (2009) have argued that the correlational methods for studying wealth and happiness underestimate the real effects of wealth. When comparing the difference in happiness among rich and poor groups, the effect size becomes quite large. Even if the absolute size of the effect is not disputed, Lucas and Dyrenforth (2005) noted that effects of similar size for marriage on happiness have been touted as important and large. Ironically, despite a newer take on income and happiness, researchers still rely on old assumptions about lay theories of the good life. Lucas and Schimmack (2009), for instance, concluded that "No psychologist or economist has proposed a value for the correlation between income and happiness that he or she believes would match people's intuition...it is possible that it is not the layperson's intuition that is flawed, but psychologists' and economists' interpretation of this effect" (p. 75). In our view, the typical correlations between income and wealth are just about on the mark for people's intuition. In this case, scientists have gotten people's intuitions wrong.

Is the good life the easy life? As a follow-up to our first set of studies, we examined the role of effort in relation to happiness, meaning, and wealth in folk theories of the good life (Scollon & King, 2004). After all, a number of scientific theories about optimal functioning include effort or hard work as a component (e.g., flow, striving). In these studies, the target life was manipulated to be high or low on happiness, meaning, and money, but also, in this case, hard work. Overall, once again, our respondents defined the good life primarily in terms of happiness and meaning and less so in terms of wealth. With regard to effort, however, many Americans tended to equate the good life with the easy life. Effort that leads to fulfillment was valued, but only if it did not compromise leisure time and was not energy depleting. Thus, in this series of studies, the folk concepts diverged from scientific theories such as flow (Csikszentmihalyi, 1990), eudaimonia (Waterman, 2008), and competence and mastery (White, 1959). In other words, lay persons and scientists alike may converge on the components of a life well-lived, but they diverge in their views of *how* to reach the good life. Lay persons, it seems, are willing to work hard and desire effortful engagement, but only if it is easy! Just as the lay notion of a good marriage may equate to a lifelong honeymoon, the lay notion of the good life may equate to a very long vacation.

Although these results seem to indicate that folk notions of the place of effort in the good life are inaccurate, it is worth noting that when hard work was portrayed as occurring in the context of happiness it was viewed as part of the good life. This notion, that positive effect is linked with the role of effort in optimal human states is certainly part and parcel of the psychological notion of states such as flow and intrinsic motivation. These states of high effort are, of course, effort paired with enjoyment.

The good life is a relational life. Although initial research using the Career Survey paradigm typically focused on life in general or the work domain, the good life might be understood as encompassing both work and, of course, social relationships. Freud famously noted that a healthy person should have the capacities for love and work, and many philosophical treatments of the good life include both active engagement in work and meaningful social relationships. Yet, modern people often complain of conflicts between these two realms of experience and often, it seems, work wins out over relationships. Popular culture exhorts us to spend more time with our families and we are reminded that no one wishes on his death bed that he had spent a little more time at work. Are these exhortations needed? Do everyday people view work as more important to evaluations of life than relationships? In a set of related studies, Twenge and King (2005) used a similar methodology to compare the relative importance of relationship versus work fulfillment in the good life. In these studies, targets were described as experiencing high or low fulfillment (defined as meaningful engagement) in either their work or their personal relationships. Targets were identified as either male or female. The dependent measures were, again, the desirability and moral goodness of those lives. The results of this work showed that, regardless of target (or participant) sex, fulfillment within the relationship realm was a robust predictor of both desirability and moral goodness. Fulfilling work, although desirable, was not seen as a strong necessity. Indeed, in college and community samples work fulfillment was largely irrelevant to ratings of the moral goodness of a life. In the absence of relationship fulfillment, a target who found enormous fulfillment in the work domain was rated as immoral and destined for hell. These results are especially notable given that the samples were drawn from Dallas, TX (certainly a hotbed of individualism) and Ann Arbor, MI. Even in US samples, meaningful relationships trumped work fulfillment as a determinant of the goodness of a life.

Twenge and King (2005) also probed the reasons why relationships might be privileged over work, incorporating the organismic needs drawn from Self Determination Theory (Ryan & Deci, 2001). They found that participants tended to see the relationship domain as the one in which needs for not only relatedness, but also autonomy and competence are most likely to be met. Thus, the results suggest that, regardless of how they spend their time, everyday Americans view social relationships as the centerpiece of the good life.

In a way, these results converge with a general sentiment that relationships are the heart of human existence. However, they also suggest that people may underestimate the role of work in the good life. Specifically, in their study of the most happy individuals, Diener and Seligman (2002) found that every single very happy individual had strong social relationships. However, not every person with good social relationships was among the most happy. In other words, good social relationships were necessary but not sufficient for high well-being. Although the effect of social relationships on well-being is undeniable, the size of this effect has more recently been disputed and is now believed to be smaller than most people think it is (Lucas et al., 2008; Lucas & Schimmack, 2009).

Whereas Diener and Seligman did not examine work fulfillment in their study, Scollon and Diener (2006) examined both changes in work and relationship fulfillment over time and their correspondence to changes in personality traits. They found that increases in work fulfillment and relationship fulfillment both correlated with increases in emotional stability. Furthermore, research has shown that loss of employment can be particularly devastating to well-being (Lucas, Clark, Georgellis, & Diener, 2004). This influence of job loss on well-being has been used as an example against the notion of recovery from negative life events. One factor in this negative response may well be the surprise that individuals feel over their own loss, because after all "it was just a job." The discrepancies among folk theories and SWB findings reveal that lay thinkers may not fully realize the high importance of work fulfillment in the good life.

The good life across cultures. In all of our studies of folk theories of the good life, we have always recognized that notions of the good life are inextricably bound by culture and time. Until recently, however, most of our samples were drawn from middle-class individuals in the United States. Scollon and Wirtz (2010) were the first to examine folk theories of the good life across cultures, comparing two societies similar in economic development, modernity, language, and exposure to Western media – Singapore and the United States. Using stimuli similar to that employed by King and Napa (1998) which examined the components of happiness, meaning, and wealth (with wealth information updated to reflect inflation), Scollon and Wirtz examined the role of culture in folk concepts of the good life.

East-West comparisons were particularly of interest because several studies in the SWB literature had shown that East Asians consistently reported lower life satisfaction and happiness than North Americans (Diener, Diener, & Diener, 1995; Rice & Steele, 2004; Scollon, Diener, Oishi, & Biswas-Diener, 2004; Suh & Koo, 2008). Our paradigm shows how folk theories of the good life can illuminate some of the observed cross-national differences in SWB. One possibility was that personal happiness is a particularly western concern and that Singaporeans would not value happiness to the same extent. Another possibility was that the Singaporean conception of the good life included wealth as well as happiness, which may have consequences for SWB given that several studies have shown that materialism can be toxic to high life satisfaction (Kasser & Ryan, 1993; Nickerson, Schwarz, Diener, & Kahneman, 2003).

In addition, the data for this investigation were collected in early 2009, providing an intriguing opportunity to see if American views toward wealth had changed after the global financial crisis that began in September 2008. After all, the late 1990s ushered in an era of extraordinary wealth for Americans, and like health which often recedes into the background of people's lives when it is good, the size of one's income may be less important in times of prosperity but more important when it is threatened. With news outlets constantly reporting the collapse of banks, foreclosures, and unemployment, financial concerns may have been looming large in American (and Singaporean) consciousness, and Scollon and Wirtz (2010) were interested to see if this would be reflected in folk theories of the good life.

Researchers interested in the good life across cultures should note that great care had to be taken to create stimuli of psychological equivalence across both samples. That is, it was not possible to take the incomes of our targets in the Career Survey and simply convert US dollar amounts to the Singaporean dollar. Through extensive research of labor statistics and pretesting of materials, Scollon and Wirtz were able to create similar stimuli across our groups (see Scollon & Wirtz for details). Even within the United States, income levels had changed in 10 years, such that the poor target would appear much poorer than intended had the income information remained the same as in 1998.

Scollon and Wirtz found both cultural similarities and differences in folk concepts of the good life. Both Singaporeans and Americans defined the good life in terms of happiness and meaning. However, whereas Americans largely discounted wealth when judging the good life, for Singaporeans, the good life included wealth. In samples of both college students and community adults, Singaporean respondents considered the wealthy life to be more desirable than the less wealthy one to the degree of half a standard deviation or more. Given that the effects of materialism on life satisfaction are negative and robust (Kasser & Ryan, 1993; Nickerson et al., 2003), a society that includes wealth as part of the good life is bound to have lower life satisfaction than one that views the good life only in terms of happiness and meaning.

Of course, uncovering cultural differences in the good life, though intriguing, does not explain *why* the Singaporean version of the good life included wealth whereas the American one did not. To address this issue, Scollon and Wirtz turned to the Suh's (2007) theory of the overly context-sensitive self. According to Suh, individuals in collectivist societies have a profound need for belongingness and social harmony that leads to a chronic tendency to view the self from the perspective of the other. This third-person, outside-in viewpoint may increase the importance of objective, external criteria in the evaluation of the good life. Whereas a person's degree of happiness can be judged on internal standards (e.g., Sue is happy because she likes her job, but Jim is happy because he has a great family life), wealth cannot (e.g., $100 will always be more than $10 no matter how you put it). Based on the idea that the third-person perspective leads to greater emphasis on objective standards, we might expect people in a third-person perspective to view wealth as more important to the good life than people in the first-person perspective.

To test this idea, Scollon and Wirtz (2010) temporarily manipulated the perspective-taking of Singaporeans either to be from the inside out or to be from the outside in by having people write either brief autobiographies (first person) or biographies (third person) of their lives. Following the perspective-taking manipulation, participants viewed the Career Survey, this time with only information about the target's happiness and wealth level (we dropped meaning as an independent variable to reduce the complexity of the design and because our other studies had shown that both cultures value meaning to nearly the same degree as happiness). As expected, viewing the self from the third person perspective heightens the role of money in conceptions of the good life. After writing about their lives from the third person perspective, respondents viewed the wealthy life as more desirable than the less wealthy one to the degree of 1 standard deviation (SD) in difference. By contrast, when individuals wrote about their lives in the first person, there was less difference in ratings of the poor versus wealthy target (only 1/3 of a SD in difference).

These studies extended past research on the good life in two important ways. First, they showed cultural differences in folk concepts of the good life that are consistent with cross-cultural differences in mean levels of SWB. Second, they demonstrated through a priming experiment how differences in at least one aspect of folk concepts of the good life emerge.

In summary, this program of research demonstrates how examining folk theories of the good life can not only illuminate the ways that everyday people view optimal functioning but also the ways that psychologists have missed the mark in their assumptions about everyday folk. Further, comparing the responses of everyday people to results in the literature demonstrates the realms of fulfillment that may be neglected in folk theories. Finally, they demonstrate how culture influences these naïve theories of optimal human functioning. While these studies are clearly provocative, they certainly do not exhaust the ways that folk theories of the good life may be studied. Next we briefly consider other strategies for exploring this important facet of experience.

Alternative Approaches to Folk Theories of the Good Life

Clearly, one alternative would be to have respondents rate real people's lives. However, unlike manipulated experimental "lives," real lives vary in complex ways, and we sacrifice experimental precision for added complexity. (After all, there are many ways in which Oprah's life differs from Angelina Jolie's, even though many would argue that both women appear to be leading happy, meaningful, and wealthy lives.) Importantly, although our approach allowed us to examine a limited number of components of the good life at a time, this limitation also served as a strength by adding experimental control to our research. We were able to examine how people weigh different characteristics of a life in judging its overall value without interference from other information such as occupation, race, or sex. All other things being equal, would a happy but poor life be considered as good as a rich one? In addition, by rating another person's life, our approach was indirect and helped minimize any defensiveness about the good life that answering questions about one's own life might introduce.

Some past studies have used qualitative approaches to understanding the good life, either through ethnography or open-ended research questions (e.g., "What is happiness?" Lu, 2001; Lu & Gilmour, 2004). While such approaches undoubtedly provide rich descriptions of local meanings, they provide limited means of assessing broad and truly shared concepts, and they do not facilitate comparisons across individuals or groups. Another approach to understanding how people define the good life is simply to ask participants directly what it is they value (e.g., Schwartz's value survey). Unfortunately, abstract ratings of values might inflate the value of desirable things. Most characteristics are important, and there is nothing to stop participants from circling the highest rating for everything (Cottrell, Neuberg, & Li, 2007; Li, Bailey, Kenrick, & Linsenmeier, 2002).

The Next Frontiers of Research on the Good Life

In many ways, research to date has merely scratched the surface of the fascinating realm of folk theories of the good life. Here we suggest a variety of potentially valuable areas for future research, including, expanding the consideration of culture, incorporating manipulations that uncover the sources of individual and national differences, further examining the role of wealth in lay theories of the good life, and expanding the net of independent variables considered. We address each of these in turn.

More cross-cultural studies. As the studies by Scollon and Wirtz (2010) demonstrate, there are cultural similarities and differences in notions of the good life. Uncovering cultural differences may help answer the question of why some societies are happier than others. In comparing two cultures, however, Scollon and Wirtz (2010) were only the first step. Folk concepts of the good life remain untapped in many more cultures which show intriguing patterns of well-being. For example, there is a great necessity for good life studies in South or Latin America because these countries typically have some of the highest levels of happiness despite levels of collectivism on par with Asian societies and economic development far below countries such as Singapore, Japan, and Hong Kong. Diener, Scollon, Oishi, Dzokoto, and Suh (2000) found that individuals in South America rated the ideal person leading the ideal life to have extremely high levels of life satisfaction whereas ideal levels of life satisfaction were considerably lower in Asian cultures. For example, the mean ideal life satisfaction in Colombia was rated as 31.02 (on a 35-point scale) whereas the mean ideal life satisfaction in China was rated 19.80 on the same scale – a difference of over 5 SDs. Clearly, not all cultures value happiness to the same extent, and whether cultures value meaning and wealth to the same degree remains an empirical question. In any case, our paradigm offers an adaptable and simple way to examine the good life across cultures.

More studies examining the construction of lay theories. At the descriptive level, studies of the good life are important in their own right, but future studies should also try to "unpack" folk concepts by examining how they are constructed. Scollon and Wirtz (2010) were the first to show how this can be done by combining context-sensitivity (Suh, 2007) with perceptions of the good life. These studies are also interesting in that they demonstrate both stability and malleability of folk theories. On the one hand, the American conception of the good life remained relatively unchanged over a decade. On the other hand, experimental manipulations can affect judgments of the goodness of a life. Future research will hopefully be able to establish the boundaries of stability and transient factors in constructions of the good life.

A deeper understanding of the role of wealth in the good life. Lay theories of the good life in North America are primarily defined in terms of happiness and meaning, not wealth. At the same time, newer research is beginning to show there may be a kernel of truth to the saying that money can buy happiness (Lucas & Schimmack, 2009). One possible explanation for why Americans may downplay the role of wealth in the good life is that the accumulation of wealth often requires hard work, and many people may be unwilling to sacrifice a life of leisure in exchange for more money. Consistent with this notion, Scollon and King (2004, Study 1) found an interaction among wealth and effort such that a wealthy life of hard work was valued just as much as a wealthy life of leisure. Thus, people are sensitive to the idea that greater income compensates for hard work. Effort, in turn, produces benefits beyond the monetary such as flow, mastery, or eudaimonia. Thus, if rich people are somewhat happier than the poor, the differences may be due to the psychological benefits confounded with a high-earning lifestyle. Future research would do well to examine interactions among wealth and effort more closely.

Other components of the good life. We might note what sorts of variables were not included in our studies, as these might be of interest in future research and would certainly provide interesting fodder for our continuing understanding of folk concepts of the good life. These variables include (but are not limited to) gender, religiosity, employment, race and ethnicity, age, living conditions, acts of service to others, etc. Again, our methodology can easily be adapted to examine these other aspects of the life well lived.

Conclusions

In conclusion, our research has shown convergence and divergence among folk theories of the good life and the scientific literature on SWB. Newer research on cultural differences in the good life provides promising avenues for understanding cultural differences in mean levels of well-being. Findings from the good life studies can be used to inform future research questions in SWB (e.g., How does wealth enhance happiness, but materialism detract from it?) as well as public policy (e.g., Should governments aim to increase the wealth or happiness of its citizens?).

In short, folk theories really are at the heart of cultural psychology, and questions about the good life are centrally important to positive psychology. Research on folk concepts of the good life remains an important part of a science that aims to bring about social change. As Aristotle noted in *Nicomachean Ethics*, "Shall we not, like archers who have a mark to aim at, be more likely to hit upon what we should? If so, we must try, in outline at least, to determine what it is." We would suggest that knowing what mark individuals are aiming at provides an important piece of information that is relevant to the question of social progress. Such data tell us about the content of the better lives and better worlds that individuals may aspire to, the sources of their discontent with present circumstances, and perhaps the inspiration for their actions toward those better lives and worlds.

References

Biswas-Diener, R., Kashdan, T., & King, L. (2009). Two traditions of happiness research, not two distinct types of happiness. *Journal of Positive Psychology, 4*, 208–211.

Bruner, J. (1990). *Acts of meaning*. Cambridge: Harvard University Press.

Chiu, C.-y, Dweck, C. S., Tong, Y.-y, & Fu, H.-y (1997). Implicit theories and conceptions of morality. *Journal of Personality and Social Psychology, 73*, 923–940.

Chiu, C.-y, Hong, Y., & Dweck, C. S. (1997). Lay dispositionism and implicit theories of personality. *Journal of Personality and Social Psychology, 73*, 19–30.

Cottrell, C. A., Neuberg, S. L., & Li, N. P. (2007). What do people desire in others? A sociofunctional perspective on the importance of different valued characteristics. *Journal of Personality and Social Psychology, 92*, 208–231.

Csikszentmihalyi, M. (1990). *Flow: The psychology of optimal experience*. New York: Harper Perennial.

Diener, E., Diener, M., & Diener, C. (1995). Factors predicting the subjective well-being of nations. *Journal of Personality and Social Psychology, 69*, 851–864.

Diener, E., Horwitz, J., & Emmons, R. A. (1985). Happiness of the very wealthy. *Social Indicators Research, 16*, 263–274.

Diener, E., Scollon, C. K., Oishi, S., Dzokoto, V., & Suh, E. M. (2000). Positivity and the construction of life satisfaction judgments: Global happiness is not the sum of its parts. *Journal of Happiness Studies, 1*, 159–176.

Diener, E., & Seligman, M. E. P. (2002). Very happy people. *Psychological Science, 13*, 80–83.

Fletcher, G. J. O. (1995). *The scientific credibility of folk psychology*. Mahwah, NJ: Lawrence Erlbaum.

Harkness, S., & Super, C. (1996). *Parents' cultural belief systems: Their origins, expressions, and consequences*. New York: Guildford Press.

Kashdan, T. B., Biswas-Diener, R., & King, L. A. (2008). Reconsidering happiness: The costs of distinguishing between hedonics and eudaimonia. *Journal of Positive Psychology, 3*, 219–233.

Kasser, T. (2004). The good life or the goods life? Positive psychology and personal well-being in the culture of consumption. In A. P. Linley & S. Joseph (Eds.), *Positive psychology in practice* (pp. 55–67). Hoboken, NJ: Wiley.

Kasser, T., & Ryan, R. M. (1993). A dark side of the American dream: Correlates of financial success as a central life aspiration. *Journal of Personality and Social Psychology, 65*, 410–422.

King, L. A., & Napa, C. K. (1998). What makes a life good? *Journal of Personality and Social Psychology, 75*, 156–165.

Li, N. P., Bailey, J. M., Kenrick, D. T., & Linsenmeier, J. A. W. (2002). The necessities and luxuries of mate preferences: Testing the tradeoffs. *Journal of Personality and Social Psychology, 82,* 947–955.

Lu, L. (2001). Understanding happiness: A look into the Chinese folk psychology. *Journal of Happiness Studies, 2,* 407–432.

Lu, L., & Gilmour, R. (2004). Culture and conceptions of happiness: Individual oriented and social oriented SWB. *Journal of Happiness Studies, 5,* 269–291.

Lucas, R. E., Clark, A. E., Georgellis, Y., & Diener, E. (2004). Unemployment alters the set-point for life satisfaction. *Psychological Science, 15,* 8–13.

Lucas, R., & Dyrenforth, P. S. (2005). The myth of marital bliss? *Psychological Inquiry, 16,* 111–115.

Lucas, R., & Dyrenforth, P. S. (2006). Does the existence of social relationships matter for subjective well-being? In K. D.Vohs and E. J.Finkel (Eds.), *Self and relationships: Connecting intrapersonal and interpersonal processes* (pp. 254–273). New York: Guilford Press.

Lucas, R. E., Dyrenforth, P. S., & Diener, E. (2008). Four myths about subjective well-being. *Social and Personality Psychology Compass, 2,* 2001–2015.

Lucas, R., & Schimmack, U. (2009). Income and well-being: How big is the gap between the rich and the poor? *Journal of Research in Personality, 43,* 75–78.

Myers, D. (2000). The funds, friends, and faith of happy people. *American Psychologist, 55,* 56–67.

Myers, D., & Diener, E. (1995). Who is happy? *Psychological Science, 6,* 10–19.

Nickerson, C., Schwarz, N., Diener, E., & Kahneman, D. (2003). Zeroing in on the dark side of the American dream: A closer look at the negative consequences of the goal for financial success. *Psychological Science, 14,* 531–536.

Rice, T. W., & Steele, B. J. (2004). Subjective well-being and culture across time and space. *Journal of Cross-Cultural Psychology, 35,* 633.

Ryan, R. M., & Deci, E. L. (2001). On happiness and human potentials: A review of research on hedonic and eudaimonic well-being. In S. Fiske (Ed.), *Annual review of psychology* (Vol. 52, pp. 141–166). Palo Alto, CA: Annual Reviews, Inc.

Ryff, C. D., & Singer, B. (2008). Know thyself and become what you are: A eudaimonic approach to psychological well-being. *Journal of Happiness Studies, 9,* 13–39.

Scollon, C. N., & Diener, E. (2006). Love, work, and changes in extraversion and neuroticism over time. *Journal of Personality and Social Psychology, 91,* 1152–1165.

Scollon, C. N., Diener, E., Oishi, S., & Biswas-Diener, R. (2004). Emotions across cultures and methods. *Journal of Cross-Cultural Psychology, 35,* 304–326.

Scollon, C. N., & King, L. A. (2004). Is the good life the easy life? *Social Indicators Research, 68,* 127–162.

Scollon, C. N., & Wirtz, D. (2010). *Is the good life happy, meaningful, or wealthy? Cultural differences and the context-sensitive self.* Manuscript under review.

Sheldon, K., & King, L. A. (2001). Why positive psychology is necessary. *American Psychologist, 56,* 216–217.

Suh, E. M. (2007). Downsides of an overly context-sensitive self: Implications from the culture and subjective well-being research. *Journal of Personality, 75,* 1321–1343.

Suh, E., & Koo, J. (2008). Comparing subjective well-being across cultures and nations: The 'what' and 'why' questions. In M. Eid & R. J. Larsen (Eds.), *The science of subjective well-being* (pp. 414–427). New York: Guilford Press.

Twenge, J. M., & King, L. A. (2005). A good life is a personal life: Relationship fulfillment and work fulfillment in judgments of life quality. *Journal of Research in Personality, 39,* 336–353.

Waterman, A. S. (2008). Reconsidering happiness: A eudaimonist's perspective. *Journal of Positive Psychology, 3,* 234–252.

White, R. (1959). Motivation reconsidered: The concept of competence. *Psychological Review, 66,* 297–333.

Seard: foll psych
foll ir œology "lay theories"
"lay notions"
"folk concepts"

Part I
Some Cautionary Thoughts

Chapter 2
Think Before You Think

Nic Marks

I work in a think tank, so perhaps it is not surprising that I am suggesting that we all think a little harder about how positive psychology could be a force for (positive) social change. The main question that we are seeking to address at the centre for well-being at *nef* (the new economics foundation) is what policy making and the economy would look like if their main aim were to promote well-being. In doing so, probably the key thing we aim to achieve is to make an impact whilst simultaneously being robust and grounded in evidence. We want to make a difference – a difference to people's lives both now and in the future. But before I try to impress upon you why I think we should all take systemic issues a lot more seriously, perhaps it is best if I tell you a little about me, the work we do at the centre for well-being, and why we do it.

You might think it a little strange for a Brit to start off talking about himself; it's all a bit personal isn't it? Well, I am of the opinion that all change starts within us. And, as this is a book about social change, it seems relevant to start with my experiences and what I have learnt from them and then move on from there. You can always skip this bit, or indeed this whole chapter, if it doesn't appeal to you – free will and all that!

Probably one of the first things to say is that I'm not really an academic. In fact, I'm a bit of a failed academic. I tried to do a PhD but simply had neither the patience nor the determination to spend 4 years of my life explaining why it was valid to think of "collective quality of life in an ecological and humanistic context" (which was the working title of my 1-year aborted attempt). Not only was the rigour of a PhD perhaps too arduous for me, but over the years, I (and others) have had to learn to accept that by nature I am a little lazy – or as I prefer to put it – I seek to be efficient with the use of my time and energy! In fact, seeking to be efficient will be a theme that runs through this contribution.

N. Marks (✉)
New Economics Foundation, London, UK
e-mail: nic.marks@neweconomics.org

R. Biswas-Diener (ed.), *Positive Psychology as Social Change*,
DOI 10.1007/978-90-481-9938-9_2, © Springer Science+Business Media B.V. 2011

Thinking

So I am not an academic as such, but that doesn't mean I don't value thinking! When I was at university, I studied mathematics, economics, and management systems, eventually specialising in what was then called "operational research" (OR). OR is basically the study of optimal solutions to complex problems and relies on the use of statistics, mathematical modelling, and simulation techniques. One of the insights I particularly liked was the 80:20 rule – getting 80% of the way to an optimal solution for 20% of the computing effort. This could be my hidden life philosophy! But the thing with the 80:20 rule is that you have to *think before you think* about "solving" the problem. You have to think about how to frame the problem, which key parameters to include in the model, and what strategies will be best employed in tackling it.

Operational research also introduced me to the concepts of algorithms and heuristics. The key difference is that an algorithm is a precise rule (or set of rules) for solving a problem whereas a heuristic is more of an experience-based technique that approaches a solution; in other words, an algorithm is more precise and formal whereas a heuristic is a bit of a rule of thumb. I'll come back to algorithms and heuristics later and to the reasons that I tend to favour the latter.

Listening

After university, for some reason, I decided that as well as working as a consultant and a statistician, I also wanted to become a psychotherapist. I am not really sure why I chose to do this, except that my mother worked in the field, but I had great fun doing the training and learnt so much about people (including myself) along the way that it has to be one of the most valuable things I have ever done. In addition to a lot of theories about personal development, the course was also very practical and taught us listening skills and intervention techniques. Therapy is very much a two-way process and one of the major challenges for the therapist is to manage his/her own biases and prejudices, the so-called "counter-transference" during the therapeutic process.

In fact, one of the reasons I have chosen to write this chapter in the first person and give an almost chronological feel to my thinking is to ensure my biases and prejudices are transparent (and challengeable). On my course, I was very struck by one teacher who identified the basic tasks of psychotherapy as three-fold: to listen to your client, to reflect back to them what you have heard, and occasionally to ask challenging questions. In a sense, if I learnt to *think before I think* from OR, then I learnt to *listen before thinking* from psychotherapy.

Intervening

The next intellectual step in my slightly random walk towards what I now do was to enroll in a masters course. It is now sadly defunct but at the time was run by the Centre for Human Potential at the University of Surrey and entitled *Change Agent*

Skills and Strategies. It was concerned with three levels of change: personal, group, and organisational. Each theme started with the personal, then later came back to treat the same issue from a group perspective, and then again from an organisational one. It isn't much of a stretch to think of the next level as social change and I chose to write about these links on many occasions during the coursework. There was quite a bit of debate amongst participants on the course as to whether it should be a Master of Arts (MA) course rather than a Master of Science (MSc) course as it actually was. Perhaps not a distinction that other parts of the world would make, but I think many participants felt that facilitating groups of people was much more of a dynamic relationship, a dance if you like, than a mechanical set of rules to follow, so more an art than a science. I was unsure; for whilst I was deeply engaged with the very experiential dimension of the course, I also loved the brain-food of models and theories!

At one stage I remember that the tension between facilitation as an art or a science came to a head in the group with many people (probably on this occasion including me) being strongly resistant to a categorisation of interventions model devised by John Heron (one of the original founders of the course who had long since left). It is strange that I was resistant to it, as in retrospect it is one of the models I find most useful. Heron (1990) really, really likes categorisations and quite possibly overuses them in a slightly pedantic way but they can be a simple way of opening up complex issues. Anyway, the one I still find useful said that when you are deliberately seeking to promote change at any level, there are two broad types of intervention – authoritative and facilitative – each with three subtypes. Table 2.1 shows the full categorisation (Heron, 1990).

Table 2.1 Heron's six categories of interventions

Authoritative	Facilitative
Prescriptive	Cathartic
(*Giving direction or advice*)	(*Expressing emotions, relieving tension*)
Informative	Catalytic
(*Providing information*)	(*Exploring or drawing out*)
Confronting	Supportive
(*Challenging*)	(*Validating, affirming, and encouraging*)

I found this categorisation helpful as it highlights the validity of many of different styles of intervention whilst encouraging me *to think carefully before intervening*.

Issues of Primary Importance

Heron's insights are useful when thinking about social change but there is another layer of complexity as, unlike individuals, social systems can't tell you what their problems are. Indeed from a personal perspective I often find myself questioning my own arrogance in thinking that I can do anything at all to make a significant difference. What right do I have to try? Yet I also have to recognise that I have a strong drive, and in some ways feel a responsibility, to try and do precisely this.

To help me steer a course through this particular minefield, I have often turned to one thinker who, over the years, has been a sort of mentor to me: Manfred Max-Neef, the Chilean Right Livelihood Award winner and so-called barefoot economist.

In a brilliantly thoughtful paper with a great title – A*bout the pruning of language (and other unusual exercises) for the understanding of social improvement* – he suggests that a lot of us spend most of our time worrying about issues of secondary importance (Max-Neef, 1988). He implores us at this time in history to concentrate on issues of primary importance. So what does he mean by "issues of primary importance"? An example he gives is that a lot of people worry about who is in power and they spend a lot of their effort trying to get someone into a position of power – basically someone more like them, someone with their sort of values – in the hope that once that person gets into power, the world will become more like the world that they want it to become. Max-Neef calls this an issue of "secondary importance" because, he argues, we have tried very many different people in power – we've tried moderates, we've tried radicals from the left and the right – but the challenges still remain. The issues of primary importance have not been solved by addressing the question of "who is in power"; instead, he suggests, they are more to do with "the structure of power", i.e., the way that we organise power in society.

Three Global Issues

So what are the issues of primary importance at this time in the early twenty-first century? Obviously different people might have different lists and emphases but quite probably at a systemic level they are all interconnected. For me, there are three main issues.

Perhaps the most obvious issue is that in an era of unprecedented plenty for the rich, more than 3 billion people – about half the world's population – live on the equivalent of less than $2.50 a day. This is 400 million more than in 1981. The average incomes of the richest 1% of the world's population are over 100 times those of the poorest 20%. During the same period, health improvement in the developing world, as measured by life expectancy and infant mortality, has slowed dramatically. As well as global inequalities, the gains made from the 1920s in reducing the income and wealth inequalities in countries such as the UK and the USA have been reversed in the last 30 years. For example, in the UK the wealthiest 10% have assets of about 100 times that of the poorest 10% (£853,000 compared to £8,800). This is a comparable level of inequality to that of the 1930s. So problem No. 1 is that we live in a world with entrenched poverty and rising global inequalities.

The second issue of primary importance, in my opinion, is that of impending climate change and the environment. In fact, it is not only my opinion. In 2009 Eurobarometer poll, 87% of Europeans considered that climate change was a serious problem, with only 10% thinking it wasn't. Nearly half (47%) said it was one of the two most serious issues facing the world today, the only issue scoring higher being poverty (69%). Whilst the details of the future impact of climate change are being endlessly debated, it seems clear that we will be entering a period of constraints on our consumption levels driven by an urgent need to reduce carbon emissions. This is without considering the huge loss of biodiversity and threats to food supplies globally due to mismanagement of the natural resources that we depend on, such as fisheries, water supplies, and agricultural land. So that's problem No. 2: we are living an unsustainable way of life.

The third issue of primary importance is that despite the fact that people in western developed countries are consuming far more material goods they are not getting any happier. For example consumer expenditure in the UK has nearly doubled since the early 1970s but levels of life satisfaction have remained resolutely flat (World Database of Happiness, 2010). This might be explained by the fact that it seems that people are becoming more materialistic in their expectations of life (Myers, 2000) and it is well known that being highly materialistic has much negative impact – for example, poorer personal relationships, lower self-esteem, and fewer good moods (Kasser, 2006). So my third issue is that despite increasing material wealth we are not becoming any happier – and I consider that to be of primary importance because I think happiness is the key to the door that will unlock the potential solutions to the first two issues.

These are my three issues of primary importance and I am very fortunate to work in an organisation whose values are aligned with these issues; all of *nef*'s work is focused on social justice, environmental sustainability, and people's well-being. You may have your own list with a different emphasis, but what I did learn from Max-Neef was to strive to *align my work with important issues*.

Wicked Problems

Now, all these issues could be described as what Rittel and Webber (1973) refer to as "wicked problems". Wicked problems are not wicked as in evil (or "cool") but wicked as in the opposite to tame. There is not a clear cause and effect about what is happening. They are systemic rather than mechanistic in their manner, and all the interconnectivity means they are not easy to solve. So when we think about changing systems that are characterised by these deep, interconnected, wicked problems, I propose that we think not so much about how we "solve" them but instead about how we can work with the energy of the system, with the tensions in the system, to shift the system onto a different path. Instead of striving for precise solutions I would suggest we seek instead to raise questions and open up new perspectives.

So if positive psychology is to become a force for positive social change, then how can it intervene in these complex spaces of interconnected wicked problems? Well, no doubt there are many ways and strategies to be formed, but if this chapter is a plea for anything then it is to *think before you think*, because otherwise you run the danger of using a lot of creative energy and not achieving much change – and remember that I am lazy and very interested in not wasting energy!

Beer and Systems

The expression "think before you think" comes from the great systems thinker Stafford Beer (Beer & Whittaker, 2009). Beer was an exceptionally interesting character and is perhaps best known for his role with the Allende government in Chile that was ousted by the US-backed coup that installed General Pinochet as President. Stafford Beer worked in a field of study called "cybernetics". He wrote several books including *Brain of the Firm, Platform for Change,* and *Heart of Enterprise.*

Cybernetics is really the study of control; not control as in oppression, but control as in self-regulation, much like a governor in the classic Watt steam engine. The governor is an automatic feedback system that decreases the flow of steam when the steam engine goes too fast and increases the flow when it slows up – thereby stabilising the engine. Beer was very interested in feedback loops and the role they play in creating conditions of circular causality – where the cause generates an effect which in turn is the cause of another effect and so on. These sorts of mechanisms can either cause a dampening of systems, such as in the steam engine, where stability is the outcome, or they can be reinforcing and thereby create expanding systems. Along with colleagues and peers, Beer took these ideas into the realm of complex human systems, such as organisations, and even whole national systems (in his work in Chile). Effectively, he was interested in how systems are able to adapt, evolve, and learn, thereby enabling them to respond to internal or external shocks. He even coined a nice phrase for this "potentiality" – *adaptive poise.*

It is probably becoming clear by now why I am interested in cybernetics in relation to the issues of primary importance I outlined earlier. My hypothesis is that as a society, or indeed as a global system, we are very low on any score of adaptive poise right now! Global inequalities are entrenched and certainly we seem unable to break the cycle of poverty. Many climatologists warn of impending runaway climate change; regardless of whether their models are right, it is clear that we are not even able to stop the increase of annual global emissions of carbon dioxide. However it is clear that future damages will flow from the already too large stock of greenhouse gases in the atmosphere not the annual additions to that stock. Meanwhile, rich western societies keep looking for happiness through the ever-increasing acquisition of material goods.

So now you know the story of my interest in this wide range of disciplines from statistics to psychology, from psychotherapy to cybernetics. Perhaps it is easier to see patterns or a *raison d'être* when you take a look backwards; somehow it all seems to make perfect sense now. Well, if not perfect sense, then at least some sense! I seem to take an insight from one field and apply it in another whilst seeking to address those issues of primary importance. To illustrate what I mean let's take a look at three examples of interventions that we have designed at *nef*; interventions that are starting to have some impact on creating positive change.

Example 1: A Societal Feedback Loop – The Happy Planet Index

The first example is the work that we are perhaps best known for – the *Happy Planet Index* (HPI; Marks, Abdallah, Simms, & Thompson, 2006). One of our principle strategies from the very beginning of the well-being work at *nef* was to "measure what matters". I was very keen to do this because I think that statistics can act as societal feedback loops. In cybernetic terms, they provide information back to the system so that it has the potential to learn and evolve. In fact, the analogy with psychotherapy is also apt, as the collection of survey data is equivalent to listening to the client (in this case a society); the publication of the statistics is the reflecting back; and the interpretation can raise challenging questions.

When creating a cybernetic feedback loop, signals have to be simple and clear to effect change. It is one of the reasons that gross domestic product (GDP) has taken such a hold on our governments – it is a single number and more is always good – it is a clear signal. GDP is actually full of complexities (and perversities) but at its headline presentation, it is pure simplicity and that is part of its power. With the HPI we have tried to mimic that simplicity whilst simultaneously trying to hold the complex tension between quality of life now and in the future.

The HPI is an indicator of how ecologically efficient a nation is at creating happy and healthy lives for its citizens. It is effectively designed to be an alternative to GDP as a measure of societal progress. Whereas GDP says progress is simply having more things, HPI points the way to a future where "good lives don't cost the Earth". Progress towards this sort of future has to be deemed as positive social change and, indeed, progress.

So how is the HPI calculated? Well, first it assesses a nation's level of well-being in terms of how happy and healthy its citizens are. Then it creates an efficiency measure by dividing this by how many ecological resources they use. So it is a "bang for your buck" index in a manner similar to how a car's fuel efficiency is measured by average miles per gallon (or kilometres per litre as we say now). The full details of calculation can be found in the reports and on the website but it is sufficient here to just show the approximate equation.

$$\text{Happy planet index} \sim \frac{\text{Happy life years}}{\text{Ecological footprint}}$$

Happy Life Years (HLY) is a neat metric: a happiness-adjusted life expectancy developed by Dutch sociologist Ruut Veenhoven (1996). It ensures that both the subjective and objective elements of well-being are captured by recognising that a satisfying life is not ideal if it is very short, but also that a long life is not ideal if it is miserable. The Ecological Footprint (EF) was developed by ecologists Mathis Wackernagel and William Rees (1996), and championed by a range of organisations including the Global Footprint Network and WWF. The EF assesses the overall environmental impact of an individual's lifestyle.

So to increase a nation's HPI score, there are two main possibilities – to enhance the population's well-being (which would lead to an increase in HLYs) or to reduce its footprint (a falling EF). These require different interventions. So, although HPI is presented as one number at a headline level, to work effectively as feedback loops, it needs to be looked at separately. Figure 2.1 is taken from the second HPI report and shows trends from 1960 to 2005 in HLY, EF, and HPI for the nations in the OECD (Organisation for Economic Co-operation and Development) – the richest nations in the world (Abdallah, Thompson, Michaelson, Marks, & Steuer, 2009). What can be clearly seen is that whilst there have been significant gains in well-being, these have been at the expense of ever-increasing pressure on the planet: we have become less ecologically efficient at delivering human well-being over this time.

The challenge that we face is to significantly reverse the trend of increasing EF whilst simultaneously maintaining the gains in human well-being. For the former, we require a set of dampening feedback loops that continuously reminds the whole of society that we need to reduce impact on the planet. A small-scale example might be so-called smart meters in people's houses that tell them how much electricity they are using right now and shows the cash they are spending – this will soon get people to turn off the lights! At a societal level, instead of the dollar to pound (sterling) exchange rate or the Dow Jones Index on the radio and TV, we could instead have information on how much energy the nation used yesterday. To make this sort of

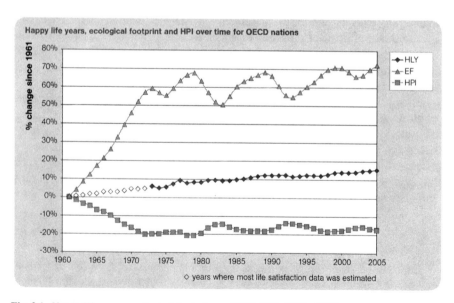

Fig. 2.1 Happy life years, ecological footprint and HPI 1960–2005; OECD countries

data more readily meaningful we could perhaps make comparisons to the same day last year and whether we have meet our 3% annual reduction target.

The HPI is an example of how we have tried to use some positive psychology research on happiness to create a fresh way of looking at the world and thereby creating some impact for positive social change. Whilst it is not a full use of all positive psychology's richness, it is certain that the happiness element with its positive vision of the future is a crucial part of the success of the HPI. This is in stark contrast to the environmental movement's normal use of apocalyptic visions of the future to scare people into engaging with the climate change agenda. The first HPI was launched in July 2006. It resonated with hundreds and thousands of people around the world – within 2 days of its launch, the report had been downloaded and read in 185 countries worldwide. Three years on, HPI 2.0 was calculated with new improved datasets for 143 countries, covering 99% of the world's population – it, too, was reported widely. The HPI is now cited most months in major international press such as *The New York Times*, *The Observer*, and the BBC World News website, all of which featured it – for example – during the month of February, 2010.

Example 2: Creating (Almost) Real-Time Feedback Loops for Organisational Change: Well-Being@Work

The HPI is directly related to all three issues of primary importance outlined earlier and uses some insights from systems theory and positive psychology to raise awareness and create some critical reflection. For the HPI to galvanise genuine positive social change, however, it faces two major challenges. First, it is, in reality, an advocacy index produced using existing data sources on very small budgets and published by a UK think tank. It has not (yet) been championed by any major international institutions or been adopted by any governmental organisations – so it is still a few steps removed from actual power structures. Secondly, from a cybernetic perspective, it suffers from lengthy time lags between the collection and reporting of data. For example, much of the data used for the second HPI was about 3 years out of date by the time we published it in the summer of 2009. These sorts of time lags are not atypical for health and environmental statistics and many times simply reflect a lack of investment in these systems. There is no theoretical reason, however, why energy data could not be collected in real time from all major suppliers – electricity companies, natural gas and oil suppliers, and renewable energy producers – then collated and supplied to the media. The only reasons are political and financial.

So whilst this second example does not address so directly my three issues of primary importance, it does start to close these two gaps. About 2 years ago, *nef* decided to launch a consulting arm, imaginatively called *nef consulting*, to put into action insights that emerged from our research. The idea is that if we can sell products and services, we can use the profits generated to cross-fund our research. I was asked if I could come up with any well-being products that we could create and immediately thought that an organisational "well-being at work" tool would be

Fig. 2.2 *nef* consulting's
well-being@work tool (©nef
consulting)

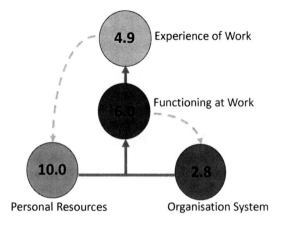

interesting. This clearly tied back to my MSc at the University of Surrey, where we looked at facilitating change at the personal, group, and organisational levels.

To be honest, I started out thinking we could simply create a measurement tool that would "inform" management of the state of well-being in the organisation. Relating back to the John Heron typology of interventions that I outlined earlier, I was imagining an authoritarian-informative intervention. This is really a classic academic intervention and indeed a classic national statistical office one, too – providing information for people to make better decisions. Because we wanted to create a product to sell rather than simply selling our time, however, we designed a software tool to do the analysis. What this means in practice is that an organisation sends a web link to its employees; they complete an online survey; and the software automatically creates the well-being at work indicators. The beauty (from a timely feedback perspective) is that the results are available as soon as the survey is closed and, as we designed a hierarchal structure of indicators, this means it is very easy to explore the data by simply clicking and discovering the results that interest you.

Figure 2.2 shows the way that we present the results to clients or, as you'll hear soon, how we encourage teams to examine their own results themselves.

The model itself is based on a project we did for the UK Government Office for Science. The office regularly runs a Foresight programme on major long-term issues; previously it has covered such diverse issues as flooding and obesity. In 2007/2008, the programme focused on *Mental Capital and Well-being. nef* managed two projects: one on creating well-being measures for public policy (Thompson & Marks, 2008) and a second on five ways to well-being that I return to later in this chapter. The model was designed for policy applications but we have adapted it slightly for organisational well-being.

The model's foundations are the Personal Resources and Organisational System domains. Here we recognise that there are two things going on: first there are the people at work – the human capital if you like that term; and second, there is a work environment, including the organisational culture, management systems, and job design. The middle domain represents how these two domains come together into what people actually do at work (called here "functioning at work"). Are they creative? Competent? How do they work as teams? Do they achieve good impact for the organisation and broader society? The top domain assesses people's actual experience of work – how interesting, stressful, and satisfying they find their jobs as well as whether they are proud to work in their organisation. I imagine this top domain – experience of work – as an emergent property of this whole organisational system of well-being at work.

The model gets its dynamic feel from the two major feedback loops that in Stafford Beer's terminology create "circular causality", with effects becoming causes of more effects. So the feedback from "functioning at work" to "organisational system" recognises that what people do within the system shapes the organisation. This can undermine the system where poor performance by (say) a manager affects the management system as a whole, or positively enhance the system where creativity stimulates innovative open structures for the organisation. The second feedback loop from "experience of work" to "personal resources" reflects Barbara Fredrickson's (2009) "broaden and build" theory of positive emotions – where the expression of positive emotions helps build resources for the future; clearly the opposite can also happen where the over expression of negativity undermines employee self-esteem.

So this is the theory and, as you can see, it is influenced by positive psychology but what I am most excited about – and this is a new product for us so at the time of writing this is very fresh – is that the tool can operate as a near-real-time feedback loop!

How does this work? Well, recently I worked with a small organisation of 25 people and on a Thursday and Friday, the employees completed the questionnaire. The following Tuesday, I ran a workshop for the whole organisation on well-being at work using the results live. It is important to note that the senior management team took the risk of not having access to the results of the survey before the whole organisation saw them – so there was no censorship or even preparation, just the pure results presented to everyone at the same time. The way the software tool works means that the results can be split by team – so at various times in the day the group split up into smaller teams huddled around a computer exploring together its own results. Then they came back to the whole group and talked about what they had discovered about themselves and their co-workers, with the indicators and model giving them a language to understand things more clearly.

Whilst the tool can still be used as authoritative-informative intervention, by using it to inform a workshop like this, the whole exercise suddenly becomes much more process orientated and facilitative. In fact, there were elements of the day that went right across all six of Heron's intervention styles (Table 2.2). At the end of the day we spent the last hour creating some action plans about how to take some of the themes forward and then ended with people voluntarily sharing something of their experience of the day. Since the workshop, the Chief Executive has described

Table 2.2 Heron's six categories of intervention: a case study for well-being@work

Authoritative	Facilitative
Prescriptive	*Cathartic*
The dynamic model itself gives direction and at times during the workshop I was asked by the group for specific advice about the relative importance of issues	There were times during the day which were releasing and indeed quite tender – as people started to empathise more with each other (especially with those in other teams)
Informative	*Catalytic*
This is the entry point for the intervention – it provides information about the organisational system to the organisational system	Breaking into teams and allowing people to explore the data for themselves was a catalyst for deeper conversation and reflections
Confronting	*Supportive*
Some results challenged senior and line managers but also the reverse was true in that senior managers challenged employees to appreciate them and the difficulty of their role more	Individuals and teams felt heard by others and their experiences were affirmed and confirmed by the data and the resulting discussions

the day as a "watershed" for the organisation and whilst she personally felt quite vulnerable during the day (it was quite a bold intervention), she is convinced it has been transformative. The HR director confirmed this and said for the first time she felt that the teams started to be empathetic to each other and really listened – she described the whole experience as her "best day at work".

We intend to go back in 6 months' time, repeat the exercise, and see the changes. But I am really excited about seeing the power of a real-time feedback loop to create dramatic change naturally by simply working with the energy of the system.

Example 3: A Prescriptive Heuristic That Is Actually Facilitative: Five Ways to Well-Being

The third example of an impactful intervention we have designed is the second project we did for the UK Government Office for Science's Foresight programme (Aked, Marks, Cordon, & Thompson, 2008). The whole Foresight programme produced a very comprehensive overview of the state of the science around the understanding and promotion of mental capital and well-being. It commissioned over 100 separate reports and involved over 300 experts from a wide range of disciplines. During a discussion with Foresight about the measurement project, I suggested that there was potential to create some public mental health messaging in a style similar to the very well-known UK public health dictum of eating "five fruit and vegetables a day".

The idea behind my suggestion, apart from being opportunistic, was to create a way for ordinary people to take action in their day-to-day lives that would improve their well-being. Having sold the idea to the Foresight Project Leader, we were given access to all the Foresight reports and used four criteria to shortlist potential actions:

1. Evidence base – whilst this was not always straightforward – as there is little epidemiological evidence examining the determinants of well-being, and what there is predominantly uses cross-sectional data – this still was the most important criteria.
2. Universal appeal – we were specifically commissioned to create actions that were suitable for the whole population and so a generic set with wide appeal was essential.
3. Target the individual – the brief was that the actions should be ones that people can do themselves without government intervention – so although we at *nef* specifically call for community and societal level interventions, they were not considered here.
4. The need for variety – there is evidence from positive psychology that any sustainable action will need to overcome the tendency for "hedonic adaptation". So we deliberately sought to have some variety so the actions could stay "fresh".

The project went through a process of creating a long list of evidence-based actions, then reducing this to a short list and finally "messaging" the chosen actions. Thus the "five ways to well-being" were born (Fig. 2.3).

Now why do I suggest that these five ways can be considered a heuristic? Well, as I mentioned at the beginning of this chapter, a heuristic is an experienced-based technique rather like a rule of thumb. The advantage from a systems point of view is that the experience allows the system (in this case an individual) to dynamically adjust and learn – the adaptive poise that Stafford Beer talked of. Not only do experience-based heuristics allow people to learn as they go along, they are also really easy to understand; whereas often, as statisticians, we can pay too much attention to the second, and sometimes third, decimal place of correlation coefficients and thereby lose the most important messages.

The five ways to well-being are now starting to gain popular momentum in the UK and even beyond (for example, we are aware of them being translated into Norwegian and Maori). An interesting example is the city of Liverpool in the UK which has recently adopted them as an overarching theme for a whole year of coordinated activities aimed at improving the lives of people in the city region and Norwich City Council is considering a similar exercise. The Department for Heath's *New Horizons* programme for promoting public mental health has also included the five ways and as part of this adoption process carried out focus group research on their suitability. Some comments from the independent research included

It seems to care about you... look after you...
It's more suggestive than instructive.
It seems more positive, it's telling you to go outside and do positive things.
It gives you a get up and go feeling, it's motivating just reading it.

It is important though to recognise the five ways' limitations: feedback from one focus group which consisted of people who have suffered from mental health problems included

These aren't going to help you through a crisis.

Connect...

With the people around you. With family, friends, colleagues and neighbours. At home, work, school or in your local community. Think of these as the cornerstones of your life and invest time in developing them. Building these connections will support and enrich you every day.

Be active...

Go for a walk or run. Step outside. Cycle. Play a game. Garden. Dance. Exercising makes you feel good. Most importantly, discover a physical activity you enjoy and that suits your level of mobility and fitness.

Take notice...

Be curious. Catch sight of the beautiful. Remark on the unusual. Notice the changing seasons. Savour the moment, whether you are walking to work, eating lunch or talking to friends. Be aware of the world around you and what you are feeling. Reflecting on your experiences will help you appreciate what matters to you.

Keep learning...

Try something new. Rediscover an old interest. Sign up for that course. Take on a different responsibility at work. Fix a bike. Learn to play an instrument or how to cook your favourite food. Set a challenge you will enjoy achieving. Learning new things will make you more confident as well as being fun.

Give...

Do something nice for a friend, or a stranger. Thank someone. Smile. Volunteer your time. Join a community group. Look out, as well as in. Seeing yourself, and your happiness, linked to the wider community can be incredibly rewarding and creates connections with the people around you.

Fig. 2.3 Five ways to well-being

So although the five ways are essentially, in Heron's categorisation, a prescriptive and informative intervention, people's actual experience of them seems to be more facilitative, particularly in a catalytic style. They are simple messages that people can understand and use in their daily lives yet they are actually grounded in a robust complex science review. Simple but not simplistic.

Conclusions

I've tried to give you some insights into how we, at the centre for well-being at *nef*, seek to stimulate social change through using insights from a broad range of disciplines. If the title of this whole book can be thought of as a question – *Can positive psychology be a force for social change?* – then my unequivocal answer would be "yes, it can". But it is also my opinion that positive psychology will not do it automatically or on its own. If I were allowed the indulgence of stretching the meaning of the five ways to well-being, then my advice to the positive psychology movement would be to

- *Connect* to other disciplines such as systems theory, economics, sociology, and the life sciences.
- *Be active* by seeking to make interventions that genuinely make a difference to people's lives.
- *Take notice* of global inequalities and entrenched poverty as well as impending climate change and the massive loss of biodiversity.
- *Keep learning* from each other and from those we seek to help (they often know so much more than we give them credit).
- *Give* something back to society and explicitly include social goals in your projects.

If positive psychology can do all these things then it will genuinely be a force for creating positive social change. However one more word of caution: the systemic forces that shape the world in which we all live are very strong. Identifying particularly ripe pressure points that might be influcnced so as to create positive social change requires that we think systematically before we think of precise interventions. In other words we need to *think before we think!*

Obviously the avenues that we are exploring at *nef* are just a few of the many possibilities we might be able to imagine. But I genuinely believe that if we apply ourselves then together we can create the world we all want, one where everyone has the opportunity to live a good life that doesn't cost the Earth.

Happy thinking.

References

Abdallah, S., Thompson, S., Michaelson, J., Marks, N., & Steuer, N. (2009). *The (un)happy planet index 2.0: Why good lives don't have to cost the Earth*. London: nef.

Aked, J., Marks, N., Cordon, C., & Thompson, S. (2008). *Five ways to well-being: The evidence*. London: *nef*. See www.fivewaystowellbeing.org for more details and postcards that are designed to communicate the five ways broadly.

Beer, S., & Whittaker, D. (2009). *Think before you think – Social complexity and knowledge of knowing*. Oxfordshire: Wavestone Press.

Eurobarometer Special Report 300. (2009). Europeans' attitudes towards climate change. http://ec.europa.eu/public_opinion/archives/ebs/ebs_300_full_en.pdf

Foresight Mental Capital and Wellbeing Project. (2008). Final project report. London: The Government Office for Science. http://www.foresight.gov.uk/OurWork/ActiveProjects/Mental%20Capital/Welcome.asp

Fredrickson, B. (2009). *Positivity*. New York: Crown.

Heron, J. (1990). *Helping the client: A creative practical guide*. London: Sage.

Kasser, T. (2006). Materialism and its alternatives. In M. Csikszentmihalyi & I. Csikszentmihalyi (Eds.), *A life worth living: Contributions to positive psychology* (pp. 200–214). Oxford, UK: Oxford University Press.

Marks, N., Abdallah, S., Simms, A., & Thompson, S. (2006). *The (un) happy planet index*. London: *nef*. (Updated as *The (un) happy planet index 2.0*, by Abdallah, S., Thompson, S., Michaelson, J., Marks, N., & Steuer, N., London: *nef*. www.happyplanetindex.org)

Max Neef, M. (1988). *About the pruning of language (and other unusual exercises) for the under-standing of social improvement*. (Reprinted in *Human scale development*, by Max M. Neef, 1991, New York: Apex Press)

Myers, D. G. (2000). The funds, friends, and faith of happy people. *American Psychologist, 55*, 56–67.

Rittel, H., & Webber, M. (1973). Dilemmas in a general theory of planning. *Policy Sciences, 4*, 155–169, Amsterdam: Elsevier. (Reprinted in *Developments in design methodology*, pp. 135–144, by N. Cross, Ed., 1984, Chichester: Wiley)

Thompson, N., & Marks, N. (2008). *Measuring well-being in policy: Issues and applications*. London: *nef*.

Veenhoven, R. (1996). Happy life expectancy. A comprehensive measure of quality-of-life in nations. *Social Indicators Research, 39*, 1–58.

Wackernagel, M., & Rees, W. (1996). *Our ecological footprint: Reducing human impact on the Earth*. Gabriola Island: New Society Publishers.

World Database of Happiness. http://worlddatabaseofhappiness.eur.nl/

Chapter 3
Socially Responsible Cheermongery: On the Sociocultural Contexts and Levels of Social Happiness Policies

Neil Thin

Cheermongers: Around the World from Birth to Death

Positive Psychology has emerged as a social and cultural movement which responds to both the comforts and the ills of modern affluence. While not entirely post-materialist (given the considerable attention to the body and the benefits of good environments), nor entirely individualistic (since a lot of attention has been paid to pro-social behaviour as a character strength, and to the importance of relationships for individual happiness), it has largely taken basic needs provision and social justice for granted. So it has located the prospects for happiness promotion at the level of the individual, and in the form of changes in personal attitudes and practices, rather than as changes in culture, society, and environment. Though not entirely a western phenomenon (since there have been happiness studies in most countries in the world, and a huge number of international and cross-cultural comparative studies) it has involved only limited attempts to engage with the world's cultural diversity so as to globalize the potential benefits of the movement.

All of us, even sociophobes, require other people for our happiness. Inversely, our life's work isn't just about our own personal happiness. It involves helping other people find theirs. It may even involve leaving happiness legacies that may ultimately matter more to future generations than our financial or architectural bequests. Positive Psychology has taught us a lot about the processes involved in getting happy, but has so far paid limited attention to the processes of generating and disseminating happiness. It has also tended to treat happiness as a private, individual-level good, to the neglect of its development and functions as a social-level public good.

Who are the key providers and spreaders of happiness in different social and cultural contexts? How do our upbeat friends, our entertainers, our barefoot therapists, our peacemakers, and other happiness brokers develop their capabilities, and how do they operate? Are they aware of this function? Are they celebrated, trained, promoted? Through what social networks, personnel, and events are happiness viruses transmitted? Could some of the knowledge generated by the Positive Psychology

N. Thin (✉)
University of Edinburgh, Edinburgh, Scotland
e-mail: n.thin@ed.ac.uk

R. Biswas-Diener (ed.), *Positive Psychology as Social Change*,
DOI 10.1007/978-90-481-9938-9_3, © Springer Science+Business Media B.V. 2011

movement help people to promote happiness more efficiently and responsibly? Could Positive Psychology itself be enriched by taking more careful account of the social processes, the cultural endorsements, and the institutions involved in joy spreading? How do the pursuits and provisioning of other goods such as wealth, knowledge, health, and status interact and intersect with the pursuit and provisioning of happiness?

Let's explore first some of the cultural diversity of the world's cheermongers, roughly in order of the life stage that they specialise in.

The Joys of Childbirth: Midwifery and Murder in Bihar

Parvati is an informal midwife in Bihar. She takes more pride and care in her work since receiving training which improved her medical skills and public recognition of her status as a life-provider. Over many years working in an area with some of the highest infant and maternal mortality rates in the world, she has saved many lives of mothers and infants, and brought untold joy to the families she serves.

As well as the direct benefits of medical services, she also facilitates happiness in other ways. Her cheerful self-assurance removes anxieties before, during, and after the birth. By taking upon herself the risks and ritual pollution of childbirth, she helps ensure that families get through both normal and traumatic births without lasting animosities.

Sadly, however, Parvati is also a serial contract killer. In several cases of unwanted daughters and babies with birth defects, she has been paid to ensure that the baby doesn't survive beyond the first few days. She has also performed abortions for unwanted female foetuses. She hates these latter tasks, but reconciles herself to them on the understanding that they cut short lives that would have been miserable. In the area she works in, male births are nearly always joyful; some female births are too, but many are not, and the best she can offer is to cut short the misery. Cultural change in favour of gender equity and socioeconomic change away from dowries and towards equitable inheritance would greatly reduce the risk that future generations of midwives are asked to double up as murderers.

Childbirth, for all its pains and risks, is among the most magical and lasting joys life has to offer. Birth personnel such as midwives thus play critical roles in facilitating happiness worldwide. But in India they are poorly rewarded, undertrained, and stigmatized due to their association with the mess and risks of childbirth. The potentially removable ills of birth are partly biological, but also take the form of adverse cultural attitudes and unfair social structures. Murthy (1998) gives a harrowing account of how the voluntary agency Adithi investigated Bihar's female: male ratio of 82:100 and found it to be mainly caused by neglect and infanticide of girls. Parents weren't prepared to talk about infanticide, but midwives were. Their actions are of course only the proximate causes, the underlying causes being centuries-old socioeconomic discrimination and cultural prejudice against women. In such circumstances, hygienic midwifery has enormous potential to save lives but rather limited potential to promote happiness. For a broader analysis of the causes and evil effects of son preference in many parts of Asia, see Das Gupta et al., 2002. For further information, see http://www.gendercide.org/case_infanticide.html

Fun at School: Circle Time, Rape, and Deworming in Kenya

Sarah is taking a gap year from her primary school teaching in the UK, and is working in a primary school in an impoverished rural area of eastern Kenya. She knew she should expect very large and ill-equipped classes, high rates of teacher and pupil absenteeism, and troubling levels of violence and sexual abuse both in and out of school. But having spent 2 years enthusiastically adopting the latest pro-happiness teaching methods under her English educational authority's Social And Emotional Learning programme in the UK, she is keen not only to provide instruction but to play some part in making her Kenyan school a happier place.

Noticing that many of her pupils are falling asleep in the afternoon, she arranges with a local health charity to make deworming tablets and a healthy lunch available to all the pupils, and within 2 months there are noticeable improvements in attendance and concentration. Sports and music are out of the question due to lack of facilities, but most seem to fit a lot of exercise in just getting to and from school, and local villages and church groups offer ample singing and dancing opportunities.

The idea of a "Circle Time" raises some eyebrows in a context where most teachers habitually teach by rote and hit pupils when they misbehave. It eventually proves a popular innovation but it takes extraordinary persistence getting a class of 100 pupils aged 6–11 organized into circles, and against her own preferences she has to agree that girls and boys can form separate circles. She also notices that many girls absent themselves from circle time as they have been sent on errands for the other teachers, and some of the girls who gain her confidence start telling her worrying stories of the prevalence of sexual abuse by both pupils and teachers.

Sarah remains dedicated to the idea that pupil happiness should be a key concern everywhere in the world, but learns that some of the finer points of social and emotional learning may take some time to reach the top of the priority list in countries like Kenya.

For better or worse, the world has launched into a radically new and unproven assumption that upbringing is largely a matter of western-style schooling. I have argued elsewhere (Thin, 2009) that the ultra-rapid universalisation of schooling as the main means for educating all of the world's young people has proceeded with pitifully inadequate analysis of how schooling affects children's well-being directly and indirectly. Regarding schooling in poorer countries, a fair amount is known about effects on knowledge, earnings, and health, but there is very little systematic assessment of its effects on happiness during and after the school years. It is widely understood that school quality is often appalling, but in most countries the research and policy priorities are to do with universalising access and attending to the basic minimum quality standards of provision, not to luxuries like pupil enjoyment, life skills, and school climate. There is a growing literature on the harms suffered by pupils (Dunne, Humphreys, & Leach, 2006) and on the persistence of corporal punishment by teachers and parents in Kenya (Human Rights Watch, 1999) and worldwide (Global Initiative to End All Corporal Punishment of Children, 2009). Regarding the priority and cost-effectiveness of attending to pupils' basic health needs, see Galal, Neumann, and Hulett (2005) and Bundy, Michael Kremer, Hoyt Bleakley, Jukes, and Miguel (2009).

Dancing: Out and About in Australia

Dominique runs a youth dance class in Victoria, Australia. Together with a pianist in a local community hall, she lights up the lives of youngsters and their parents by offering technical instruction and putting on the occasional public performance. Seeing herself primarily as a technical instructor, she doesn't think of herself as someone who also facilitates healthy exercise, intersex relationships, musical appreciation, the ability to enjoy public performance, and opportunities to escape humdrum or conflict-ridden home life. But what she produces is not just a peculiarly specialised kind of bodily grace, it is also a wide variety of personal and collective happiness.

Dance, among other forms of ritualized movement and collective experimentation with the beauties of sound and light, affords vital opportunities for transcending and escaping the self and for engaging with other people in various ways. Findings from an ethnographic study of the experiences and benefits of Australian youth dance classes have been published by Gardner, Komesaroff, and Fensham (2008), who argue that state support for such activities would not only help fight the obesity epidemic but promote a wide range of other social and cultural benefits. Before joining the merry band of anti-happiness curmudgeons and turning her guns on the North American cult of positivity (Ehrenreich, 2009), the pop sociologist Barbara Ehrenreich was strongly in favour of the culture of merriment. She wrote an excellent book on festive joy through the ages which extolled the virtues of dancing and all the exciting and therapeutic socialising that goes with it (Ehrenreich, 2006). For a quick overview of the neuroscience of dancing, love, and happiness, see Freeman, 1997. For further discussion of the therapeutic benefits of dance, see the *American Journal of Dance Therapy*.

Dance, like exercise, allows people to enjoy their bodies, but there are always risks that these activities become reduced to instrumental means of bodily improvement. This is dangerous, as it can lead to bodily paranoia, something which is whipped up in modern societies by moral panic about childhood obesity. Google Scholar, for example, today (January 2010) finds just 28 items with "child" and "happiness" in the title, but replace "happiness" with "obesity" and you get 624. So fat children are 20 times as interesting to scholars as happy children are. I was mightily relieved to find there was one article on "the happy obese child", to remind us that the traditional association between plumpness and jollity hasn't been buried forever.

Love and Marriage: Stars, Contracts, and Love Pioneers in Kerala

Kannan is a marriage broker in Kerala who uses astrological information to help families decide on suitable matches for their offspring. He knows that it isn't just individuals that will be joined in marriage, but families and extended kin networks too. Reputations, wealth, and the future well-being of many people are at stake. Kannan recognizes that blunt and hasty conversations about personal qualities and livelihoods could quickly turn sour. So he allows them to learn about each other through the safer medium of conversations about stars, planets, and birthdates. He also generates a calm and respectful atmosphere by exuding fascination and confidence in his profession. Astrological consultations aren't just perfunctory necessities in the marriage-arranging process. When you get a good astrologer like Kannan, they are fun to be with and they take some of the terror out of the potentially horrific process of negotiating the lives and debating the qualities of loved ones with strangers.

Most probably he genuinely believes that astrological charts give directly useful information about human characters and relationships. So he has limited understanding of how, if at all, his advice affects people's lives. He is probably not at all conscious of the fact that he is picking up vital cues about prospects for his clients' interpersonal and social compatibility, and is unaware that he is, essentially, an interfamily therapist. In the UK, Kannan would be legally obliged to advertise his astrological services as "for entertainment purposes only", but he would be free to set up as a life coach or marriage guidance counsellor without any such regulatory constraint.

Increasingly, his work is complicated by the encroachments of a new generation of love pioneers who not only want to engage in premarital romances, but want to marry their partners. This tests Kannan's mind-reading and face-saving skills to the limit. But if he performs well by deflecting attention from no-win arguments and nudging people towards decisions that may actually be in their interest, he can help the families through what is inevitably a life-threatening crisis period. He may play a key role in building social acceptability of love marriage, a strange and unwelcome form of intimacy that in India today still tends to be hidden or labelled as "abduction".

A core part of Positive Psychology's ideology is that it will lead to morally superior, more happiness-inducing forms of decision-making. Evidence about happiness outcomes will gradually replace authoritarianism, traditionalism, superstition, and mistaken common sense as the basis for decisions. Decisions about love and marriage are everywhere of vital importance for people's life outcomes, but for the most part of the world decisions about marriage are not seen as primarily the responsibility of young individuals. Indeed, for most people in the world the idea of young people making decisions about life partners on their own, and on the basis of something so fickle as romantic inspiration, is horrific and/or ludicrous. In India, parents see it as their responsibility to protect their offspring from the worries and risks of such an important decision, and even they tend to be sufficiently nervous to consult with astrologers about the match and the date, in addition to the multiple social consulting about the qualities of the potential spouse, their family, and their wider kin group. Like the midwife, the astrologer relieves kin of some of the pressures of risky responsibility, and distracts from anxieties and crude interpersonal and interfamily evaluations by introducing a degree of randomness in the decision.

There is no definitive research showing whether marital outcomes are better or worse under autonomous or parentally guided mate selection, but several studies have found that marital satisfaction levels are similar with either system (Myers, Madathil, & Tingle, 2005), and others have shown that many marriage arrangement processes increasingly occupy a middle ground between autonomy and parental arrangement (Donner, 2002). There can be no doubt that arranging marriages, along with related matters of negotiating dowries and inheritances, is a focus of appalling levels of anxiety and family strife in India. But it would be smug and naive for westerners to recommend a quick transition to "love marriage" as a eudaimonically and ethically superior solution.

In the West, happiness research has shown that having a stable long-term relationship, perhaps involving marriage, correlates moderately well with self-reported happiness. In a situation where marriage and long-term relationships are seen as optional, this information might conceivably have some influence on personal decisions, or, more likely, it might be used as an argument for governmental and nongovernmental support that would help people achieve lasting forms of intimacy. But in India as in much of the world, however, marriage isn't an option, and decisions about partners are made by parents and kin networks (Medora, 2003). Romantic love exists in most cultural contexts, but often is seen as having little or no relevance to marriage (Jankowiak, 1995; Hatfield & Rapson, 1996). Perhaps one day, love-based marriage decisions, informed by happiness research, will be shown to lead to better and more lasting relationships than parental decisions and astrologically guided decisions. So far, though, it is hard to see what relevance western research on marriage and love has in nonwestern contexts.

Health Seeking, Peace Making, and Hate-Mongery in Africa

Zodani is a traditional healer, village council leader, and family therapist in the Limpopo Province of south Africa. Though not overtly rich or powerful, he is nonetheless recognized as pivotal to the well-being and survival of many hundreds of people. Every day, individuals and families consult him about their personal health and about family and village politics such as interpersonal vendettas and disputes. Therapeutic pluralism flourishes here, and Zodani is eclectic in the range of remedies he offers and advocates. In many cases, he appears to help people return to health and happiness, providing a rich mixture of herbal medicines, peacemaking opportunities, and practical advice. Often, he plays a vital therapeutic role in allaying people's everyday fears and helping them make important life decisions or nudging them towards health simply by giving them confidence. Occasionally,

however, particularly during periods of economic or political turmoil, his practical advice has involved naming specific individuals as witches. In effect, he orders
assassinations: the named individuals either hear of the accusation and flee the village permanently, or they are caught and typically burned alive. With economic
change, the frequency of these occurrences is increasing. He is both admired and
feared for this important role: most people see witch-sniffing as a vital role in the
fight against evil, but anyone who can sniff witches is in touch with dark forces
himself.

Zodani's former friend and school classmate Sidney has a very different approach
to the witchcraft problem. Having joined the provincial government and espoused
modern western anti-superstitious views, he sees witchcraft as a disruptive fantasy
which must be fought by rational education and where necessary in the law courts.
For many years he tried to scare people like Zodani by taking them to court for
incitement to murder whenever evidence could be found that they had accused people of witchcraft. He found, however, that many of his governmental colleagues
weren't interested in joining that crusade for fear of being accused of siding with
the witches. Indeed, in a cultural context where the majority of people believe in
and fear witchcraft, many of his colleagues unsurprisingly felt that the law courts
would better serve the well-being of citizens by bringing witches, not medicine-men
and harassers, to justice. Some saw this as the broader issue of defending the value
and dignity of "African science" and "African justice" in the face of creeping west-
ernization. Recently, Sidney's efforts have gone towards establishing state-financed
old-age pension schemes and support for micro-credit, in the hope that by strengthening the financial position of older people, especially women, he will in the long
run give them sufficient power and status to be able to avoid or fight back against
witchcraft accusations.

The role of "traditional healers", often government sponsored, in exacerbating
the AIDS crisis in southern Africa, is now recognized worldwide as a grotesque
source of avoidable death and suffering. But their role in promoting, though also
sometimes abating, witch-hunt frenzies has received less international attention.
Witchcraft-related killings, harassment, and fears remain pervasive in many countries today, including most African countries. Though informed by cultural beliefs
about occult forces, they are also often strongly linked with social inequalities
and social tension such as intergenerational cultural differences and conflicts over
resources. Getting on in life has always been a mixture of effort and luck. Humans
are not very good at accepting luck for what it is, and when others are lucky or
we are unlucky, we have always tended to imagine others using illegitimate occult
forces to gain their advantage. Witchcraft shows that this is as much a cultural and
social problem as a psychological one.

Patterns of witchcraft accusation and retribution vary, but in many parts of
Africa old women are particularly vulnerable, and the risk can sometimes be effectively combated by strengthening the rights and resources of vulnerable people
(Schnoebelen, 2009). Miguel, having shown persuasive evidence that outbreaks of
witch-killing in Tanzania and elsewhere are linked with environmental adversity and
consequential economic shocks, has proposed old-age pensions as a way of saving

elderly women from the threat of being singled out as witches and expelled or killed by their kin (Miguel, 2005, p. 1170). Witchcraft is far too varied and complex for any simple solution to address, but economic empowerment might help African policy makers to avoid the minefield of trying to combat witch harassment and witchcraft beliefs by more direct opposition – a failed civilising mission inherited from the previous colonial regimes. In many areas, though, new economic opportunities have exacerbated witchcraft, since the two key categories of accused people tend to be the new rich and the people who envy them (Golooba-Mutebi, 2005).

Witchcraft is "real". It is an important influence on people's well-being in many parts of the world today. Now you and I, dear reader, probably don't believe that witches are real occult attackers. Indeed, I would urge you not to adopt the ethically and intellectually implausible stance of "postmodern" anthropologists who simply shrug and declare that lots of realities are possible, witchcraft among them (e.g. Geschiere, 2008, p. 334) or who say that "the validity of witchcraft beliefs is not at issue here" (Schnoebelen, 2009, p. 2). It seems to me very much to the point to assert, loudly and repeatedly, the invalidity of belief in witches and in "witch-sniffing", as indeed many brave Traditional Healers' Associations have done throughout Africa in recent years. Not that this will necessarily change stubborn people's minds, but when people hold beliefs that are both morally and scientifically wrong, we should tell them so. That said, as a set of cultural beliefs, and responses to those beliefs, witches have the same kind of "reality" that God, Heaven, Santa Claus, and homoeopathic medicine have, except that they are mainly "negative" rather than "positive" illusions.

It might be argued that belief in witchcraft, like belief in God or the Devil, can have good effects and so is in that respect a "positive" illusion and hence a potential ally of "positive" social policy. Anthropologists of the past have assured us that in general, witch beliefs serve as crucial reinforcers of social virtues such as sharing, cooperation, and even love (Gluckman, 1955). But in the modern era there are better ways of promoting pro-social behaviour than scaring people with witch fantasies, and for the most part the costs in terms of fear, mistrust, and violence seem hard to justify. God and Heaven, of course, aren't above suspicion: they have often served "negative" purposes such as justifying wars and making people accept unfair forms of this-worldly suffering. But although I see both witches and benign deities as illusions, I have no qualms about asserting that the world would be happier without witchcraft whereas I would be hard pressed to defend atheism on eudaimonic grounds.

As many anthropologists and historians have shown (e.g. Geschiere, 2008), naive assumptions that modern enlightenment would brush away the superstitions and injustices of witchcraft have proved unfounded. Several African states as well as local justice institutions remain strongly implicated in the assumption that the "victims" of witchcraft are the bewitched and that witches (not just those who make accusations and punish "witches") need to be identified and punished. When the fear of witchcraft and of accusations of witchcraft remains pervasive, everyone suffers and many are killed. The anthropologist Unni Wikan has argued (1987) that behind the fabled and romanticised grace and smiles of the Balinese lies a desperate lack of trust in even the closest of kin and friends, with everyone required to put on a show of equanimity to avoid both occult attacks and suspicions that you are an occult attacker.

Witchcraft hasn't featured much in the literature on Positive Psychology so far, perhaps because North Americans don't in general believe in witchcraft, but it is salutary to bear in mind that if the Positive Psychology were a predominantly European movement, it would have paid much less heed to religion and so-called spirituality than has been the case. A balanced approach would recognize that around the world, people tend to entertain a range of occult beliefs, some of which may help them at least some of the time, and others which can easily turn pathological and deadly.

On the Ethnocentric Roots and Countercultural Ambitions of Positive Psychology

You will have noticed that a lot of the above doesn't seem to fit with the idea of focusing on the good life. Instead, in our search for cheermongery we have encountered a variety of social and cultural pathologies which for vast numbers of people worldwide present enormous obstacles to the pursuit of good lives: son preference and gender discrimination; "pollution" beliefs and witchcraft beliefs; intergenerational inequities and misunderstandings; violence, mistrust, and fear; and of course the physical laziness, obesity, and social disruptions that come with modern affluence and economic change. For social scientists and social activists, it is all too tempting to give way to righteous indignation, to reject the positivity of happiness studies as irrelevant or even damaging to development, and to see the struggle for progress largely as one of fighting these sociocultural pathologies head-on.

As a polemical and radical movement, Positive Psychology has sometimes been misdiagnosed as a "negative to positive" movement, from an emphasis on harm to an emphasis on goodness. But it is better described as a shift *from pathological to holistic* approaches to the good life. That is, the movement doesn't ask us to stop being concerned with harm and its reduction, but rather to adopt more balanced, integrated approaches to human betterment, which try to complement pathological and clinical concerns with understanding and promotion of things that go well with people's lives (Tennen & Affleck, 2003; Held, 2004; Linley et al., 2006). The trouble is, for many people in rough parts of the world, harms are so constantly threatening that asking people to shift attention towards happiness might seem irresponsible.

In defence of positivity, though, two things must be noted. First, it is almost never the case that suffering is the only valid story to tell about the lives of poor people in poor countries, so it is crucial that we learn about how people manage to enjoy themselves and find a sense of meaning or purpose despite adversity. After all, women worldwide suffer appalling discrimination, yet they say they are as happy as men or happier, and in most countries live longer too (Diener, Suh, Lucas, & Smith, 1999). Second, direct confrontation of sociocultural pathologies has rarely worked, and most social progress occurs indirectly, by enabling people to enjoy comfortable, safe, happy lives (Lyubomirsky, King, & Diener, 2005). Happy people aren't always virtuous, but there are important synergies between happiness and pro-social behaviour.

Contributors to this book are also proposing a second kind of shift that will move the attention of positive psychologists *from individual to social levels* of change. This will implement the movement's emphasis on individual-level, "inside-out" approaches to attitudinal self-help (Outhwaite & Bettridge, 2009; Sheldon & Lyubomirsky, 2009) with stronger attention to the need for changes in the social conditions for happiness. These two pathological-to-holistic and individual-to-social movements are good, but I propose here that they could both be strengthened by a third kind of shift which positive psychologists have so far only occasionally and for the most part insubstantially addressed: *from ethnocentric and culture-blind to multicultural and culturally inflected approaches to social progress.* Considered radically, this doesn't just mean making occasional forays into non-western cultures. Even within any one local community, western or otherwise, happiness promoters must recognise that everyone's beliefs, theories, empirical knowledge, and actions, including their own, are cultural. And this *always* means that we are "multicultural" (Goodenough, 1976, p. 4).

Everyone in the world learns through multiple channels, though some channels are more dominant than others. There are no discrete "cultures," although as with languages, it's sometimes useful to imagine them as discrete entities. But unlike written languages, culture exists fluidly, in learning and interaction. A common concern among those who question the ethnocentrism of happiness studies is to worry about whether "happiness" means the same as "felicidad" or "ikigai", and if not whether international survey comparisons are possible. But this is somewhat beside the point, since one use of "happiness" doesn't translate to another use of "happiness" anyway. Everyone worldwide uses various happiness concepts and evaluates their life variously according to mood and contexts. It's not just that different people, due to "cultural" differences, mean different things by "happiness": you and I use it with radically different meanings in our everyday lives because the concepts it conjures up derive from a complex assortment of cultural streams.

We are all "ethnocentric" to the extent that our beliefs, values, and practices are strongly rooted in particular cultural influences. There's nothing intrinsically wrong with this, provided that we are aware of it and recognise two possible problems associated with strong cultural themes. First some of our dominant themes won't go down so well with people who are more persuaded by other cultural themes. Second, strong cultural themes tend to be associated with the failure to recognize our ideologies as ideologies, and to perceive them – if we notice them at all – as natural. This leads to misguided universalist assumptions that distort science.

Individualism, positivity, self-esteem, and self-fulfilment happen to be dominant beliefs and values in Positive Psychology and in contemporary North American ideology, but there are people in every culture, including North America, who question these values (Crocker & Park, 2004; Ehrenreich, 2009; Christopher & Hickinbottom, 2008). But the Positive Psychology movement has also been creatively countercultural: it has challenged some cultural themes that were dominant in Psychology, such as pathologism and cognitivism, and has avoided being led by some broader North American cultural themes such as economism, consumerism, Christian monotheism, and belief in an afterlife. It could move further to engage in a wider range of cross-cultural dialogues to pursue its ambitions to bring about substantial improvements to well-being and social justice worldwide.

At the individual level, some positive psychologists have, of course, begun addressing cross-cultural issues, but mostly this has been restricted to broad-brushed international or inter-regional contrasts. Moving to social levels, it becomes much harder to ignore the fact that happiness is always culturally inflected: each individual in every society learns how to aspire, how to communicate, and how to reflect on life through a variety of cultural influences which often conflict with one another. At supra-individual levels of analysis it is also harder to ignore the ecological implications of happiness pursuits. We become happy or unhappy through *society* (relationships and institutions), through *culture* (learning processes), and through *ecological* engagement (accommodating to and modifying biophysical environments). Some people also consider "spiritual" engagement to be a further dimension, but this I think can comfortably be accommodated within the social and cultural categories. Changes in quality of life involve all of these dimensions, but specific approaches to change tend to emphasise some more than others:

- *Individual-focused* approaches proceed as if the most important changes are within the control of the individual: changes in bodies, minds, and behaviour systems (e.g. safer childbirth practices, deworming schoolchildren, dancing for health, personal choice of marriage partner).
- *Social* approaches emphasise changes in relationships, organisations, and institutionalised patterns such as roles (e.g. the status and remuneration of midwives, teachers, and traditional healers; the role of inheritance in intergenerational relationships, and the effects of marriage "gifts" on interfamily and intrafamilial relationships; the promotion and maintenance of community trust).
- *Cultural* approaches emphasise changes in learning processes, knowledge transmission, and cultural artefacts (e.g. attitudes to birth pollution and to the value of girls and women; young people's autonomy and voice in school and in choosing marriage partners; witchcraft beliefs).
- *Ecological* approaches emphasise individual and collective changes in our accommodations to and adaptations of the physical environment (not foregrounded in the above examples, but environmental improvements could clearly make a difference to the joys and safety of schooling, and to the uncertainties and economic shocks that perpetuate fear of witches).

Cultural diversity may entail major differences in the contexts for happiness-promoting interventions. These differences don't map neatly onto discrete national, ethnic, or regional "cultures"; they emerge from the multiple ways in which we learn and transmit knowledge and values. These multiple flows aren't just patterned by geography and time, but attach to categories of people and to social positions.

Within countries, there may be crucial cultural differences associated with gender, age, class, ethnicity, or occupation. The following are some of the critically important issues in cultural analysis of happiness prospects:

- *The self:* understanding the concept of personal happiness must start by thinking about what kinds of self might be deemed happy or otherwise. All cultures require multiple self concepts, including the concept of a discrete individual as well as temporary or permanent roles, and socially or cosmologically embedded selves. Some cultures and some individuals put most emphasis and value on the autonomous individual who lives one this-worldly life. Others see the self – and therefore happiness and associated concepts such as life satisfaction – in much more fluid social, ecological, cosmological, and cross-temporal terms. Happiness may be mainly about social connections, or about embeddedness in a wider ecological environment, or about relations with spirits and deities. And it may be at least as much about previous and future lives as it is about this life.
- *Conceptual:* there may be no conceptual or linguistic equivalent to the catch-all term "happiness", but rather a multiplicity of terms relating to different kinds of good feeling and good living at individual and collective levels. To pursue happiness, we don't require a single all-purpose "happiness" concept.
- *Value:* whatever concepts may translate roughly as "happiness", they may not have prime position as the ultimate value, but may be ranked lower than other values such as virtue, religious merit, wisdom, status, or excellence. Nor is it likely that we will find that most people in the world can draw neat contrasts between "positive" and "negative" experiences as North American Positive Psychologists would have us do.
- *Emotion and character norms and display rules:* expectations of what a good character ought to feel, and how and when they ought to display and communicate their feelings, are strongly influenced by cultural traditions. Being gleefully happy in public isn't necessarily a wise move in a low-trust culture where witchcraft suspicions are rife.
- *Somatization (embodiment):* there is wide cultural variety in the degree to which emotional experience is manifested in the body, and the ways in which this happens and in which it is experienced, displayed, and thought about. The western idea of distinguishing "mental health" from bodily health is of limited relevance to most people in the world.

Towards Social Happiness Policies

> Human progress is toward greater mutual dependence, as well as toward greater individuation (Herbert Spencer, 1851).

Two really good kinds of change might be taken a step further by this book. First, specialists in Positive Psychology might become more socially and culturally engaged, promoting social change and embracing cultural diversity. Second, inversely, specialists in social transformation might become more positive, recognizing that social progress must be about living well in good societies rather than just about reducing harms such as poverty and crime, and promoting "justice" and "rights" through better access to interim goods such as money, land, and schooling.

Thinking about Positive Psychology as a "mechanism for social change" is promising but we might do better without the metaphorical implication of science being applied to society in a mechanistic way. Social transformation happens, if at all, organically and not mechanistically, and often by accident rather than design. Change occurs through relatively unpredictable iteration between individual and social levels. Social engineering programmes tend to fail, and can have disastrous consequences if pushed too hard by authoritarian states. But we still need happiness-aware approaches to social policy, and we should ensure that our personal or collective plans are informed by the best evidence we have about happiness.

Similarly, we must avoid framing the proposed interactions in terms of "Psychology" as the agent acting on "Society". Society doesn't sit around waiting to be instructed by psychology on how to change. Psychology is part of society, it is itself cultural. Change will involve mutual, iterative influences between psychology and society. Positive Psychology will be transformed as new knowledge emerges from social experiments and studies in different parts of the world. Lots of the self-help recommendations coming out of the Positive Psychology movement require social transformation, not just individual willpower, to become effective, and the science of positivity will in turn change as it observes the effects of those changes.

It is true that the primary referent of happiness is individuals' feelings. Even when extended to cover various virtues and existential meanings, it typically refers to individual subjectivity. We won't get very far with our wonderful project of globalizing cheermongery if we don't start by recognizing these default meanings as cultural products. Despite paying substantial attention to social aspects of personal happiness pursuits, psychology has emphasised the feeling individual, and has shown less interest in happiness as an evaluative lens through which to view society. Happiness has been seen as an *emotional state, mood, or disposition;* as a *character trait;* as a form of *self-evaluation* or *judgement of others;* as a personal *motive;* or as an interpersonal *display,* something individuals try to communicate. It hasn't, generally, been treated as a *social quality:* as a form of interpersonal contagion; as an expected property of events, times, or spaces; as an evaluation of groups or of institutions; as a virus that travels through social networks (but see Fowler & Christakis, 2008). Yet our everyday discourse shows that we are well aware that happiness has all of these social, supra-individual, relational meanings. We talk of happy birthdays, joyful atmospheres, happy hours, cheerful organisations, and so on.

Because humans are social, happiness is at least as much about giving and communicating as it is about receiving and feeling. If we want positive psychology to become a major force for the good worldwide, we have to identify and nurture some of the implementers and transmitters, and consider the social and cultural contexts in which they operate as well as their different levels of influence. Positive psychology's core personal-level tenet, that individuals should play to their strengths emphasising positive aspects of our characters, is just as valid as a social policy principle. Social happiness policy must be based on recognising and nurturing the kinds of people and institutions that make the most positive contributions to social happiness. We must also consider the cultural and social embeddedness of our evidence-based advice, recognising positive psychology to be more of a culturally and socially motivated movement than a detached science.

Application of positive psychology involves deliberate cultural and social change, not just providing individuals with options for self-betterment. There are already lots of joy-spreading specialists who make a difference to lots of other people's happiness. They do so directly and indirectly, intentionally and unintentionally, in the name of happiness or via some other objective, and with or without a formal licence. What will they do differently, and how will they be facilitated and rewarded differently, in the light of knowledge gained from happiness studies? What cultural and social changes are being envisaged, and on the basis of what kinds of cross-cultural dialogue and comparison?

Conclusions: Social Development as if Happiness Mattered

Modern international development cooperation has shifted from an obsession with "growth" and "take-off" in the 1950s and 1960s to concerns about "human capital", then distributional equity and environmental sustainability, participatory "people-first" approaches, human rights, poverty reduction, and now the Millennium Development Goals which focus largely on measurable changes in pathological indicators. Post-materialist concerns with the existentially and hedonically good life still seem remote from some aspects of development planning, but it is possible that in the current decade well-being and happiness could at last become major themes in international development planning.

Just as positive psychology had long-term antecedents in humanistic psychology and self-help and therapeutic movements dating back to the previous century, so too there have been movements for positive social change that have yet to crystallise into a high-profile "positive social policy" or "social happiness policy" movements. While many commentators have linked happiness studies with nineteenth-century interest in political utilitarianism, they have for the most part focused on rather detached philosophical and macro-level theorising about the purposes and responsibilities of governments, rather than going into any detail on the deliberate or unplanned social changes that might promote mass-scale happiness or other desired ultimate goods (see e.g. Layard, 2005; Bok, 2010).

In 2002, commissioned by the World Bank and UK Government to collate the "social development" policies of a wide range of international development agencies, I noted the worrying absence of coherent and positive policies for social progress. But I also noted, among agencies ranging from community organisations to international NGOs, businesses, governments, and multilateral development institutions, a consensus on four categories of quality that can meaningfully be labelled both "social" (in that they pertain to society) and "positive" (in that they are about well-being and social goods rather than just about efforts to combat social pathologies): *social justice, solidarity, participation,* and *security* (Thin, 2002, Chapter 5). This offers a minimalist classification of the desirable social processes that socially responsible cheermongery must engage with. All of these are also culturally inflected, in that we learn culturally about what is fair, whom we should love or respect, what we can participate in, and who or what guarantees our safety. Indeed, in some cultural contexts these social values may be more prominent in conceptions of the good life and happiness than personal emotions are (Uchida & Kitayama, 2009; Iyengar & DeVoe, 2003). There is endless room for debate as to what these social desiderata mean; nonetheless they are more realistic candidates as universal social goals than, for example, choice, freedom, multiculturalism, or equality.

These social qualities are interdependent with the "character strengths" which psychologists have identified as morally approved worldwide, such as kindness, justice, honesty, gratitude, and courage (Park, Peterson & Seligman, 2006) and are similar to Sissela Bok's "minimalist" set of universal basic values even though she claims that "solidarity" can't be included in such a list (Bok, 1995/2002, pp. ix, 13–15). Socially responsible efforts to develop positive psychology as a force for good change worldwide will address these social qualities at all levels, from individual and family, through local communities, wider social networks, businesses and civil institutions, to national and global levels. This process will help people rethink "justice" as being about the distribution and sharing of well-being, not only about access to resources. We will think about solidarity less in the dry sociological terms of "associations", "social capital", and "social cohesion", and more in terms of love and contagious happiness. Participation will not just be about formal public voice and the right to vote, but about creative public engagement and the optimism that encourages it. Security will not just be about crime, punishment, and deterrence, but about the active enjoyment of peace, and about the freedoms that ensue from predictable social and economic relations.

References

Bok, S. (1995/2002). *Common values.* Columbia, MO: University of Missouri Press.

Bok, D. (2010). *The politics of happiness: What government can learn from the new research on well-being.* Princeton: Princeton University Press.

Bundy, D. A., Michael Kremer, P., Hoyt Bleakley, M. C., Jukes, H., & Miguel, E. (2009). Deworming and development: Asking the right questions, asking the questions right. http://www.research4development.info/PDF/Outputs/Ehca_RPC/BundyCommentary0000362.pdf

Christopher, J. C., & Hickinbottom, S. (2008). Positive psychology, ethnocentrism, and the disguised ideology of individualism. *Theory and Psychology, 18*(5), 563–589.

Crocker, J., & Park, L. E. (2004). The costly pursuit of self-esteem. *Psychological Bulletin, 130*(3), 322–414.

Das Gupta, M., Zhenghua, J., Bohua, Li., Zhenming, X., Chung, W., & Hwa-Ok, B. (2002). *Why is son preference so persistent in East and South Asia? A cross-country study of China, India, and the Republic of Korea* (Research Working Paper WPS 2942). Washington, DC: World Bank.

Diener, Ed., Suh, E. M., Lucas, R. E., & Smith, H. L. (1999). Subjective well-being: Three decades of progress. *Psychological Bulletin, 125*(2), 276 302.

Donner, H. (2002). "One's own marriage": Love marriages in a Calcutta neighbourhood. *South Asia Research, 22*(1), 79–94.

Dunne, M., Humphreys, S., & Leach, F. (2006). Gender violence in schools in the developing world. *Gender and Education, 18*(1), 75–98.

Ehrenreich, B. (2006). *Dancing in the streets: A history of collective joy.* Cambridge: Granta.

Ehrenreich, B. (2009). *Smile or Die: How positive thinking fooled America and the world* [USA title: *Bright-sided: How the relentless promotion of positive thinking has undermined America*]. London: Granta.

Fowler, J. H., & Christakis, N. A. (2008). Dynamic spread of happiness in a large social network: Longitudinal analysis over 20 years. *British Medical Journal, 337*(2338), 1–9.

Freeman, W. (1997). Happiness doesn't come in bottles: Neuroscientists learn that joy comes through dancing, not drugs. *Journal of Consciousness Studies, 4*(1), 67–70.

Galal, O. M., Neumann, C. G., & Hulett, J. (2005). Proceedings of the international workshop on articulating the impact of nutritional deficits on the education for all agenda. *Food and Nutrition Bulletin, 26*(2), Supplement 2.

Gardner, S. M., Komesaroff, P., & Fensham, R. (2008). Dancing beyond exercise: Young people's experiences in dance classes. *Journal of Youth Studies, 11*(6), 701–709.

Geschiere, P. (2008). Witchcraft and the state: Cameroon and South Africa ambiguities of 'reality' and 'superstition'. *Past & Present, 199*(3), 313–335.

Global Initiative to End All Corporal Punishment of Children. (2009). Ending legalised violence against children. Save the Children Sweden. http://www.endcorporalpunishment.org/pages/pdfs/reports/GlobalReport2009.pdf

Gluckman, M. (1955). *Custom and conflict in Africa.* Oxford: Oxford University Press.

Golooba-Mutebi, F. (2005). Witchcraft, social cohesion and participation in a South African Village. *Development and Change, 36*(5), 937–958.

Goodenough, W. H. (1976). Multiculturalism as the normal human experience. *Anthropology and Education, 7*(4), 4–7.

Hatfield, E., & Rapson, R. L. (1996). *Love and sex: Cross-cultural perspectives.* Needham Heights, MA: Allyn and Bacon.

Held, B. S. (2004). The negative side of positive psychology. *Journal of Humanistic Psychology, 44*, 9–46.

Human Rights Watch. (1999). *Spare the child: Corporal punishment in Kenyan schools.* Washington, DC: Human Rights Watch. www.hrw.org/reports/1999/kenya/index.htm

Iyengar, S. S., & DeVoe, S. E. (2003). Rethinking the value of choice: Considering cultural mediators of intrinsic motivation. In V. Murphy-Berman & J. J. Berman (Eds.), *Cross-cultural differences in perspectives on the self.* Lincoln, NE: University of Nebraska Press.

Jankowiak, W. (Ed.). (1995). *Romantic passion: The universal experience?* New York: Columbia University Press.

Layard, R. (2005). *Happiness: Lessons from a new science.* Harmondsworth: Penguin.

Linley, P. A., Joseph, S., Harrington, S., & Wood, A. M. (2006, January). Positive psychology: Past, present, and (possible) future. *The Journal of Positive Psychology, 1*(1), 3–16.

Lyubomirsky, S., King, L., & Diener, Ed. (2005). The benefits of frequent positive affect: Does happiness lead to success. *Psychological Bulletin, 131*(6), 803–855.

Medora, N. P. (2003). Mate selection in contemporary India: Love marriages vs. arranged marriages. In R. R. Hamon & B. B. Ingoldsby (Eds.), *Mate selection across cultures.* London: Sage.

Miguel, E. (2005). Poverty and witch killing. *The Review of Economic Studies, 72*(4), 1153–1172.

Murthy, R. (1998). Learning about participation from gender relations of female infanticide. In I. Guijt & M. K. Shah (Eds.), *The myth of community: Gender issues in participatory development* (pp. 78–92). London: Intermediate Technology Publications.

Myers, J. E., Madathil, J., & Tingle, L. R. (2005). Marriage satisfaction and wellness in India and the United States: A preliminary comparison of arranged marriages and marriages of choice. *Journal of Counseling & Development, 83*(2), 183–190.

Outhwaite, A., & Bettridge, N. (2009). From the inside out: Coaching's role in transformation. *The Coaching Psychologist, 5*(2), 76–89.

Park, N., Peterson, C., & Seligman, M. E. P. (2006, July). Character strengths in fifty-four nations and the fifty US states. *The Journal of Positive Psychology, 1*(3), 118–129.

Schnoebelen, J. (2009). *Witchcraft allegations, refugee protection and human rights: A review of the evidence.* UNHCR Policy Development and Evaluation Service, Research Paper No. 169. http://www.humansecuritygateway.com/documents/UNHCR_WtichcraftAllegationsRefugee ProtectionHumanRights_Africa.pdf

Sheldon, K. M., & Lyubomirsky, S. (2009). Change your actions, not your circumstances: An experimental test of the Sustainable Happiness model. In A. K. Dutt & B. Radcliff (Eds.), *Happiness, economics, and politics: Towards a multi-disciplinary approach* (pp. 324–342). Cheltenham: Edward Elgar.

Spencer, H. (1851). *Social statics: Or the conditions essential to human happiness specified, and the first of them developed.* London: John Chapman.

Tennen, H., & Affleck, G. (2003). While accentuating the positive, don't eliminate the negative or Mr. in-between. *Psychological Inquiry, 14,* 163–169.

Thin, N. (2002). *Social progress and sustainable development.* London: ITDG Publications.

Thin, N. (2009). *Schoolchildren's wellbeing and life prospects: Justifying the universal tax on childhood.* University of Bath Well-Being in Developing Countries Working Paper 09/46. http://www.bath.ac.uk/econ-dev/wellbeing/wedworkingpapers.htm

Uchida, Y., & Kitayama, S. (2009). Happiness and unhappiness in east and west: Themes and variations. *Emotion, 9*(4), 441–456.

Wikan, U. (1987). Public grace and private fears: Gaiety, offense and sorcery in Northern Bali. *Ethos, 15*(4), 337–365.

Part II
Positive Psychology and Public Policy

Chapter 4
Monitoring Psychosocial Prosperity for Social Change

Ed Diener and Carol Diener

A portrait of the good life has emerged among social and behavioral scientists based on factors that have been found to lead to health, effective functioning, and happiness. Several elements of "psychosocial prosperity" are now well supported by research evidence, and have achieved consensus among scientists. Furthermore, these elements have cross-national generality. Therefore, it is time to clearly articulate this vision to the societies of the world, with the goal of moving beyond economic wealth as the overarching aim of nations. A broad definition of psychosocial prosperity, including elements such as supportive social relationships, competence and mastery, subjective well-being, and community trust, in addition to material sufficiency, will provide societies with valuable standards in addition to materialistic ones against which to evaluate progress. Social scientists should be highly involved in defining prosperity, creating national measures of it, and implementing organizational structures and interventions to enhance it. Importantly, social scientists must play a central role in determining how potential policies and laws will influence psychosocial well-being. Unless a clear vision of psychosocial prosperity that can inspire people is offered, the current economic paradigm is likely to continue to dominate national policies and individual choices. A major step toward policy makers considering psychosocial prosperity is the implementation of national measures of it.

Behavioral scientists should be more ambitious in their goals for helping their societies set policy priorities because they have in the past century uncovered a number of the central elements of positive human functioning. Although their efforts have been primarily educational, conveying their vision of the "good life" to the public, social scientists should now work more actively to implement their findings at the policy level. This vision of psychosocial prosperity needs to be articulated to the public, and measures implemented that reveal how groups are faring. These measures will indicate the influence of societal policies and trends

E. Diener (✉)
University of Illinois, Urbana-Champaign, IL, USA; The Gallup Organization,
Washington, DC, USA
e-mail: ediener@uiuc.edu

R. Biswas-Diener (ed.), *Positive Psychology as Social Change*,
DOI 10.1007/978-90-481-9938-9_4, © Springer Science+Business Media B.V. 2011

on psychosocial prosperity. "Well-being" recently has become a common theme in the work of health professionals, nongovernmental organizations, and international agencies, and social scientists must move to the center of discussions about what it entails.

Social and behavioral scientists, of course, have already been involved in the formation and implementation of societal policies. However, this role has often been one of helping societies attain goals that are set by others rather than aiding societies to set their primary objectives. Social scientists have made substantial contributions to human welfare in diverse areas such as physical and mental health, education, and organizational effectiveness. They have been involved in helping people discover the vocation that best suits them, quit smoking, and in designing safer cockpits, for example. Social scientists must now play a central role in helping societies to create their overarching goals in the area of quality of life.

There is a golden opportunity at this time to help societies create a broad vision of psychosocial prosperity that will make life around the world more rewarding. Current questioning about how consumerism can hamper well-being, issues of economic sustainability, and analyses of how psychosocial factors influence health are converging forces that create a unique opportunity to offer a clear vision about what societies should be. No longer should behavioral scientists be content to accept the societal goals given to them by politicians, but they should move to the center of discussions of what national priorities should be. This does not mean that they must take a partisan conservative or liberal stance on policies, but that they should provide the framework, data, and interventions on which more informed discussions of policies can occur. The most economically developed nations of the world are now capable of offering food, clothing, and housing to all citizens, and the important issue is what direction societies should take next. Monitoring psychosocial prosperity will be the first step in instituting social change.

In the list below we present eight elements of psychosocial prosperity. We believe that there is a consensus among social scientists, as well as supportive data, that these elements help individuals and societies function more effectively, allowing citizens to live longer and healthier lives, and experience greater feelings of well-being. For each of the eight elements, four in the social domain and four in the psychological domain, we have listed an example of an item from the Gallup World Poll (described later) to assess the psychosocial prosperity of nations. The items used by the Gallup Organization can be refined and extended, but we list them here to give an idea of the content of each category.

Social Prosperity
1. Social support
   Have family and friends you can count on in an emergency
2. Public trust
   Government officials are corrupt (reverse scored)
3. Safety and security
   Had money or property stolen in past year (reverse scored)
4. Tolerance
   Your city or area is a good place for racial and ethnic minorities to live

Psychological Prosperity
5. Competence and growth
   You learned something new yesterday
6. Positive evaluations of life and life satisfaction
   You are satisfied with health, standard of living, and job (three separate items)
7. Positive engagement
   You would like more days like yesterday
8. Low levels of chronic negative feelings
   You felt depressed a lot yesterday (reverse scored).

These eight elements are desirable in all cultures of the world. An intolerant society with corruption, crime, and lack of social support will not fulfill human needs as well as one with the characteristics we list. Similarly, a society in which the citizens are incompetent in their skills and in reaching their goals, who view their lives as terrible, and who experience more anger and depression than joy and contentment is one in which few would choose to live. Importantly, economic growth can abet psychosocial prosperity, but it does not guarantee it.

Our list is meant to be a starting point rather than a definitive inventory. The list is consistent with general accounts of well-being (e.g., Ryan & Deci, 2000; Ryff, 1989; Ryff & Singer, 1998), evolutionary accounts (e.g., Kenrick, Griskevicius, Neuberg, & Schaller, 2010), and more specific theories as well (e.g., Csikszentmihalyi, 1988). There are a number of additional candidates for the list of psychosocial prosperity, for example, creativity, spirituality, meaning and purpose, resilience and coping, and effective self-regulation. In some cases we omitted possible elements because there is less agreement or research on them, or because measures are still being developed. Other elements can be added to our list and valid measures of them developed as needed. We intend our list to be illustrative of attributes of psychosocial prosperity about which there is sufficient evidence to support measures at the societal level. A broad panel of experts is needed to examine existing findings and create a more complete list of the components of psychosocial prosperity for which supportive evidence is now substantial, compile adequate measures of them, and make recommendations about the weighting of components of indexes.

Elements of Psychosocial Prosperity

Although there may be cultural differences in the emphasis on various elements, value is placed on each of our eight elements in all societies. Although volumes would be needed to review the extensive evidence confirming that the psychosocial factors in our list are beneficial, the description below is meant to give a brief introduction in this regard.

Social Prosperity

Social support. People have been described as "social animals," (Aronson, 2004), and psychologists have confirmed that humans function best with the support of others (Myers, 1999). Baumeister and Leary (1995) review the research showing that people have an inherent need to belong to social groups, and pay a price when this is thwarted. People who are isolated do not live as long (House, Landis, & Umberson, 1988), and loneliness has many bad outcomes for people (Cacioppo & Patrick, 2008).

Lucas (2007) reviews evidence that the dissolution of relationships, as in divorce or widowhood, is associated with long-term decreases in the experience of well-being. One of the worst things that can happen to a person is to be ostracized from his or her group (Williams, 2009), and a number of social groups impose shunning, excommunication, or solitary confinement as the ultimate punishment. Specific social factors such as human touching have been shown to reduce stress (Coan, Schaefer, & Davison, 2006). Individuals who help others seem to experience greater longevity than people who do so less (Brown, Nesse, Vinokur, & Smith, 2003; Dillard, Schiavone, & Brown, 2008). Diener and Seligman (2002) found that all of the extremely happy people they studied perceived their social relationships to be strong, without exception.

Public trust. Not only do people function better when surrounded by supportive family and friends, but they thrive in societies that are also supportive. Putnam (2000) coined the term "social capital" to capture the idea that societies thrive when people can rely on and trust others. Halpern (2005) reviews the evidence showing the multiple positive benefits of "social capital." If people have a wide circle of people they can rely on to help them and treat them fairly, they are likely to prosper. When corruption and crime are widespread, people cannot feel entirely safe, and they cannot rely on others in times of peril. There is now ample evidence to show that corruption and crime decrease the quality of life in societies, and are associated with poorer health and lower subjective well-being. For example, Veenhoven (2005) found that corruption has a strong negative association with the "happy-life-years" in nations. Similarly, Bobak, Murphy, Rose, and Marmot (2007) found that corruption in nations is related to poorer health. Political trust is related to higher well-being and lower corruption across societies (Catterberg & Moreno, 2006).

Helliwell and his colleagues (Helliwell, Barrington-Leigh, Harris, & Huang, 2010) found in a global survey that being able to count on others is as strongly associated with life satisfaction as is income, and that trusting others and public officials also predicts life satisfaction. Bjornskov (2008) found across states of the USA that social trust was related to higher reports of happiness, and that changes in trust over time tracked changes in happiness. Furthermore, Helliwell et al., found that a positive social context in the society benefited life satisfaction even controlling for the respondent's own personal social support. In addition, the researchers found that the effects were relatively consistent across regions of the world.

Tolerance. All societies are composed of diverse groups, whether they are based on age, gender, ethnicity, religion, political party, region, or occupation. To the extent that these groups respect and tolerate each other, and have peaceful ways to mediate disagreements, the society will be more likely to flourish. Where people are intolerant of other groups, there will be more conflict and tension in the society.

Where there is intolerance and prejudice, discrimination and conflict are likely to follow. People who are the targets of prejudice and discrimination tend to have poorer health (Okazaki, 2009; Mays, Cochran, & Barnes, 2007; Williams & Mohammed, 2009). People who are stigmatized by society can come to devalue the domains of activity that involve the stereotype in order to protect their self-esteem (Major & Schmader, 1998). This can lead to disengagement from activities that are valued by the broader society, and the resulting lowered motivation can have a negative impact on achievement. As Major and Schmader write, "If success in the domain is highly central to important life outcomes,... the price tag of disengagement can be steep" (p. 238). Discrimination is thus bad both for the target and for society as a whole, depriving the nation of valuable human resources.

Thus there are a number of social characteristics that describe the good society, including social support, trust and lack of corruption, security and safety, and tolerance. People living in societies with these characteristics are more likely to be happy, healthy, and function more effectively. Indeed, the findings that behavioral and social scientists have collected on the effects of positive versus negative social environments indicate that these effects are profound across diverse outcomes.

Psychological Prosperity

Just as with social prosperity, a large body of evidence points to the manifold benefits of psychological prosperity. A core element of such prosperity is that people themselves like their lives – they enjoy life, believe their lives are successful and rewarding, and do not suffer from chronic negative feelings about their lives. In addition, factors such as feelings of mastery, competence, and control are beneficial to humans for quality of life.

Mastery, competence, and growth. In light of the fact that humans have large brains and are very flexible in their behavior, it is not surprising that evolution has gifted them the ability to enjoy learning new things, improving skills, and using skilled behaviors. Several theories suggest that humans are programmed to find both control of the world and learning to be rewarding. White (1959) advanced the notion of "effectance motivation," a universal need of all humans to feel effective in their world. Another early proponent of a need for mastery was De Charms (1968), who believed that people have a need to feel that they are the origin of their own behavior rather than being coerced. Deci and Ryan (1985) argued that people develop "intrinsic motivation," doing tasks for their own sake, in part because of a need for competence. In Deci and Ryan's "Self-determination Theory," competence refers to the need to experience oneself as being capable of controlling and predicting one's environment.

Csikszentmihalyi (1988) suggested that intrinsic motivation and "flow" are associated with using one's skills to meet challenges. Skill acquisition and mastery allow humans to be prepared for future environmental challenges, and to learn behaviors that solve current problems. Learning new skills through practice, social interactions, and observation serves to provide knowledge and skills that can be adaptive in future situations. Thus, the acquisition of skills and knowledge is not only useful in terms of adaptive behavior, but is pleasant as an end in itself.

Positive evaluations of life. When offering satisfaction judgments people indicate the degree to which their life approaches what they view as the desirable life. This form of well-being has the advantage of not imposing the values of others on people, but instead allowing individuals to use the criteria they believe are important for a good life. Thus, the goal of high life satisfaction for all citizens is consistent with democratic ideals.

An added advantage of assessing life satisfaction is that respondents can take multiple facets of life into account, including those that leaders and experts might not have considered. In addition to global judgments of life, people can evaluate various aspects of their lives such as health, income, social relationships, and recreation. Such evaluations can be especially helpful in the policy context because they can specifically focus on areas of policy interest.

Positive engagement. Enjoyment and pleasure in interaction with the world have been seen as the highest good by philosophers from the hedonists to the Epicureans to the utilitarians. Whether or not pleasant feelings are the highest good, they certainly enhance quality of life. Furthermore, positive moods and emotions are a signal that individuals perceive the events and circumstances in their lives as desirable.

Adding to the importance of positive feelings is evidence suggesting that "happiness" can in many circumstances enhance effective functioning. From the groundbreaking work of Isen (2009) on creativity, to the broaden-and-build model of Fredrickson (2001), and the effects of mood on perceptions of difficulty in tasks (Proffitt, 2006), there are reasons to believe that people in positive moods often function effectively. Tice, Baumeister, Shmueli, and Muraven (2007) found that positive emotions help "recharge" self-regulatory ability.

Fredrickson's theory suggests that the purpose of positive feelings is to broaden and build a person's skills and resources in successful times when there are no imminent threats. In this model people often play and socialize, for example, when they are in a positive mood because this allows them to learn new skills and strengthen social bonds. Taken together, research findings suggest that people in a good mood are likely to be more creative, approach-oriented, and will over time accumulate needed resources for future challenges. Fredrickson, Tugade, Waugh, and Larkin (2003) found that people high in positive moods were more resilient after the September 11 attacks in the USA, being less likely to become depressed. Work in organizations has shown that workers who experience more positive emotions are more creative (Amabile, Barsade, Mueller, & Staw, 2005; George & Zhou, 2007). Because positive moods are related to creativity, supporting others, and task persistence, it is not surprising that they precede measures of success in the workplace (Boehm & Lyubomirsky, 2008; Tsai, Chen, & Liu, 2007).

People in a positive mood on average experience better health, owing to fewer cardiovascular problems, greater immune function, and perhaps slower aging (Diener & Biswas-Diener, 2008). Cohen, Doyle, Turner, Alper, and Skoner (2003) found that positive emotions at the beginning of a study predicted less illness and stronger immune function when people were exposed to viruses. In experimental work, Burton and King (2008) found that participants who had written about positive experiences in their lives visited the health center less over the ensuing months. Fredrickson and her colleagues found that induced positive emotions helped laboratory participants recover more quickly when exposed to negative stimuli, and improved cardiovascular recovery after an anxiety induction (Fredrickson, Mancuso, Branigan, & Tugade, 2000; Fredrickson & Levenson, 1998).

The health benefits of positive moods might even extend to life expectancy. The well-known study on nuns by Danner, Snowdon, and Friesen (2001) found that positive feelings were a predictor of longevity, and this finding was replicated by Pressman and Cohen (2007) for a sample of eminent psychologists. Xu and Roberts (2010) found that positive feelings and life satisfaction both predicted mortality from natural and unnatural causes, and this effect was especially strong in their healthy subsample. In a meta-analysis Chida and Steptoe (2008) found that positive affect reduced risk of mortality, and that this association was independent of the effects of negative affect.

Low levels of chronic negative feelings. Negative emotions signal to people that there are problems in their lives. They signify circumstances such as loss, threat, and feelings that one is being treated unfairly. In other words, negative emotions result when a person perceives that something bad is happening, and therefore they are indicative of undesirable circumstances from the person's perspective. Although negative feelings can be functional in terms of helping the person adjust and cope with a situation (Tamir, 2009), they can be harmful when they become chronic or long-lasting. Furthermore, even when helpful, they point to a problem situation that requires solving, and thus, the more of them there are, the more problems people perceive in their lives. Thus, negative feelings serve as an indicator that people experience problems in their lives. At the societal level the goal is to eliminate those problems rather than only to reduce the feelings without altering the problems themselves.

Negative feelings can have deleterious health and behavioral consequences when they are long-lasting. For example, chronic anger has been related to risk of cardiovascular problems (Smith, Glazer, Ruiz, & Gallo, 2004), and depression increases the risk of heart disease and death when a myocardial infarction does occur (Musselman, Evans, & Nemeroff, 1998; Roose, 2003). Depression is also a risk factor for noncompliance with medical treatment (DiMatteo, Lepper, & Croghan, 2000), diabetes (Musselman et al., 2007), and obesity (Blaine, 2008). Many of these undesirable consequences of negative feelings might derive from the fact that negative emotions can undermine self-regulation (Tice, Baumeister, & Zhang, 2004).

Negative affect is predictive of earlier onset of lung cancer among those predisposed to it, for example smokers (Augustine, Larsen, Walker, & Fisher, 2008). Also, Diener and Biswas-Diener (2008) describe evidence suggesting that stress might induce more rapid aging by shortening the telomere caps at the ends of DNA (Epel, Daubenmier, Moskowitz, Folkman, & Blackburn, 2009). In a recent study, Choi, Fauce, and Effros (2008) found that cortisol reduces telomerase, which is a protective factor for the telomeres that help protect the integrity of DNA.

Whatever processes are involved, chronic negative emotions are clearly related to many undesirable outcomes.

Not only do chronic negative emotions affect health, but they can be toxic to people's relationships with others. The children of depressed mothers are more likely to exhibit a variety of problems, for example, accidental injuries (Phelan, Khoury, Atherton, & Kahn, 2007), poorer academic performance, and antisocial behaviors (Wright, George, Burke, Gelfand, & Teti, 2000). Maternal depression can be associated with aggressiveness in children (Burk et al., 2008). Rat mothers exposed to stress later licked and groomed their offspring less, even offspring conceived after the stress had ended (Champagne & Meaney, 2006).

Depression is a risk factor for separation and divorce as well as longer hospitalizations (Beck & Koenig, 1996). Importantly, Beck and Koenig found that minor depression accounts for 9–16% of disability days. Furthermore, people tend to dislike interacting with depressed individuals and perceive them in more negative terms (Hoffman, 1996).

Benefits of Psychosocial Prosperity

Psychological prosperity helps the individual and also benefits societies. People who feel capable and positive, and not chronically negative, are likely to have better social relationships, perform better at work, and live longer. Frisch et al., (2005) created a quality of life measure that includes most of the elements of psychosocial prosperity we propose, and this measure predicted important life outcomes such as retention in college. Taken together, social and psychological prosperity reinforce each other, and are just as important as economic prosperity in defining "flourishing." Furthermore, there are benefits to the individual when others in the society are flourishing (Diener & Tay, 2009).

Across 360,000 representative respondents in 145 nations in the Gallup World Poll, the eight psychosocial prosperity variables correlated with each other at the societal level. Our analyses indicate that the elements of psychosocial prosperity at both the individual and societal levels are positively associated with each other, and may be due to what Inglehart and Welzel (2009) describe as the democratization and modernization process.

In Table 4.1 we present the association across societies of the eight elements of psychosocial prosperity with each other. Only one correlation – between safety and mastery – was in an unexpected direction. When societal income was controlled, a majority of the correlations remained significant. Thus, the eight elements of psychosocial prosperity tend to co-occur in nations. Furthermore, the subjective measures converge at the societal level with objective measures.

Social support, life evaluations, and safety predict life expectancy in nations even after controlling for per capita income. Social support as assessed by items such as "I can count on others in an emergency" is strongly related both to life expectancy and high evaluations of life. In Table 4.2 we present the correlations of these psychosocial variables with life expectancy of nations. The life expectancy

Table 4.1 Correlations of the psychosocial variables at the societal level

	Social				Psychological		
	Social support	Public trust	Safety and security	Tolerance	Competence and mastery	Life evalua-tions	Positive engagement
Public trust	0.25						
Safety/security	0.26	0.27					
Tolerance	0.34	0.35					
Mastery	0.52		−0.31	0.22			
Life evaluations	0.74	0.50	0.35	0.25	0.49		
Positive engagement	0.60	0.29		0.26	0.75	0.67	
Low negative feelings	0.24	0.36	0.27	0.28	0.22	0.33	0.45

Note: 123 nations. All correlations shown are $p < 0.05$ or less.

Table 4.2 Correlations of psychosocial variables with the longevity in nations

	Zero-order correlations	Partial correlations controlling GDP/capita
Social support	0.68**	0.19*
Safety	0.62**	0.47**
Life evaluations	0.76**	0.29**
GDP/capita	0.85**	

Note: *, $p < 0.05$; **, $p < 0.01$.
N = 123 nations.

figures were derived from the United Nations' figures on the Human Development Index. As can be seen, even though GDP per capita is very strongly related to average longevity in societies, the psychosocial variables were associated with life expectancy even controlling for income. Thus, a strong argument in support of the elements we list is that each is associated with many other desirable societal features.

Do the subjective measures we advocate add anything to the objective social indicators that are already available to policy makers? Several of the psychosocial variables such as positive feelings and life satisfaction can be most readily assessed by self-report surveys. Other variables such as tolerance, safety, competence, and social support can be assessed by both objective and subjective indicators, although the latter add valuable information to the former, and sometimes are more accurate and valid than "objective" indicators. For example, it is found that subjective reports of health add in the prediction of longevity beyond objective measures (e.g., Singh-Manoux et al., 2007). Surveys of crime victimization are imperfect but have strengths that complement police reports of crime. Because a large percentage of crime goes unreported to the police, surveys often give a more complete picture of crime frequency and have adequate validity (e.g., Hindelang, Hirschi, & Weiss, 1979). It should be noted that the psychosocial prosperity and GDP of societies correlate 0.57 in our sample of nations. Thus, there is a large amount of variance in psychosocial prosperity that is not accounted for by income.

Global Psychosocial Prosperity

What would national accounts of psychosocial resources look like, based on the above list, and what might they tell us that other accounts do not tell us? The Gallup World Poll provides an opportunity to answer these questions on a global basis because the survey is the first representative sample of virtually the entire world. Descriptive statistics for the survey are shown in Table 4.3.

Several important facts are evident in the table. First, nations differ enormously in their psychosocial prosperity. For instance, in the nation lowest on public trust, 13% of the population believe they can trust the police, and government and business leaders, whereas in the highest nation over 90% trust officials. The crime numbers reveal that in the most fortunate nation 3% of the population were assaulted or were victims of theft, whereas in the worst nation this figure was 38%. Further, the table reveals that even in the best nations there is room for improvement, and in the average nation there is much room for improvement. For instance, low social support was reported by 17% of people in the world, and only 36% of people think that government and business leaders can be trusted.

Twenty-nine percent of respondents across the globe felt that their area was not a good place for ethnic, religious, or immigrant minorities, and 12% were assaulted

Table 4.3 Descriptive statistics for nations on psychosocial prosperity

	Lowest nation	Highest nation	Mean	USA
Social prosperity	35	85	53	67
1. Social support	50	96	83	93
2. Public trust	13	92	36	51
3. Safety	62	97	88	92
4. Tolerance	29	92	71	85
Psychological prosperity	51	82	68	77
5. Competence and mastery	36	83	63	73
6. Positive evaluations of life	34	86	63	79
7. Positive engagement	40	85	70	79
8. Low levels of negative feelings	61	87	78	79
Overall psychosocial prosperity	47	83	61	72

Note: Scores vary from 0 to 100, where zero indicates that all respondents answer in the negative direction on all items for that characteristic, and 100 denotes that all respondents answer all items in a positive direction.

or robbed during the past year. Thus, despite the fact that the world is developing economically, there is much room for improvement in the psychosocial realm. Because we do not have longitudinal data yet, we cannot be sure whether social support, tolerance, and so forth are increasing or decreasing. The large differences between societies indicate that psychosocial prosperity is not simply an individual matter. Although some elements of psychosocial prosperity are undoubtedly personal (Peterson & Seligman, 2004), the enormous differences shown in Table 4.1 suggest that societies can strongly influence them.

In examining societies around the globe, how do they score? Below we list some nations that score in dire poverty (scores at 50 and less on the 0–100 scale), poor (51–55), midlevel (56–64), moderately (65–74), and flourishing (75 and greater):

Dire psychosocial poverty		Poor psychosocially		Midlevel psychosocial prosperity		Moderate psychosocial prosperity		Psychosocial prosperity	
Palestine	0.48	Pakistan	0.51	Poland	0.58	Mexico	0.65	Netherlands	0.75
Chad	0.48	Georgia	0.52	Greece	0.60	Austria	0.71	Switzerland	0.76
Cambodia	0.47	India	0.55	Argentina	0.62	USA	0.72	Sweden	0.80

Nations in the Dire Psychosocial Poverty category have scores indicating that across the eight categories as many respondents are doing badly as are doing well. In the Flourishing category the scores indicate that across respondents and the eight categories at least three-fourths of responses are positive. Seligman (2009) recently suggested that a goal of positive psychology should be that by 2050, at least 50% of the world is flourishing. However, this threshold for flourishing is undoubtedly much higher than the level reported in the measures we analyzed.

Does economic development fully capture the psychosocial prosperity of nations, making the psychosocial measures unnecessary? Although psychosocial prosperity and gross domestic product per capita are positively associated at both the individual and societal levels, there are clear discrepancies between the two. For instance, Costa Rica and Russia both have per capita GDP of about US $10,000 a year, and yet psychosocial prosperity in Costa Rica is much higher. Similarly, New Zealand and South Korea have about equal incomes, approximately US $25,000 a year, and yet the former is much higher in psychosocial prosperity. The nation often thought of as the most economically prosperous in the world, the United States, scored relatively well in social support but fared badly in public trust, and does not have the highest score in any of the eight categories.

Below is a list of nations that are higher in psychosocial prosperity than would be predicted by their average incomes, and others that are lower than predicted by their wealth, as well as the psychosocial prosperity scores of these societies.

Higher in psychosocial prosperity than predicted by income		Lower in psychosocial prosperity than predicted by income	
Norway	0.78	Armenia	0.50
Australia	0.77	Palestine	0.48
Canada	0.78	Japan	0.59
Singapore	0.79	Russia	0.54
Costa Rica	0.68	Iran	0.53
Ireland	0.77	Cambodia	0.47
New Zealand	0.81	South Korea	0.55

Note that there are both wealthy and developing nations in both lists. Some relatively wealthy nations are even more psychosocially prosperous than we would expect based on their incomes, but some poorer nations are as well. A prosperous nation such as Japan on the lower list might also surprise readers. The Gallup World Poll showed that it scores relatively low on tolerance and on public trust.

Aggregated psychosocial scores are informative, but scores of individual characteristics from the Gallup World Poll are also revealing. Some nations score much lower on one of the eight scores than they do on the others, pointing to places where improvements are most needed. Public trust and mastery are lower in many nations that otherwise score well on psychosocial prosperity. Singapore, Switzerland, and Finland score lower on tolerance than other nations in the most prosperous category. Hong Kong scores lower in mastery and satisfaction than it does in other categories, such as crime, where it scores very well, second only to Singapore. Thus, the individual scores reveal where even successful nations can improve. At the low end of psychosocial prosperity, a nation such as Pakistan scores relatively well on absence of crime, but extremely low on public trust.

The Policy Role of Positive Psychology

Psychosocial Measures and Policy

Creating a list of agreed-upon psychosocial indicators of well-being is a first step in gaining more attention to these factors, and insights into ways to enhance them. Currently, many or most of them fall largely outside the awareness of policy makers when they make important decisions. National accounts of psychosocial well-being, published periodically over time, and linked to various groups, regions, and activities, would help educate leaders and ordinary citizens about a broader vision of the good life.

In the book *Well-Being and Public Policy* (2009), Ed Diener, Richard Lucas, Ulrich Schimmack, and John Helliwell describe how national measures of subjective well-being could be used in diverse areas of policy by business and organizational leaders. In areas varying from the environment, to health, to the economy, the authors describe how measures of subjective well-being can shed light on policy alternatives. Although they focus on measures of subjective well-being rather than the broader view of psychosocial well-being presented here, many of their same arguments and policy considerations apply. For example, concerns about government paternalism are equally unfounded for both types of measures. The psychosocial measures give a voice to the views of ordinary citizens. Furthermore, the society shapes the degree to which the policies will influence individual lives, and this will occur even in the absence of the psychosocial measures. The elements of psychosocial prosperity we describe here represent a broad vision of quality of life, and a set of elements that represents diverse fields. Jowell and Gillian (2009) argue in a similar fashion that trust, tolerance, social cohesion, and security are needed to supplement economic measures and indicators of subjective well-being.

Social and behavioral science should be at the core of each stage of implementing policies to enhance well-being. First, they provide the foundations for understanding the key elements of well-being. Second, positive psychologists should be leaders in developing and validating measures of well-being. These measures will undoubtedly include both survey assessments and other types of behavioral measures. Third, positive psychologists and other behavioral scientists will play a key role in creating and assessing interventions to enhance well-being. Indeed, it will be crucial to demonstrate to policy makers that we have effective interventions for improving psychosocial prosperity in order to convince them to measure it. No matter how desirable psychosocial prosperity is, policy makers will be interested only if they can believe their actions could improve it. Thus, it is imperative that measures of psychosocial prosperity be accompanied by rigorous research on how it can be raised at a societal level. Finally, social and behavioral scientists should have a central role in assessing the influence that various policy changes might have on well-being, in terms of theory and empirical assessments.

Economics and Well-Being

Positive psychologists can learn much by studying the success of law and economics in the public arena. When one examines the highest levels of governments, they are peopled by lawyers, executives, and economists (The Economist, 2009). Most governments and organizations include economists at the highest levels of decision and policy making. National governments have cabinet-level posts for commerce and treasury matters, directly under the chief executive, and these positions are often held by economists and business leaders. Although other social scientists are sometimes consulted, they rarely are posted at the top levels of government. For example, US President Barrack Obama has a number of economists who work as his immediate advisors.

Of the various scholarly disciplines, economists possibly have exerted the largest influence on policy in recent years. Economists have a clearly articulated vision of well-being and quality of life, based on ideas about the production and consumption of goods and services. How societies can further material development is expressed in economic theories, and is presented to societies as a way to evaluate policies.

Importantly, economists guide the measurement of many aspects of societies, and these numbers are published in high-profile outlets. Despite the huge success that economists have had in influencing public policies, there are clear limitations to the vision they advance for quality of life.

If positive psychologists believe that they have important knowledge that is useful to policy makers, they must ask why they do not have a greater role in high government positions. We advocate national measures of psychosocial prosperity as the first step in greater involvement for social scientists in policy roles. We do not advocate abandoning economic measures or ignoring them; they have been of value to societies. What we propose is the systematic collection of measures on other areas of prosperity in order to give politicians a broader view of how their policies affect well-being. A major way of gaining attention to phenomena in the modern world is to measure them and publicize the findings.

Implementing the Vision

Timing for National Psychosocial Accounts

The list we offer, and the measures collected by Gallup, are meant to be illustrative and preliminary rather than a final product. At the same time, we caution that social scientists ought to proceed rapidly because there is now a window of opportunity for action. Environmental and health organizations have become increasingly interested in well-being. Institutions such as the Center for Disease Control and Prevention in the United States are taking active steps to assess well-being as part of health promotion, for instance. The Organization of Economic Cooperation and Development and the statistical agencies in several nations are implementing or considering instituting measures of well-being. Environmental groups such as NEF (New Economics Foundation) in the United Kingdom suggest measures similar to those we propose here to evaluate how societies, organizations, and groups are faring. Thus, the time is auspicious for a broad effort to convince leaders of the benefits of psychosocial measures.

Implementation of National Psychosocial Accounts

How can we implement an agenda based on the idea of psychosocial well-being, and insure that it is considered by policy makers? Measuring psychosocial prosperity in a valid way will be necessary, and in a way that is seen as politically neutral, not as taking a partisan stance. As mentioned above, a number of agencies and nongovernmental organizations have become interested in well-being more broadly defined than economic growth, and therefore it will not be as difficult to implement measures as it would have been a decade ago. Second, we need to offer a clear and concrete vision of how societies would be different if such measures are in place. In what ways would psychosocial measures complement economic measures? What tradeoffs are there that are not obvious in the economic measures taken in isolation? What problems exist that are largely missed by economic measures, and even by other social indicators?

One aspect of convincing those in power to implement psychosocial measures is to demonstrate that we have some effective ways of improving each of the areas in groups that are found not to be thriving. If outcomes are seen to be largely due to temperament or individual choices, policy makers will see the psychosocial outcomes as falling outside their purview. Thus, we must show that societal characteristics and programs can influence psychosocial prosperity. It will also be useful to search for natural allies, groups that will benefit from the measures of psychosocial well-being. For example, environmental groups, groups representing minorities, and church groups might be natural allies. However, the formation of alliances must occur while insuring the objectivity of our measures. Social scientists cannot afford the appearance of offering biased advice.

A blue-ribbon panel should create the list of psychosocial elements that contribute to well-being, and examine the adequacy of current measures to validly assess these characteristics. The panel could also provide analyses of several policy issues where measures could provide useful insights. The panel should analyze the benefits of raising the average psychosocial prosperity of societies versus policies aimed at helping those who are suffering the most. Although the measures will eventually shed light on a wide range of topics, including controversial ones, it would be folly to emphasize the most controversial topics from the outset because politically it would doom the project from the start.

The measurement of psychosocial prosperity and interventions to increase this type of wealth is an ambitious one. If we examine what economists have accomplished, however, the project is possible. The measures could provide a system that would assist many areas of the social scientists to be more active in policy. Because the measures would reflect diverse forms of well-being, most areas of the social sciences could contribute, and make policy recommendations based on the measures. This is a project for all of the social and behavioral sciences, and care must be taken to avoid partisanship and rancorous debate.

Conclusions

In a recent interview (2009) Nancy Cantor, who is President and Chancellor at Syracuse University, suggested that psychologists should be at the table when the most pressing issues of the day are discussed, and that the highest level policy makers such as the president and Supreme Court need to consult psychologists about the big issues facing the nation and world. Next on her wish list, Cantor said, is that psychologists would be engaged in the big issues of the time, and that the reward system would reinforce such work. We echo this call for a more ambitious policy role for social scientists!

How can positive psychologists and other social scientists become more involved in policy discussions? Policy makers must believe that we have something useful to say. We can accomplish this in part by approaching policy makers with the relevant knowledge we have about various issues. The societal measures of psychosocial prosperity would have several beneficial effects. For one thing, they would serve the purpose of making social and psychological prosperity salient to both policy makers and the public. For another, they would begin making obvious the places where societies are flourishing or floundering. The measures would not simply score the society as a whole, but would reveal the groups, regions, roles, and activities where citizens are floundering versus flourishing. Thus, the measures of psychosocial prosperity could provide an overarching system for specific recommendations. National accounts of psychosocial well-being could provide an effective stimulus for policy makers and organizations to more heavily rely on the important knowledge social scientists have gained over the past century.

References

Amabile, T. M., Barsade, S. G., Mueller, J. S., & Staw, B. M. (2005). Affect and creativity at work. *Administrative Science Quarterly, 50*, 367–403.

Aronson, E. (2004). *The social animal.* New York: Worth Publishers.

Augustine, A. A., Larsen, R. J., Walker, M. S., & Fisher, E. B. (2008). Personality predictors of the time course for lung cancer onset. *Journal of Research in Personality, 42*, 1448–1455.

Baumeister, R. F., & Leary, M. R. (1995). The need to belong: Desire for interpersonal attachments as a fundamental human motivation. *Psychological Bulletin, 117*, 497–529.

Beck, D. A., & Koenig, H. G. (1996). Minor depression: A review of the literature. *International Journal of Psychiatry and Medicine, 26*, 177–209.

Bjornskov, C. (2008). Social capital and happiness in the United States. *Applied Research in Quality of Life, 3*, 43–62.

Blaine, B. (2008). Does depression cause obesity? A meta-analysis of longitudinal studies of depression and weight control. *Journal of Health Psychology, 13*, 1190–1197.

Bobak, M., Murphy, M., Rose, R., & Marmot, M. (2007). Societal characteristics and health in the former communist countries of Central and Eastern Europe and the former Soviet Union: A multilevel analysis. *Journal of Epidemiology and Community Health, 61*, 990–996.

Boehm, J. K., & Lyubomirsky, S. (2008). Does happiness promote career success? *Journal of Career Assessment, 16*, 101–116.

Brown, S. L., Nesse, R. M., Vinokur, A. D., & Smith, D. M. (2003). Providing social support may be more beneficial than receiving it: Results from a prospective study of mortality. *Psychological Science, 14*, 320–327.

Burk, L. R., Park, J., Armstrong, J. M., Klein, M. H., Goldsmith, H. H., Zahn-Waxler, C., et al., (2008). Identification of early child and family risk factors for aggressive victim status in first grade. *Journal of Abnormal Child Psychology, 36*, 513–526.

Burton, C. M., & King, L. A. (2008). Effects of (very) brief writing on health: The two-minute miracle. *British Journal of Health Psychology, 13*, 9–14.

Cacioppo, J. T., & Patrick, W. (2008). *Loneliness: Human nature and the need for social connection.* New York: W. W. Norton & Company.

Cantor, N. (2009). Nancy Cantor: A view from the chancellor's office. (An interview with Walter Mischel). *Observer, 22*, 13–16.

Catterberg, G., & Moreno, A. (2006). The individual bases of political trust: Trends in new and established democracies. *International Journal of Public Opinion Research, 18*, 31–48.

Champagne, F. A., & Meaney, M. J. (2006). Stress during gestation alters postpartum maternal care and the development of the offspring in a rodent model. *Biological Psychiatry, 59*, 1227–1235.

Chida, Y., & Steptoe, A. (2008). Positive psychological well-being and mortality: A quantitative review of prospective observational studies. *Psychosomatic Medicine, 70*, 741–756.

Choi, J., Fauce, S. R., & Effros, R. B. (2008). Reduced telomerase activity in human T lymphocytes exposed to cortisol. *Brain, Behavior, and Immunity, 22*, 600–605.

Coan, J. A., Schaefer, H. S., & Davison, R. J. (2006). Lending a hand: Social regulation of the neural response to threat. *Psychological Science, 17*, 1032–1039.

Cohen, S., Doyle, W. J., Turner, R. B., Alper, C. M., & Skoner, D. P. (2003). Emotional style and susceptibility to the common cold. *Psychosomatic Medicine, 65*, 652–657.

Csikszentmihalyi, M. (1988). *Optimal experience*. New York: Cambridge University Press.

Danner, D. D., Snowdon, D. A., & Friesen, W. V. (2001). Positive emotions in early life and longevity: Findings from the nun study. *Journal of Personality and Social Psychology, 80*, 804–813.

De Charms, R. (1968). *Personal causation: The internal affective determinants of behavior*. New York: Academic Press.

Deci, E. L., & Ryan, R. M. (1985). *Intrinsic motivation and self-determination in human behavior*. New York: Plenum Press.

DiMatteo, M. R., Lepper, H. S., & Croghan, T. W. (2000). Depression is a risk factor for noncompliance with medical treatment. *Archives of Internal Medicine, 160*, 2101–2107.

Diener, E., & Biswas-Diener, R. (2008). *Happiness: Unlocking the mysteries of psychological wealth*. Malden, MA: Blackwell Publishing.

Diener, E., Lucas, R., Schimmack, U., & Helliwell, J. (2009). *Well-being for public policy*. Oxford: Oxford University Press.

Diener, E., & Seligman, M. E. P. (2002). Very happy people. *Psychological Science, 13*, 81–84.

Diener, E., & Tay, L. (2009). Universal needs and subjective well-being. In preparation.

Dillard, A. J., Schiavone, A., & Brown, S. L. (2008). Helping behavior and positive emotions: Implications for health and well-being. In S. J. Lopez (Ed.), *Positive psychology: Exploring the best in people, Vol 2: Capitalizing on emotional experiences*. Westport, CT: Praeger Publishers/Greenwood Publishing Group.

Epel, E., Daubenmier, J., Moskowitz, J. T., Folkman, S., & Blackburn, E. (2009). Can meditation slow rate of cellular aging? Cognitive stress, mindfulness, and telomeres. *Annals of the New York Academy of Sciences, 1172*, 34–53.

Fredrickson, B. L. (2001). The role of positive emotions in positive psychology: The broaden-and-build theory of positive emotions. *American Psychologist, 56*, 218–226.

Fredrickson, B. L., & Levenson, R. W. (1998). Positive emotions speed recovery from the cardiovascular sequelae of negative emotions. *Cognition and Emotion, 12*, 191–220.

Fredrickson, B. L., Mancuso, R. A., Branigan, C., & Tugade, M. M. (2000). The undoing effect of positive emotions. *Motivation and Emotion, 24*, 237–258.

Fredrickson, B. L., Tugarde, M. M., Waugh, C. E., & Larkin, G. (2003). What good are positive emotions in crises? A prospective study of resilience and emotions following terrorist attacks on the United States on September 11th, 2001. *Journal of Personality and Social Psychology, 84*(2), 365–376.

Frisch, M. B., Clark, M. P., Rouse, S. V., Rudd, D. M., Paweleck, J. K., Greenstone, A., et al. (2005). Predictive and treatment validity of life satisfaction and quality of life inventory. *Assessment, 12*, 66–78.

George, J. M., & Zhou, J. (2007). Dual tuning in a supportive context: Joint contributions of positive mood, negative mood, and supervisory behaviors to employee creativity. *Academy of Management Journal, 50*, 605–622.

Halpern, D. (2005). *Social capital*. Cambridge, UK: Polity Press.

Helliwell, J. F., Barrington-Leigh, C., Harris, C., & Huang, H. (2010). International evidence on the social context of well-being. In E. Diener, D. Kahneman, & J. F. Helliwell (Eds.), *International differences in well-being*. Oxford, UK: Oxford University Press.

Hindelang, M. J., Hirschi, T., & Weiss, J. G. (1979). Correlates of delinquency: The illusion of discrepancy between self-report and official measures. *American Sociological Review, 44*, 995–1014.

Hoffman, D. M. (1996). Psychological and physiological responses to depressed others. *Dissertation Abstracts International, Section B, The Sciences and Engineering, 57*, 4030.

House, J. S., Landis, K. R., & Umberson, D. (1988). Social relationships and health. *Science, 241*, 540–545.

Inglehart, R., & Welzel, C. (2009). *Human beliefs and values: The link between modernization and democracy*. University of Michigan. Submitted for publication.

Isen, A. (2009). A role for neuropsychology in understanding the facilitating influence of positive affect on social behavior and cognitive processes. In S. J. Lopez & C. R. Snyder (Eds.), *Oxford handbook of positive psychology* (pp. 503–518). New York: Oxford University Press.

Jowell, R., & Gillian, E. (2009). Happiness is not enough: Cognitive judgments as indicators of national well-being. *Social Indicators Research, 91*, 317–328.

Kenrick, D., Griskevicius, V., Neuberg, S., & Schaller, M. (2010). Renovating the pyramid of needs: Contemporary extensions built upon ancient foundations. *Perspectives on Psychological Science, 5*, 292–314.

Lucas, R. E. (2007). Adaptation and the set-point model of subjective well-being: Does happiness change after major life events? *Current Directions in Psychological Science, 16*, 75–79.

Major, B., & Schmader, T. (1998). Coping with stigma through psychological disengagement. In J. K. Swim & C. Stangor (Eds.), *Prejudice: The target's perspective* (pp. 219–241). San Diego, CA: Academic Press.

Mays, V. M., Cochran, S. D., & Barnes, N. W. (2007). Race, race-based discrimination, and health outcomes among African Americans. *Annual Review of Psychology, 58*, 201–225.

Musselman, D. J., Bowling, A., Giles, N., Larsen, H., Betan, E., & Phillips, L. S. (2007). The interrelationship of depression and diabetes. In A. Steptoe (Ed.), *Depression and physical illness* (pp. 165–194). New York: Cambridge University Press.

Musselman, D. L., Evans, D. L., & Nemeroff, C. B. (1998). The relationship of depression to cardiovascular disease: Epidemiology, biology, and treatment. *Archives of General Psychiatry, 55*, 580–592.

Myers, D. G. (1999). Close relationships and quality of life. In D. Kahneman, E. Diener, & N. Schwartz (Eds.), *Well-being: The foundations of hedonic psychology* (pp. 374–391). New York: Russell Sage.

Okazaki, S. (2009). Impact of racism on ethnic minority mental health. *Perspectives on Psychological Science, 4*, 103–107.

Peterson, C., & Seligman, M. (Eds.). (2004). *Character strength and virtues*. New York: Oxford University Press.

Phelan, K., Khoury, J., Atherton, H., & Kahn, R. S. (2007). Maternal depression, child behavior, and injury. *Injury Prevention, 13*, 403–408.

Pressman, S. D., & Cohen, S. (2007). Use of social words in autobiographies and longevity. *Psychosomatic Medicine, 69*, 262–269.

Proffitt, D. (2006). Embodied perception and the economy of action. *Perspectives on Psychological Science, 1*, 110–122.

Putnam, R. (2000). *Bowling alone: Collapse and revival of American community*. New York: Simon & Schuster.

Roose, S. P. (2003). Depression: Links with ischemic heart disease and erectile dysfunction. *Journal of Clinical Psychiatry, 64*, 26–30.

Ryan, R. M., & Deci, E. L. (2000). Self-determination theory and the facilitation of intrinsic motivation, social development, and well-being. *American Psychologist, 55*, 68–78.

Ryff, C. D. (1989). Happiness is everything, or is it? Explorations on the meaning of psychological well-being. *Journal of Personality and Social Psychology, 57*, 1069–1081.

Ryff, C. D., & Singer, B. (1998). The contours of positive human health. *Psychological Inquiry, 9*, 1–28.

Seligman, M. E. P. (2009, June 18–21). *Positive psychology and positive education*. International Positive Psychology Association first world congress on Positive Psychology, Philadelphia.

Singh-Manoux, A., Gueguen, A., Martikainen, P., Ferrie, J., Marmot, M., & Shipley, M. (2007). Self-related health and mortality: Short- and long-term associations in the Whitehall II study. *Psychosomatic medicine, 69*, 138–143.

Smith, T. W., Glazer, K., Ruiz, J. M., & Gallo, L. C. (2004). Hostility, anger, aggressiveness, and coronary heart disease: An interpersonal perspective on personality, emotion, and health. *Journal of Personality, 72*, 1217–1270.

Tamir, M. (2009). Why do people want to feel and why? *Current Directions in Psychological Science, 18*, 101–105.

The Economist. (2009, April 18). There was a lawyer, an engineer, and a politician. . .., 64–65.

Tice, D. M., Baumeister, R. F., & Zhang, L. (2004). In P. Philippot & R. S. Feldman (Eds.), *The regulation of emotion* (pp. 213–226). Mahwah, NJ: Lawrence Erlbaum Associates Publishers.

Tice, D. M., Baumesiter, R. F., Shmueli, D., & Muraven, M. (2007). Restoring the self: Positive affect helps improve self-regulation following ego depletion. *Journal of Experimental Social Psychology, 43*, 379–384.

Tsai, W. C., Chen, C. C., & Liu, H. L. (2007). Test of a model linking employee positive moods and task performance. *Journal of Applied Psychology, 92*, 1570–1583.

Veenhoven, R. (2005). Apparent quality-of-life in nations: How long and happy people live. *Social Indicators Research, 71*, 61–86.

White, R. W. (1959). Motivation reconsidered: The concept of competence. *Psychological Review, 66*, 297–333.

Williams, K. D. (2009). Ostracism: Effects of being excluded and ignored. *Advances in Experimental Social Psychology, 41*, 279–314.

Williams, D. R., & Mohammed, S. A. (2009). Discrimination and racial disparities in health: Evidence and needed research. *Journal of Behavioral Medicine, 32*, 20–47.

Wright, C. A., George, T. P., Burke, R., Gelfand, D. M., & Teti, D. M. (2000). Early maternal depression and children's adjustment to school. *Child Study Journal, 30*, 153–168.

Xu, J., & Roberts, R. E. (2010). The power of positive emotions: It's a matter of life or death – Subjective well-being and the longevity over 28 years in a general population. *Health Psychology, 29*, 9–19.

Chapter 5
Gross National Happiness: A Gift from Bhutan to the World

George W. Burns

"Gross National Happiness is more important than Gross National Product." These now famous words by the fourth king of Bhutan, Jigme Singye Wangchuck, have formed the basis for the country's political philosophy, have been written into its democratic constitution, are measured by a series of established indicators, and have attracted the interest of multidisciplinary scientists.

When I found myself in the privileged position of having lunch with his son, the newly crowned fifth King of Bhutan, Jigme Khesar Namgyel Wangchuck (locally called King Khesar) here was an opportunity I did not want to miss. This was probably a once-in-a-lifetime opportunity to learn from the son of the originator and architect of Gross National Happiness (GNH).

I hasten to add that I was not alone. All the international presenters at the Fourth Gross National Happiness Conference had been introduced to King Khesar and now, in traditional style, were seated around low tables sharing a smorgasbord lunch with His Highness in the Royal Banquet Hall in Bhutan's capital city, Thimphu. Crowned at the age of 28, he is a tall and handsome young man who attended two colleges in Massachusetts, United States, before graduating from Magdalen College, University of Oxford, United Kingdom, where he completed a Master of Philosophy degree in politics. His integrity and humanity were evidenced in his actions. He invited us as guests to select our fare from the tables before he took his own. He moved from table to table, giving guests the opportunity to meet and talk with him.

In his coronation address, just a couple of weeks before our luncheon, King Khesar had made it clear that he intended to follow his father's footsteps with regard to GNH. He said, "... whatever goals we have – and no matter how these may change in this changing world – ultimately without peace, security and happiness we have nothing. That is the essence of the philosophy of gross national happiness... I shall give you everything and keep nothing; I shall live such a life as a good human being that you find it worthy to serve as an example for your children. ... I also pray that while I am but king of a small Himalayan nation, I may in my time be able to do

G.W. Burns (✉)
Hypnotherapy Centre, Milton H. Erickson Institute, Western Australia, Australia
e-mail: georgeburns@iinet.net.au

R. Biswas-Diener (ed.), *Positive Psychology as Social Change*,
DOI 10.1007/978-90-481-9938-9_5, © Springer Science+Business Media B.V. 2011

much to promote the greater well-being and happiness of all people in this world – of all sentient beings."

Five years earlier, then in his role as Crown Prince, King Khesar had opened the world's First Conference on Gross National Happiness, saying, "I believe that while Gross National Happiness is inherently Bhutanese, its ideas may have a positive relevance to any nation, peoples, or communities – wherever they may be. I also believe that there must be some convergence among nations on the idea of what the end objective of development and progress should be. There cannot be enduring peace, prosperity, equality and brotherhood in this world if our aims are so separate and divergent – if we do not accept that in the end we are people, all alike, sharing the earth among ourselves and also with other sentient beings, all of whom have an equal role and state of this planet and its players" (Ura & Galey, 2004, p. ix).

Gross National Happiness

What is Gross National Happiness? How did it develop? And how is it applied?

To understand GNH it helps to understand a little of the recent history of Bhutan. Bhutan is a landlocked Buddhist nation that follows a religious, cultural and linguistic tradition similar to Tibet but, in many ways, is also uniquely individual. The country at its widest measures just 190 miles (300 km) from east to west and 95 miles (150 km) from north to south. In that 95 miles it rises from a mere 330 feet (100 m) on the Indian plains to 24,800 feet (7,540 m) on the northern border with Tibet – a tiny wedge between the world's two most populous nations: democratic India and communist China. It is a contorted geography of valleys and mountains that have isolated people into 19 different language groups and is thus one of the most language-dense countries on the planet. For centuries its economy and culture have been based on subsistence rather than consumerism.

The royal lineage is relatively recent in comparison to European monarchies. The first king was crowned little more than a century ago on 17 December 1907. It was under the third king, who was educated in India and England, that Bhutan began a programme of modernisation. In 1961 it emerged from centuries of self-imposed isolation, opened itself to the outside world, and began a process of planned development. When the third king died prematurely at the age of 44 in 1972, his 16-year old son, Jigme Singye Wangchuck, ascended the throne and was crowned in 1974. King Jigme promised to continue his father's programme of modernisation and economic self-reliance. This programme emphasised education, health services, rural development, and communication, as well as conservation of the natural environment. In the mid-1980s it became apparent that some reflection on and reconsideration of these objectives was essential if Bhutanese values were to be preserved from the influence of external factors. The king began to explore and speak about a specific Bhutanese path to development that would be consistent with Bhutanese values, culture, institutions, and spiritual beliefs. He wanted to discriminatively take from developed countries the things that had worked for the benefit of a population's well-being while preserving the centuries old traditions that had worked for the well-being of the Bhutanese. It is in this context that he made his now-famed state-ment: "Gross National Happiness is more important than Gross National Product." While this may have been refreshingly new to many Western ears, for Bhutanese the concept and term were not so novel. They had long been known in local parlance.

It is easy for us to think of positive psychology as something new but the search for happiness is probably as old as humankind itself and the inclusion of the con-cept of happiness in social and political policies dates further back in history than most people realize. In seventh century Tibet (from where the Bhutanese culture largely originated), King Songsten Gampo (ca. 617–650) ruled with a military suc-cess that subjugated Nepal, invaded northern India, threatened the western borders of China, and extended as far as Turkey. To appease him, neighbouring China and Nepal each offered him a princess in marriage – political manoeuvres that heralded a significant change in policy. Love can alter a person, and this seemed to happen to Songsten Gampo. Influenced by his wives' Buddhist beliefs, he relinquished his military career and set about creating social reforms with the introduction of a new legal system, the building of schools and temples, the establishment of a medical system, and, of specific interest to us, the invitation for Indian spiritual and philo-sophical teachers to educate his people in how to be happy. His political changes that held happiness at their core were primarily responsible for the transformation of Tibet from a warring nation to a civilization that would become renowned for its peace, serenity, contemplative practices, and spirituality (Chan, 1994; Murdoch & Oldershaw, 2008).

Over the intervening centuries, the provision of a political and social environ-ment that facilitated happiness has been seen as a core political objective in most Buddhist cultures. Though not new to a country like Bhutan, what King Jigme's statement did was to directly juxtapose the concept of GNH against Gross National Product (GNP). It challenged orthodox Western developmental theory that tends to see development purely in material terms. Increasing Gross National Product (GNP), or Gross Domestic Product (GDP) as it is now more commonly known, alone meant increasing material development as an end in itself, and that, King Jigme foresaw, would come at a cost to the other values dear to his people. In posit-ing the concept of GNH, material development was perceived *not* as an end in itself but as *one* means to enhance the overall well-being of his people and his nation. Gross National Happiness was based on the premise that the principal goal of soci-ety should be the attainment of material progress hand-in-glove with psychological, cultural, and spiritual development while still maintaining harmony with the natural environment.

The principle describes development as a continuous process towards a balance between material and non-material needs of individuals and society. The country's philosophy of development, while recognizing the importance of economic growth as essential to support and nurture the spiritual and social needs of the community, is not an end in itself, but one among many means of achieving holistic development.

Gross National Happiness is based on the ideology that the pursuit of happiness is found in all people and is the strongest force of desires. Included in the concept of

GNH, and characteristic of Bhutan's Buddhist heritage, is a "middle path" approach in which spiritual and material pursuits are balanced.

At its core GNH holds the belief that development should promote happiness as its primary value. Equal importance must be placed on socioeconomic development, along with the spiritual, cultural, and emotional needs of the people. Economic growth, far from being the dominating force in development, is seen as just one aspect of the multi-armed developmental programme that aims to improve the social requirements of society and not just the financial balance sheet. Thus, GNH has become the philosophical foundation for the policy-making process and implementation of development in Bhutan.

A major political change occurred in 2008 when Bhutan became the world's newest democracy. It came about peacefully: interestingly, not from the will of the people but from the persuasion and personal efforts of the fourth king. In his address to the United Nations, the newly elected Prime Minister of Bhutan, Jigmi Y. Thinley, said, "Gross National Happiness is based on the belief that happiness is the single most important goal and purpose in life for every individual and that the end of development must be the promotion and enhancement of happiness. It must, therefore, we believe, be the responsibility of the State to create an enabling environment within which its citizens can pursue happiness. The concept emphasises a balanced life – matching material needs of the body with the spiritual, psychological, and emotional needs of the mind. To this end the Royal Government of Bhutan has structured its development programmes on four broad themes or "pillars" that constitute a paradigm of holistic and sustainable development" (Thinley, 2008).

The Pillars of GNH

Following the king's statement almost three decades ago, Bhutan's government leaders immersed themselves in discussions about developing GNH and its applications in their forward movement as a nation. This led to the definition of the four pillars of GNH referred to by Prime Minister Thinley:

- Sustainable and equitable socioeconomic development
- Environmental conservation
- Promotion of culture
- Good governance

Sustainable and Equitable Socioeconomic Development

While economic growth and development are included in the pillar of sustainable and equitable socioeconomic development, they are not the whole picture. Within this pillar, Bhutan gives priority to sustainable and equitable development in the health and education sectors where services are offered free of cost to all citizens. Over 30% of the national budget of Bhutan is given to this social sector, providing tangible evidence of the government's commitment to a population that is healthy and educated. Capacity building in the development of professional skills to manage development has also received high priority.

Environmental Conservation

Environmental conservation is valued widely throughout Bhutanese society as many citizens' sources of livelihood are directly dependent on their natural environment, especially those working in agriculture. Because it is a common belief that irresponsible activities in nature will lead to negative and therefore unhappy outcomes, most Bhutanese accept the fact that the environment should be preserved for future generations. This in turn has limited severe environmental degradation such as seen in neighbouring countries like Nepal where the denuding of forests on the slopes of the Himalaya has led to landslides that have destroyed villages and taken lives. Environmental benefits that have derived from this pillar of GNH include the listing of Bhutan as a world biodiversity hotspot, increased preservation policies, and constitutional protection of the environment.

While all four pillars of GNH are incorporated into Bhutan's democratic constitution that was adopted on 18 July 2008, the constitution makes the following specific statement about the environment: "The Government shall ensure that, in order to conserve the country's natural resources and to prevent degradation of the ecosystem, a minimum of 60% of Bhutan's total land shall be maintained under forest cover for all time" (The Constitution of the Kingdom of Bhutan, 2008, p. 12).

Promotion of Culture

Preserving and promoting Bhutan's unique cultural heritage is another factor in developmental policy and GNH strategy. Based on the widely held belief that a decline in traditional heritage and culture will lead to a general dissatisfaction in society, Bhutan zealously guards its culture and the government sees the preservation of culture as a high priority. This is observed in the school system where all children are taught Bhutanese cultural values and language, side by side with science, mathematics, and English language.

Good Governance

Good governance is apparent through the government's dedication to promoting the happiness and well-being of its citizens first and foremost. The fourth king has long advocated and steered his people towards democracy. He has gradually abdicated himself from power, withdrawing from the executive function of government in 1998, introducing universal voting rights in 2002, and overseeing the establishment of an elected democratic government in 2008. Interestingly, the people considered they had good governance under the king and were perhaps the world's most reluctant country to move to democratic government. When I visited in the year prior to the first elections, people were asking, "Why is the king forsaking us?" "Why is he forcing us into a democracy?" In general, they saw little need to change the benevolent form of monarchical governance that was working well.

In contrast to the four pillars of GNH, Gross Domestic Product – the most common measure of most countries "health" – is solely an economic or materialist measure, taking into account nothing more than the total quantity of goods and services produced and sold on the domestic market economy. Coleman claims that GDP is not an indicator of national well-being but simply an accounting system (Coleman, 2009, p. 17).

This view, perhaps surprisingly, has found support among economists who might be expected to show strong preferences for economic indicators. United Kingdom economist Richard Layard, for example, has argued that a primarily economic model is far too limited and restricted in its approach. He takes a stance similar to that long held by the Bhutanese government, claiming that happiness should be the goal of a country's political philosophy and that progress towards it should be studied and measured with the same level of scrutiny as GDP (Layard, 2005).

American Nobel Prize-winning economist Joseph Stiglitz chaired a panel of 37 economic experts set up by French President Nicolas Sarkozy to work on a set of proposals for a new system to measure economic growth with more emphasis on the environment and a nation's social well-being (Isensen, 2009). Stiglitz's conclusions recommended a shift away from using GDP as the sole focus for gauging prosperity. He claimed that GDP was an antiquated standard open to the criticism of being an overly narrow indicator. The well-being of any society is diverse, complex, and multifactorial, not just economic. Some wealthy nations and societies do not rate any better on happiness scales than poorer nations or societies, while the poor, in the absence of factors such as poverty and war, can be equally as happy. GDP alone does not measure this and often ignores wider factors, such as environmental degradation, people's health, workplace safety, job security, vacation time, and a population's general degree of happiness. It is simply problematic to attempt to assess the multifactorial variables that determine the well-being of a society with a single unitary measure.

Stiglitz stressed that there was "no single indicator that can capture something as complex as our society. But because what we choose to measure and how we construct our measures can have such an important role in the decisions that are made, it is important that there be an open and public discussion of our system of metrics" (Isensen, 2009).

One of a number of problems is that ultimately harmful economic activity actually raises a nation's GDP. A country that cuts down all its trees and sells the wood increases its gross domestic product, but over the long term it is destroying its natural resources to the detriment of its citizens and the environment.

Until now, this has never been measured. The same is true for wasting energy.

Sarkozy said his intention was "to put this report on the agenda of all international meetings, and to fight for all international organizations to modify their statistical systems based on the recommendations of the commission" (Isensen, 2009).

The French president has been one of the most vocal critics calling for an over-haul of the global economic system. He has repeatedly demanded tighter controls for financial markets and an end to the big bonuses which have been blamed for the excessive risk-taking that led to the recent global economic crisis.

"For years, we have been telling people that their living standards are getting better, while at the same time their lives were growing more difficult," Sarkozy said. "We must understand the people who have lost their homes, their jobs and some of their pensions in the wake of the financial crisis and who feel they have been cheated, although it is not their fault" (Isensen, 2009).

Professor Jean-Paul Fitoussi, one of the 37 economic experts who worked on the Stiglitz report, summed up the problem with the GDP measurement, saying that "when numbers tell us we are doing well, while people feel the floor collapsing under their feet, then either the measurement standard is wrong, or we are using the wrong numbers" (Isensen, 2009).

Developing Indicators to Measure GNH

If we are to expand our ways of viewing the well-being of society and its members, the next question becomes how we can measure if this new system is working. Here Bhutan can provide us with a case study as it is perhaps the only country in the world to have already explored this and other related questions. Through the Centre for Bhutan Studies, the country asked itself, "If GNH is our political goal, how can progress towards it be measured? How can the country know if it is on track or achieving its objective? What indicators can provide feedback and help shape ongoing policy?"

Measuring progress in GDP is a relatively simple process. If the economic balance sheet is in the blue, progress is happening, at least at a financial level. The indicators of this are the dollar figures at the bottom of a column. It works much like we all manage our household budget. If your income exceeds your expenses, all is well but if expenses extend beyond income then you are in trouble. However, every family, hopefully, is aware that, though important, their happiness and well-being relate to more than just the balance of the budget.

In developing a new political philosophy, Bhutan faced the challenge of also developing indicators to operationalise GNH, measuring progress towards it, and ensuring the continuing implementation of its values. The task of doing this fell to the Centre for Bhutan Studies that has defined nine indicators, pilot tested them, and conducted the first ever nationally representative GNH survey (Ura & Penjore, 2009).

Indicators are a way for a nation to objectively measure progress and are intimately connected with social and political policy. They provide policy makers and the population with information on which to make informed decisions. Indicators can reveal which areas of development are progressing and which may need attention, which programmes are being effective and which are not, or which efforts need to be abandoned and which need to be expanded.

Speaking of Bhutan's indicators, Coleman says, "Good evidence is essential for informed decision-making. Without such measures, policy making would be blind, and have no understanding where the greatest needs are, and which population groups need to be targeted with which programs. They can also send early warning signals to policy makers if key indicators begin to trend downward, and thus allow and encourage timely remedial action" (Coleman, 2009, p. 15).

Bhutan's nine indicators of GNH include

- Health
- Education
- Living standards
- Time use
- Environmental quality
- Culture
- Community vitality
- Governance
- Psychological well-being

As space does not permit me to cover all of these indicators, let me provide examples from four areas.

Health

In the last 50 years Bhutan has transformed itself from a medieval community to a modern state and at the same time has also transformed its health care system from one that was based solely on traditional medicine systems to one that offers modern health care programmes integrating both Western and traditional systems. While it may not have some of the state-of-the-art facilities such as are available in the wealthiest, developed countries, Bhutan's health indicators show that it has surpassed many other developing countries that commenced their development programmes far earlier. Maternal mortality rates have fallen from 380/100,000 childbirths in the 1980s to 260 in 2000. The infant death rate, previously one of the highest in the world, has plummeted from 120/1,000 live births in the 1980s to 40/1,000 in 2005. Over a similar period life expectancy has climbed to about 70 years (Dorji, 2009). These indicators inform health care workers, provide positive feedback on existing programmes, and offer data on which planners can build future health care services. Building on the health indicator of GNH, Bhutan has forged a health care system that encompasses three unique features.

1. Both modern and traditional systems of medical care are offered side by side in the same building in all district hospitals. This enables patients to choose which therapy they prefer, or whether to engage both in their healing. It also allows practitioners to work collaboratively in the interests of the patient.

2. The prevention and control of diseases is integrated into a well-developed, primary health network that extends into quite remote areas where motorable roads have not yet arrived – and this includes most Bhutanese villages. Incorporated into this network is a national community-based mental health program.

3. All aspects of health care are delivered to every citizen free of charge by the government. This also includes medical treatment for Bhutanese citizens who have to seek treatment outside the country if it is not available within Bhutan. Such a free and egalitarian health service cannot be found in most developed countries (Dorji, 2009).

Time Use

Time use was chosen as one of the indicators of GNH for several reasons. First, time use studies provide information that is often missed in conventional economic accounts like GDP. Second, without an understanding of how people use their time, governments may fail to recognise the total productive capacities of its people. This in turn could lead to the implementation of misinformed policy that may not only be non-productive but may also be harmful. Third, policy makers need to be aware not only of the paid work in which people are engaged but also the unpaid productive activities in society such as child care, household duties, care of the sick and aged, and volunteer work that helps maintain the various institutions within any society. These activities are fundamental not only to the well-being of people who receive the service but also to the people who provide the caring service (Schwartz, 2010) and to the community as a whole. Galay says, "A true picture of well-being can be obtained only if these activities are taken into account. Time use studies provide information on such activities that are fundamental to the well-being of society" (Galay, 2009, p. 170).

Most readers of this book, working in professional areas, will be aware of the issue of the work-life balance. As people (including ourselves) devote more time to work they generally have less time to do the things they enjoy. As the scales tip towards a greater amount of work time, people are not only less happy but also more stressed (Kahneman, Grueger, Schkade, Schwartz, & Stone, 2006). The European Quality of Life Survey of 2003 found a strong correlation between time use and subjective well-being, with people who worked long hours and reported a poor work-life balance generally having lower levels of subjective well-being (Böhnke, 2005).

Environmental Quality

Bhutan's approach to conservation of the natural environment is not only a bold and advanced move but it is also one that recognises the close relationship between human happiness and our environment. I don't know of any other country in the world that has written it into law that 60% of the country will remain under forest forever.

The Western world has long been aware of the impact of human activities – especially activities assessed solely in terms of economic development – on the environment. In fact it is hard not to be aware of issues such as climate change that face us almost every day on television and in the press. The product of many factors including deforestation and the consumption of fossil fuels, climate change is causing glaciers to retreat, food chains to break down, ocean levels to rise, and human suffering to increase. Governments are now taking notice (mainly because the consequences are being predicted in financial terms) while scientists such as David Suzuki have approached the issues as what he calls "a matter of survival".

Bhutan's actions to preserve the environment on such a large scale has high-lighted something a lot more subtle but, nonetheless, crucially important: Long before the loss of nature becomes a matter of survival it will have an impact on our happiness and psychological well-being. Already many researchers and authors have claimed that the more detached people become from nature, the more their health suffers both physically and mentally (Nesse & Williams, 1996; Nesse, 2005). On the other side of the coin, there is much evidence to show that contact with nature has a very positive correlation with physical, psychological, social, and spiritual well-being (for reviews of the literature see Burns, 2005, 2009).

Psychological Well-Being

While economic and social indicators of well-being are widely available and fre-quently updated in Bhutan, the Centre for Bhutan Studies recently undertook a countrywide survey to assess psychological well-being. No national measure had previously existed in this area (Zangmo, 2008). Zangmo points out that a society with a philosophy of GNH calls for the inclusion of psychological well-being indica-tors at least on a par with economic ones. She says, "Media should provide attention to how a society is progressing in terms of psychological well-being and politi-cians should base their campaigns on their plans for reducing distress, increasing life satisfaction and happiness level" (Zangmo, 2008).

Probably the acid test of a country taking a GNH approach to politics is the happiness of its citizens. GNH proponents are quick to point out that it is the gov-ernment's responsibility to ensure an environment and facilities conducive to the attainment of happiness but the individual's responsibility to ensure his/her own personal well-being. Local businessman and author, Tshering Tashi, said in personal correspondence, "I believe it is not the responsibility of the state to make every one of its citizens happy. The pursuit of happiness is not only personal but subjective. However, the state shoulders the responsibility of creating a healthy atmosphere to pursue happiness." The government may have a philosophy of GNH but this should not be seen as a promise of happiness to each or every individual.

Nonetheless, a frequently asked question is "Are the Bhutanese people happy or happier than people from other countries?" Has GNH facilitated the attain-ment of greater happiness? The Centre for Bhutan Studies undertook a survey of average happiness levels for seven member nations of the South Asia Association of Regional Cooperation (SAARC). The eighth member, The Maldives, was not included as no data was available. The countries are comparable at some levels in that they are in the same region and most would be considered "developing" countries. They are also diverse in several ways in that India is one of the most populous countries in the world while Bhutan is comparatively tiny in size and population. Overall, differences on an 11-point scale (0–10) were small but Bhutan did rank at the top of the list (Zangmo, 2008).

An Example of Applying GNH in Social Policy

In summing up what I have presented so far, Bhutan has a philosophy of GNH. It has established four pillars on which this philosophy is based. In addition, it has defined nine indicators that have been rigorously studied throughout the country and closely analysed. These indicators give feedback to the public and politicians about what programmes are facilitating a development towards happiness and what might need to be modified. Based on this strong foundation, the next questions become, "How is this philosophy and knowledge translated into happiness-oriented policies?" and "How is this process different from one based on GDP?"

To any mountaineer Bhutan has an enticing array of virgin Himalayan summits including Gangkar Puensum, the world's highest unclimbed peak. If assessed from a solely GDP approach, the sport of mountaineering could certainly make a significant contribution to a relatively poor country's coffers. With one alpine club alone already offering the Bhutan government one million US dollars for the privilege of attempting to summit Gangkar Puensum, the economics must be as tempting to the government as the peaks are to the climbers (Tashi, 2009).

By comparison, mountaineering makes a significant contribution to neighbouring Nepal's national income. In 2007 the fee for a team climbing Mt Everest – just one of the 325 peaks open for climbing – was US $50,000. Mountaineering has become the highest per capita income generating sector in the Nepali economy with each mountaineer spending 27 times more than an ordinary tourist (Dhakal, 2009).

Bhutan is an economically poor country. The United Nation's Human Development Index (HDI) – a quantified score that is calculated by averaging three indicators of income, educational attainment, and life expectancy – placed Bhutan as 130 on a list of 160 countries (Carpenter & Carpenter, 2002). Many of its people, particularly in rural areas, still live in poverty. Many countries in a similar situation would probably rate their choice about whether to permit mountaineering or not solely on a financial decision – perhaps with the luxury of an environmental impact assessment. Mountaineering has previously been permitted in Bhutan and, indeed, several of its important peaks have been climbed. However, Tshering Tashi explains, "We, the Bhutanese, consider our mountains to be sacred. For centuries they have been home to our most well renowned hermits and sites of religious pilgrimages. Like our ancestors we continue to worship and protect the mountains which have also protected us, serving as a natural barrier that has helped keep out invaders. Today, the snow from the mountains feeds the glacial lakes which provide the water that not only irrigates our rice fields but also runs the turbines to generate the electricity that drives the Bhutanese economy.

"We, the Bhutanese also believe that the mountains are the abodes of local deities that protect us. People living in the mountains said that after people (mountaineers) climbed to the top of the mountains, the mountain vultures would not descend to the sky burial sites to eat the corpses. This was considered a bad omen. The people living in the mountainous regions recollect unusual stories. Some of them remember unusual weather such as heavy hail storms and flash floods, which they attribute to the disturbance caused by outside mountaineer climbers" (Tashi, 2009. p. 114).

As a result the people approached the king with their concerns. The National Assembly looked at it from the perspective of the four GNH pillars. It took into account the economic factors along with the cultural and religious sentiments of the people, the desire to maintain the pristine nature of the region, the potential costs of ecological imbalances created by such expeditions, and the need to provide good governance to the people. The non-economic pillars of GNH were considered to be far greater than the potential revenue that might be generated. As a result the National Assembly placed a total ban on mountaineering perhaps becoming the only country in the world where it is completely prohibited. Gangkar Puensum to this day remains the world's highest unclimbed peak.

As well as having the principles on which such decisions can be made, policy makers also need appropriate processes by which decisions such as those on mountaineering can be brought into practice. In Bhutan's case, there has been a long established Planning Commission charged with overseeing the country's development in accord with the principles of GNH. On 18 January 2007, the Royal Government announced the establishment of the GNH Commission to revamp and rename the former Planning Commission (www.bbs.com.bt/GNH%20Commission%20formed.html). Simultaneously the Centre for Bhutan Studies (CBS) was directed to develop practical and target-oriented indicators for GNH as well as provide feedback on issues under consideration by the GNH Commission. All development projects, including funding, have to be processed by the GNH Commission to ensure they meet both the pillars and indicators for national happiness and well-being.

Gross International Happiness?

Does Bhutan's GNH have applicability for the rest of the world? Do people want governments to be more involved in happiness than in just keeping the nation's accounts balanced? Do citizens desire, as Bhutan's prime minister, Jigmi Thinley, indicated, the state to be responsible for creating and enabling an environment in which its citizens can pursue happiness? Nic Marks claims that there is indeed "considerable support among the public for governments to use broader measures of progress" (2009, p. 103). A poll conducted in the United Kingdom in fact found that 81% of people endorsed the idea that a government's prime objective should be "greatest happiness" rather than the "greatest wealth". By comparison, only

13% considered government should focus primarily on wealth and forget the happiness issue (BBC, 2006).

During the luncheon I had with King Khesar, I took the opportunity to ask him, "How do you see your own continuing role in regards to the promotion of Gross National Happiness? Do you see yourself as an ambassador taking GNH to the rest of the world?" I guess I was wondering how this concept, originating from a tiny Himalayan kingdom – that perhaps the majority of the people in the world have never heard of – could influence global policy change to fulfil the king's dream of promoting greater well-being and happiness of all people.

He replied, "I would like to travel. The opportunity was there while I was in England but I was too busy with my studies. I would also like to promote the concept of GNH internationally but as my first commitment is to my people, I plan to devote the next 2 years visiting every village and meeting every person in my own country. I want to see what we can do to further people's happiness here first."

As he spoke I was mindful he was not setting himself an easy challenge. In a country where only one road dissects it east to west and where there are no internal air services, most villages are several days' walk from the nearest road head. The only way to visit these village people is to hike through the tallest mountain range in the world.

In addition, the king seemed to say that happiness begins at home, with each and every individual. This reflected the comments of Prime Minister Jigmi Thinley to the United Nations when he said that happiness is the single most important goal and purpose in life for every individual and that it is the responsibility of the State to create an enabling, facilitating environment in which individual citizens can pursue happiness (Thinley, 2008).

Bhutan thus offers us a case example, not of an idealized philosophy, but of a practical, scientific approach for creating a political environment conducive to the pursuit of happiness. Over the last few decades Bhutan has undertaken a political experiment that has recently culminated in a national survey. It has measures, indicators and feedback systems in place to assess progress towards its goals – factors that will remain in place and continue to monitor progress.

From this tiny Buddhist Himalayan kingdom, wedged between the great population giants of China and India, the concept of Gross National Happiness has spread. Indeed, the world's newest democracy seems to be offering the world important political and personal philosophies. At the time of writing there have now been five conferences on GNH; two in Bhutan, one in Nova Scotia, Canada, one in Thailand, and one in Brazil. These conferences attract a multidisciplinary group of international presenters and participants, including researchers, economists, philosophers, psychiatrists, psychologists, health workers, United Nations representatives, educationalists, politicians, and many others.

How the concept of GNH has expanded onto the international arena can be seen in other initiatives. In the United States, the Gross National Happiness American Project has been formed with the purpose of organising conferences to explore changing social policy measures from wealth to well-being, and more broadly promote the concept of GNH. In France, as already mentioned, President

Nicolas Sarkozy has drawn a group of leading economists into a think tank to re-examine the validity of continuing with GDP as a sole or primary measure of a nation's well-being. In a ground-breaking initiative in September 2009 Sarkozy raised the idea of a GNH-type model of development at the G20 meeting in Pittsburgh. This is a clear example of how a concept like GNH can engender sci-entific investigation that then informs policy makers and, hopefully, builds into strategies and approaches that enhance the potential well-being of all.

As I mentioned, Bhutan offers us an illustrative case example but this may not necessarily apply as a template of social policy for all cultures, all societies and all nations. Bhutan is a relatively monoracial, monocultural country with a small pop-ulation compared to more populous, multiracial, multicultural nations such as the United States and Australia. Social and political policies based on the enhancement of happiness might look different from country to country. Indeed, the nine indi-cators defined by Bhutan (and described earlier in this chapter) are different from the eight candidate psychological and social indicators based in Western research and described by Ed Diener in the preceding chapter. While such differences are to be expected, and perhaps even encouraged, the big picture issue here is a paradigm question: Do we want our development – individually, nationally, and globally – to be based primarily on a measure of greatest wealth or one of greatest happi-ness? Already there seems to be some evidence to answer this in favour of the latter (BBC, 2006; Marks, 2009). If we answer this first question in the affirmative, this leads us to further questions: How do we want such policies for happiness to look? What are the values and evidence on which they can be based? How can we develop indicators to measure our progress? How can we provide feedback to policy makers? And it is here that Bhutan offers us an illustrative example.

Gross National Happiness, Bhutan's gift to the world, is not only coming to the awareness of the world's politicians and policy makers but also seems to be emerg-ing as a basis to shift political and social philosophy from wealth to well-being. As nations of the world begin to explore whether GDP should or will remain an adequate measure of their current and future well-being and the well-being of the whole planet, can we hope that Gross National Happiness will grow into Gross International Happiness?

References

BBC. (2006). *Britain's Happiness in Decline*. http://news.bbc.co.uk/2/hi/programmes/happiness formula/4771908.stm. Accessed December 5, 2009.

Burns, G. W. (2005). Naturally happy, naturally healthy: The role of the natural environment in well-being. In F. A. Huppert, N. Baylis, & B. Keverne (Eds.), *The science of well-being* (pp. 405–431). Oxford: Oxford University Press.

Burns, G. W. (2009). Can we have both psychological and ecological well-being? In K. Ura & D. Penjore (Eds.), *Gross national happiness: Practice and measurement* (pp. 127–148). Thimphu: Centre for Bhutan Studies.

Böhnke, P. (2005). *First European quality of life survey: Life satisfaction, happiness and sense of belonging*. Luxembourg: Office of Official Publications of the European Communities.

Carpenter, R., & Carpenter, B. (2002). *The blessings of Bhutan*. Honolulu, HI: University of Hawaii Press.

Chan, V. (1994). *Tibet handbook: A pilgrimage guide*. Chico, CA: Moon Publications.

Coleman, R. (2009). Measuring progress towards gross national happiness: From GNH indicators to GNH national accounts. In K. Ura & D. Penjore (Eds.), *Gross national happiness: Practice and measurement* (pp. 15–48). Thimpu: Centre for Bhutan Studies.

Dhakal, D. P. (2009). *Mountain tourism and mountaineers*. Accessed August 17, 2009, from http://news.visitingnepal.com/archives/129

Dorji, C. (2009). Bhutanese healthcare reform: A paradigm shift in health care to increase gross national happiness. In K. Ura & D. Penjore (Eds.), *Gross national happiness: Practice and measurement* (pp. 413–435). Thimpu: Centre for Bhutan Studies.

Galay, K. (2009). Time use and happiness. In K. Ura & D. Penjore (Eds.), *Gross national happiness: Practice and measurement* (pp. 169–206). Thimpu: Centre for Bhutan Studies.

Isensen, N. (2009). *Sarkozy calls for a new international prosperity barometer*. Accessed December 5, 2009, from http://www.dw-world.de/dw/article/0,,4692507,00.html

Kahneman, D., Grueger, A. B., Schkade, D., Swartz, N., & Stone, A. (2006). *Would you be happier if you were richer? A focussing illusion* (A CEPS working paper no. 125). Accessed December 5, 2009, from http://www.princeton.edu/ceps/workingpapers/125krueger.pdf

Layard, R. (2005). *Happiness: Lessons from a new science*. London: Allen Lane.

Marks, N. (2009). Creating national accounts of well-being: A parallel process to GNH. In K. Ura & D. Penjore (Eds.), *Gross national happiness: Practice and measurement* (pp. 102–123). Thimpu: Centre for Bhutan Studies.

Murdoch, A., & Oldershaw, D. (2008). *16 Guidelines for a happy life: The basics*. London: Essential Education.

Nesse, R. M. (2005). Natural selection and the elusiveness of happiness. In F. A. Huppert, N. Baylis, & B. Keverne (Eds.), *The science of well-being* (pp. 3–32). Oxford: Oxford University Press.

Nesse, R. M., & Williams, G. C. (1996). *Evolution and healing: The new science of Darwinian medicine*. London: Phoenix.

Schwartz, C. (2010). Can helping others help oneself? In G. W. Burns (Eds.), *Happiness, healing, enhancement: Your casebook collection for applying positive therapy* (pp. 151–162). Hoboken, NJ: Wiley.

Tashi, T. (2009). The tallest virgin mountain in the world. In T. Fisher & T. Tashi (Eds.), *From Jesuits to jetsetters: Bold Bhutan beckons: Inhaling gross national happiness* (pp. 114–125). Brisbane: CopyRight Publishing.

The Constitution of the Kingdom of Bhutan. (2008). Accessed October 4, 2010, from http://www.constitution.bt

Thinley, L. J. (2008, September 26). A statement to the 63rd session of the General Assembly of the United Nations, New York.

Ura, K., & Galey, K. (Eds.) (2004). *Gross national happiness and development*. Thimpu: Centre for Bhutan Studies.

Ura, K., & Penjore, D. (Eds.) (2009). *Gross national happiness: Practice and measurement*. Thimpu: Centre for Bhutan Studies.

Zangmo, T. (2008, November 24–26). *Psychological wellbeing: Findings of the gross national happiness survey*. Paper presented at the 4th international conference on Gross National Happiness, Thimphu.

Chapter 6
Ecological Challenges, Materialistic Values, and Social Change

Tim Kasser

The environmental sciences have increasingly warned informed citizens and political leaders about the multiple crises affecting our one and only home planet. The percentage of species expected to go extinct in the next couple of decades is on par with the massive die-offs historically due to cataclysms such as asteroids. The levels of pollution in our air and of garbage in our water are so extensive that babies are born with toxic chemicals in their blood-streams and huge areas of the Pacific Ocean and the Gulf of Mexico can no longer support sea life. And the rise in atmospheric carbon dioxide levels foretells extensive climate disruptions that threaten to create massive numbers of refugees whose homes will be underwater, shortages in food and potable water, and international conflicts over the resources necessary to sustain life.

The response to these data by citizens and leaders in wealthy countries has thus far not risen to the challenges ahead for humanity. Citizens continue to place environmental problems relatively low in their rank-orderings of national priorities. Politicos' negotiations about climate disruption at international conferences are still often derailed by concerns about their nations' economic growth (such as occurred in Copenhagen in the winter of 2009), and continue to be influenced largely by the idea that businesses have a "right" to pollute (i.e., cap-and-trade policies). To the extent a consistent message regarding social change has been promoted, it is that "consumers" (nee citizens) can do their part to save the Earth by switching their light bulbs from incandescents to compact fluorescents or by driving hybrid automobiles. Unfortunately, most environmental research does not suggest that these approaches will come close to meeting the environmental challenges ahead, or that such small behavioral changes will generalize to the types of life style changes that are likely to be required of the citizenry (Thogerson & Crompton, 2009).

From the perspective of a psychologist interested in social change, it seems to me that what remains largely unspoken, but ultimately necessary, is to recognize that our world's ecological crisis is a deeply *internal* crisis of *values*. Values

T. Kasser (✉)
Knox College, Galesburg, IL, USA
e-mail: tkasser@knox.edu

R. Biswas-Diener (ed.), *Positive Psychology as Social Change*,
DOI 10.1007/978-90-481-9938-9_6, © Springer Science+Business Media B.V. 2011

are the psychological representations of what people believe is important in life (Rokeach, 1973), and one particular set of values is clearly relevant to the ecological crises humanity faces: the self-enhancing, materialistic concerns for money, wealth, possessions, status, and an appealing image.

Self-Enhancing, Materialistic Values

Substantial cross-cultural psychological research documents that self-enhancing, materialistic values are indeed a crucial component of people's motivational systems. In these studies, individuals around the world have been presented with a variety of different aims they might value or goals they might have, and have been asked to rate how important these values and goals are to them. Using statistical techniques such as factor analysis, smallest space analysis, multidimensional scaling analysis, and circular stochastic modeling, researchers have been able to identify smaller subsets of particular values and goals that cluster together as coherent groups. For example, Shalom Schwartz's (1992, 2006) seminal work has identified 10 types of basic priorities held by people in dozens of nations around the world. Two of these types of priorities cluster together as what Schwartz calls the "self-enhancement" values, for they concern the attempt to stand out from others through the acquisition of money, status, and the like. Specifically, the first self-enhancement value, *power*, concerns the desire to obtain resources and wealth, whereas the second, *achievement*, concerns the desire to stand out as particularly excellent and successful by the definitions of one's society. The cross-cultural research my colleagues and I have conducted (Grouzet et al., 2005; Kasser & Ryan, 1996; Ryan et al., 1999; Schmuck, Kasser, & Ryan, 2000) similarly yields an "extrinsic" or "materialistic" cluster consisting of three types of goals: *financial success*, which concerns the desire for money and possessions; *image*, which concerns the desire to have an appealing appearance; and *status*, which concerns the desire to be popular and admired by others.

In addition to documenting the existence of these self-enhancing, materialistic values, a variety of types of studies support the proposal that these types of aims in life contribute to the environmental difficulties that humanity now faces.

For example, studies show that the more people care about self-enhancing, materialistic values and goals, the more likely they are to hold attitudes and values that are inconsistent with good environmental stewardship. Studies in Australia (Saunders & Munro, 2000) and the United States (Good, 2007) document that materialistic values and a strong consumer orientation are associated with lower biophilia (i.e., the love of all living things; Kellert & Wilson, 1993) and worse environmental attitudes. The cross-cultural research of Schwartz (1992, 2006) similarly reveals that the self-enhancing values of *power* and *achievement* are associated with caring less about values such as "protecting the environment," "attaining unity with nature," and having "a world of beauty." Additionally, a study of almost 1,000 undergraduates from Brazil, the Czech Republic, Germany, India, New Zealand, and Russia showed that worse environmental attitudes were associated with high power values in five nations and with higher achievement values in two nations (Schultz et al., 2005).

Self-enhancing, materialistic values have also been associated with *behaving in less ecologically sustainable ways*. Materialistic values have been negatively correlated with how much American adults engage in ecologically friendly behaviors such as buying second-hand, recycling, riding a bicycle, reusing paper, etc. (Richins & Dawson, 1992; Brown & Kasser, 2005); such results have been replicated in samples of US and UK adolescents (Gatersleben, Meadows, Abrahamse, & Jackson, 2008; Kasser, 2005). Brown and Kasser (2005) also examined how materialistic values are associated with ecological footprints, a measure that quantifies the amount of ecological resources necessary to support one's lifestyle via self-reports of one's behaviors in the realms of transportation (e.g., riding a bicycle vs. driving an SUV), housing (e.g., living in a small vs. large home), and food (e.g., eating a vegetarian diet vs. eating a meat-based one). The findings from 400 North American adults showed that those who cared more about materialistic values had substantially higher ecological footprints than did those who were less focused on such aims.

The role of materialistic values in ecological destruction is also supported by research using resource dilemma games (Dechesne et al., 2003; Kasser & Sheldon, 2000; Sheldon & McGregor, 2000). For example, Sheldon and McGregor assessed college students' values and then assigned them to one of three kinds of groups based on their scores: a group with four subjects who all scored high in materialism, a group with four subjects who all scored low in materialism, or a group with two members who scored high and two who scored low in materialism. Subjects then played a "forest-management game" in which they were asked to imagine that they were in charge of a company that would bid against three other companies (i.e., their other group members) to harvest timber from a state forest. All subjects in a group made an initial bid for how much they wanted to harvest; the total amount of the four bids in the group was then subtracted from the existing forest acreage, another 10% was added back (to represent regrowth in the forest), and then a second year of bidding commenced. This process continued either until 25 "years" of bidding had passed or until no forest remained. Sheldon and McGregor found that materialistic individuals reported being more motivated by "greed," or the desire to profit more than other companies, and, importantly, that the groups composed of four materialistic individuals were significantly less likely to have a forest remaining at the 25th year of bidding.

Similar dynamics appear to play out on a national scale. Kasser (in press) obtained measures of the CO_2 emissions (per capita) of 20 wealthy, capitalistic nations and correlated these with how much the citizens in those nations cared about *mastery* values, which are aimed at manipulating the world to serve one's own interest. Even after controlling for a nation's Gross Domestic Product (per capita), the more mastery was valued by citizens of a nation, the more CO_2 that nation emitted, and thus the more it was contributing to climate disruption.

To summarize, the body of literature just reviewed suggests that to the extent individuals value self-enhancing, materialistic aims in life, they are more likely to have negative attitudes about the environment, are less likely to engage in relatively simple behaviors that benefit the environment, and are more likely to make behavioral choices that contribute to environmental degradation. Further, evidence suggests that when nations strongly value self-enhancing, materialistic values, they emit more greenhouse gases. Such findings, although admittedly correlational, are consistent with the proposal that society's focus on the acquisition of more and more wealth and consumer goods, on economic growth, and on financial profit contribute both to the environmental degradation threatening humanity's only liveable habitat and to the thus far weak responses of citizens, businesses, and politicians to this threat.

A Strategy to Enhance Sustainability by Decreasing Materialistic Values

In this section, I lay out a two-armed strategy for social change that is aimed at promoting sustainability by decreasing the extent to which people and society focus on the self-enhancing, materialistic values known to be associated with ecological degradation. The first arm of this strategy is to identify and remove the root causes of self-enhancing, materialistic values, thereby decreasing the likelihood that people will focus on the kinds of aims in life that interfere with an ecologically sustainable world. The second arm of the strategy is to encourage alternative values that both oppose the self-enhancing, materialistic values and that promote ecological sustainability. The remainder of this section provides a brief overview of each of these two approaches and the empirical basis for them.

Addressing the Causes of Self-enhancing, Materialistic Values

The research suggests that there are two primary pathways that lead individuals to place a relatively high importance on materialistic values (Kasser, Ryan, Couchman, & Sheldon, 2004). The first pathway is the rather obvious influence of social modeling and the second is the subtler route of responses to felt threats and insecurity.

Social modeling occurs when individuals are exposed to people or messages in their environment suggesting that money, power, possessions, achievement, image, and status are important aims to strive for in life. The empirical evidence clearly documents that people's levels of materialism are positively associated with the extent that their parents, friends, and peers also espouse such values (Ahuvia & Wong, 2002; Banerjee & Dittmar, 2008; Kasser, Ryan, Zax, & Sameroff, 1995). Television also plays an important role in encouraging materialistic values, as documented by numerous studies (Cheung & Chan, 1996; Good, 2007; Kasser & Ryan, 2001; Rahtz, Sirgy, & Meadow, 1989; Schor, 2004). Another piece of evidence supporting a social modeling explanation is that children exposed to advertising in school have a stronger materialistic orientation (Brand & Greenberg, 1994).

The second pathway that tends to increase materialism is that of insecurity. When people experience threats to their survival, their safety and security, and their perceived likelihood of satisfying their psychological needs, the empirical literature suggests that they tend to orient toward materialistic aims. For example, children's materialism is higher when they grow up in a family with a cold, controlling mother, when their parents divorce, and when they experience poverty (Cohen & Cohen, 1996; Kasser et al., 1995; Rindfleisch, Burroughs, & Denton, 1997; Williams, Cox, Hedberg, & Deci, 2000). Experimental manipulations also support a causal role of insecurity in increasing materialistic values. For example, when people consider economic hardship, poor interpersonal relationships, and even their own death, they increase the priority they place on materialistic aims and they tend to act in more ecologically destructive ways (Dechesne et al., 2003; Kasser & Sheldon, 2000; Kasser & Sheldon, 2008). Further, experimental manipulations that have induced feelings of hunger (Briers, Pandelaere, Dewitte, & Warlop, 2006), personal self-doubt (Chang & Arkin, 2002), and social exclusion (Twenge, Baumeister, DeWall, Ciarocco, & Bartels, 2007) have also resulted in increases in selfish, materialistic behavior.

Thus, one means of promoting sustainability is to decrease the factors known to encourage self-interested, materialistic values and behaviors. This might be done by (a) reducing the extent to which self-enhancing, materialistic values are modeled in society; (b) increasing the extent to which people feel secure; and/or (c) helping people respond to feelings of threat and insecurity in ways other than orienting toward self-enhancing, materialistic values.

Promoting an Alternative Set of Values

The second arm of the theoretical strategy for promoting sustainability relies on the fact that self-enhancing, materialistic values and goals exist within broader systems of personal goals and values. That is, people strive for a variety of different aims, some of which are materialistic and self-enhancing, and some of which concern other values and goals. Cross-cultural research provides a fairly consistent picture of the organization of these goal systems, showing that some values and goals are typically experienced as psychologically consistent with each other, whereas other values and goals are experienced by most people as in opposition to each other. The extent of consistency or conflict among value and goal types can be statistically represented by a "circumplex" structure, in which goals that are psychologically consistent are placed next to each other in a circular arrangement whereas goals that are in psychological conflict are placed on opposite sides of the circumplex; Figs. 6.1 and 6.2 present two such circumplex models of values and goals that have been well-validated cross-culturally.

Schwartz's (1992, 2006) model, presented in Fig. 6.1, shows that the self-enhancing values of *achievement* and *power* lie next to each other, representing their psychological compatibility; similarly my colleagues and I have shown that

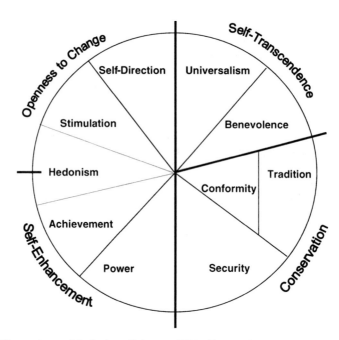

Fig. 6.1 Circumplex model of values (Schwartz, 2006). Figure printed with the permission of the publisher

the materialistic aims of financial success, image, and popularity cluster together as a consistent set of goals (Grouzet et al., 2005; see Fig. 6.2).

Importantly, these circumplex models also reveal the values and goals that lie in opposition to the self-enhancing, materialistic values. Figure 6.1 shows that the self-enhancing values are opposed by two "self-transcendent" values, *benevolence*, which concerns acting in ways that help the people to whom one is especially close, and *universalism*, which concerns acting in ways that improve the broader world. Figure 6.2 similarly shows that materialistic goals are opposed by a set of three "intrinsic" goals: *self-acceptance* (or understanding one's self and striving to feel free), *affiliation* (or having good relationships with family and friends), and *community feeling* (or trying to make the wider world a better place).

These models, based on data from thousands of individuals across dozens of nations, thus suggest another strategy for reducing self-enhancing, materialistic values: encourage the values that stand in psychological opposition to the ecologically destructive values of self-enhancement and materialism. Because it is relatively difficult for people to simultaneously pursue both sets of values (Schwartz, 1992) and because activating one set of values diminishes the likelihood of behaving on the basis of opposing sets of values (Maio, Pakizeh, Cheung, & Rees, 2009), efforts to increase the importance people place on values such as benevolence and universalism and goals such as self-acceptance, affiliation, and community feeling should

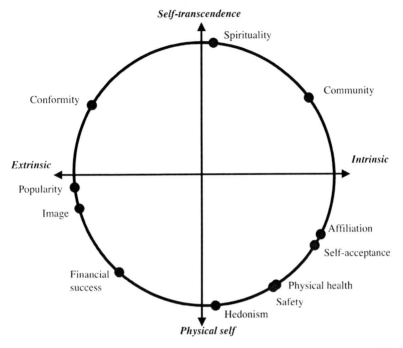

Fig. 6.2 Circumplex model of goals (Grouzet et al., 2005). Figure printed with the permission of the publisher

result in a relative de-emphasis on the self-enhancing, materialistic aims that are associated with ecological degradation.

The potential usefulness of encouraging these alternative values is further bolstered by the fact that empirical research demonstrates that the self-transcendent, intrinsic values are associated with more positive ecological outcomes. For example, Schultz et al.'s (2005) cross-cultural study documented that in each of the six nations studied, self-transcendent values such as benevolence and universalism were significant positive predictors of having engaged in a set of 12 environmentally helpful behaviors (ranging from recycling to picking up litter to environmental political actions). Generosity (which is akin to the *universalism* and *community feeling* values) also predicts more positive environmental attitudes and behaviors in UK and US adolescents (Gatersleben et al., 2008; Kasser, 2005). Further, the more people focus on intrinsic values (relative to materialistic values), the more sustainable and less greedy their behaviors are in both resource dilemma games (Sheldon & McGregor, 2000) and in their own lives (Brown & Kasser, 2005). Finally, nations have significantly lower CO_2 emissions when their citizens place a strong importance on *harmony* values (which are akin to the universalism values and community feeling goals; Kasser, in press).

Encouraging intrinsic goals can have other salutary effects as well. The research consistently shows, for example, that people who place a relatively high value on intrinsic goals in comparison to extrinsic, materialistic goals report higher personal well-being (e.g., more self-actualization and vitality) and lower personal distress (e.g., less depression and anxiety; see Kasser, 2002 for a review, and see Twenge et al., 2010, for evidence across time in the United States). And people who place a relatively high value on intrinsic goals in comparison to extrinsic, materialistic goals behave in more cooperative, pro-social ways, sharing more and being more empathic and less manipulative (see Kasser et al., 2004). Thus, not only do the self-transcendent, intrinsic values oppose self-enhancing, materialistic values, and not only do they support more positive ecological behaviors, but they also seem to provide greater personal well-being and promote the kinds of cooperative, pro-social behaviors that will be necessary to solve the social and ecological crises humanity is likely to face.

Four Applications of the Strategy for Social Change

The values-based perspective I have been describing here suggests that our present ecological difficulties derive in part from the fact that people often give high priority to a set of self-enhancing, materialistic values that contribute to ecologically destructive attitudes and behaviors. This diagnosis, in combination with empirical research and psychological theorizing, yields two basic approaches for promoting the types of social changes that will support ecological sustainability. First, because people act in more materialistic ways when they are exposed to social models that encourage materialism and when they feel threatened and insecure, it may be useful to remove the social models and to diminish the feelings of insecurity that create and maintain self-enhancing, materialistic values, and to help people find other, less ecologically destructive means of responding to threats when they feel insecure. Second, because self-enhancing, materialistic values exist in broader value systems and are opposed by transcendent, intrinsic values that promote pro-ecological attitudes and behaviors, it may be useful to develop means of encouraging people to prioritize and act consistently with these values.

In the four sections that follow, I describe more concrete avenues for applying this strategy.

Voluntary Simplicity

American history has been dominated by the dream of material prosperity and consequent attempts to "tame" (i.e., economically develop) a vast continent. At the same time, however, some Americans have questioned the nation's focus on economic growth, consumption, and material acquisition, and instead have tried to live a "simpler" life. The historian David Shi (1985) has documented this countervailing trend from the time of the early Puritans and Quakers, through the American Revolution and Transcendentalism, and into the counter-cultural movement of the 1960s. These days, individuals who pursue such alternative lifestyles have been labeled "cultural creatives," "downshifters," and, probably most widely, "voluntary simplifiers" (VSrs). The commonality across these various labels is the conscious decision to reject the mainstream work-spend-work-some-more lifestyle and instead focus on obtaining "inner riches," by prioritizing personal growth, family, volunteering, and spiritual development (see the qualitative interviews of Elgin, 1993 and Pierce, 2000). What's more, many VSrs report that they are highly motivated by ecological concerns.

One of the first quantitative scientific studies on VS was conducted by Brown & Kasser (2005), who obtained a sample of 200 self-identified VSrs (through a variety of list-servs and publications) and matched them with 200 mainstream Americans on gender, age, and zip code. Several interesting differences between the groups emerged. First, compared to the mainstream group, the VS group was significantly more likely to report engaging in positive environmental behaviors and to be living in ways that decreased their ecological footprints. Second, compared to the mainstream group, the VS group reported significantly higher levels of life satisfaction and a preponderance of pleasant versus unpleasant emotion in their daily lives. (This finding is particularly noteworthy given that the VS group's average annual income was about two-thirds that of the mainstream group's). Third, structural equation modeling demonstrated that the VS group's greater happiness and more ecologically responsible behavior could be partially explained by the fact that the VS group had a value system that was significantly more oriented toward intrinsic goals and less oriented toward extrinsic, materialistic goals than that of the mainstream Americans.

These results suggest that part of the promise of the VS lifestyle concerns the second arm of the strategy described above. That is, VS seems to promote (or at least be consistent with) the kinds of intrinsic goals that oppose ecologically damaging extrinsic, materialistic goals. But a VS lifestyle might also help to work against the factors known to cause materialistic values. For example, interviews (Elgin, 1993; Pierce, 2000) and first-person accounts (Holst, 2007), reveal that many VSrs eliminate television and other sources of advertising from their families' lives, choose friends who support their values, and work for and with organizations that do not pressure them to prioritize financial profit and work excessively long hours. All of these behaviors would limit how much VSrs are exposed to the social models that encourage materialistic values. Other anecdotal data suggest that a VS lifestyle might enhance a sense of personal security by encouraging self-sufficiency. VSrs often learn how to make their own clothes, grow their own food, repair their own possessions, entertain themselves without reliance on costly electronic equipment, and even build their own homes; such skills surely promote a sense of personal security and confidence that one can deal with various types of hassles and threats. What's more, some evidence suggests that VSrs are especially interested in pursuing the types of meditative and spiritual practices known to be effective ways of addressing one's own personal insecurities (Elgin, 1993). The fact that Brown and Kasser (2005) found that the VS group was significantly happier than mainstream Americans suggests that such efforts may have met with some success. Future research might follow up on these qualitative, anecdotal findings to more systematically determine the role these factors might play both in sustaining the VS lifestyle and in promoting ecologically responsible behavior.

Only about 10–20% of the American population seems to pursue anything approaching a VS lifestyle (Brown & Kasser, 2005; Elgin, 1993; Ray, 1997). Given the promise that VS might hold for promoting intrinsic values, ecologically sustainable behavior, and happiness, how might those interested in social change work to increase this percentage?

First, my conversations with many people suggest that one of the clear barriers to pursuing a VS lifestyle in the United States is the concerns people have about living without health insurance if they only have a part-time job, or do not work for pay at all; this anecdotal evidence is consistent with the findings that death anxiety can shift people away from intrinsic values and towards materialistic values (e.g., Kasser & Sheldon, 2008). More formal studies are needed to determine whether concerns about health care access do indeed lead people to give up on desires for a more materially simple lifestyle, but if such evidence is forthcoming, it would be another reason for having reformed the US health care system so that health insurance is not provided primarily through one's full time employer.

Another roadblock to the adoption of a VS lifestyle is likely the stress of living "outside the mainstream." Current American social norms suggest that a happy, successful, meaningful, and even patriotic life entails working long hours and consuming at high levels, and some VSrs have indeed reported feeling ostracized by friends and families who do not understand their lifestyle choices; others have even been called "subversive" for refusing to follow the standard American work-hard-and-consume lifestyle (Elgin, 1993; Pierce, 2000). Another effect of these social norms is that some people have a rather distorted view of what VS might entail; I've met more than a few people who say that while a simpler life appeals to them, they can't imagine "becoming Amish" or "living like the Unabomber." If these are people's primary understanding of what it means to live more simply, and if they worry that they will be seen as "odd" by their neighbors and friends for even considering such a lifestyle, it is no wonder that many people interested in simplifying their lives go no further than subscribing to magazines such as *Simple Living* where they can view hundreds of advertisements and articles about products aimed at this "market segment." Thus, such individuals are channeled back into the mainstream norms of consumption rather than toward the kinds of fundamental lifestyle changes necessary to reach ecological sustainability.

These norms could of course be addressed through concerted public education efforts designed to change social perceptions about what "the good life" is and what "simplicity" means. Another educational approach could entail the creation of community-sponsored "simplicity circles" (Andrews, 1998), which are small groups that meet to provide members with information about and support for living in materially simpler ways. Having the opportunity to read such material and talk with others who are attempting to live a lifestyle more consistent with intrinsic values is likely to help establish new sets of norms that make it somewhat easier to live in a materially simpler manner.

Time Affluence

As we have seen, contemporary culture encourages a conception of "the good life" that is defined largely via a concept of "material affluence," i.e., whether one has wealth and the high levels of possessions and consumption that accompany wealth. Creating a more ecologically sustainable world will be difficult so long as this materialistically dominant definition of the good life holds sway, especially since material affluence is one of the three primary factors known to influence ecological degradation (see Ehrlich & Holdren's (1971) classic *IPAT* model). As such, it seems necessary to develop other, less ecologically damaging conceptions of the good life around which people can orient their lives. One promising alternative is to decrease work hours and maximize "time affluence" (deGraaf, 2003; Jackson, 2009; Kasser & Sheldon, 2008; Schor, 2010). That is, rather than attempting to become as wealthy as possible (which often entails working more), people might instead strive to reduce their work hours and have more time available to pursue other, less materialistically oriented, interests.

At least three empirical studies support the promise that time affluence holds for reducing ecological degradation. At the level of the individual person, Kasser and Brown (2003) found that people had lower ecological footprints and engaged in more beneficial environmental behaviors when they worked fewer hours per week. Hayden and Shandra (2009) replicated these results in a sample of 50 nations: after controlling for other nation-level variables (such as work output per hour, population, and urbanization), nations whose citizens worked fewer hours per year had lower ecological footprints. Finally, among economically developed nations, average work hours are associated with lower energy use, thus diminishing CO_2 emissions (Rosnick & Weisbrot, 2006). Indeed, analyses from this study suggested that if the United States were to follow the European Union's model of lowered work hours, its energy usage would decline about 20% and its carbon emissions would decline about 3%. In contrast, "a worldwide choice of American work hours over European levels could result in 1–2 degrees Celsius of additional warming..." (p. 7).

Schor (2010) provides two primary explanations for why lowering work hours can promote ecological sustainability. First, working fewer hours results in lower income levels, and thus less consumption, especially of the kinds that are particularly bad for the environment (e.g., taking luxury vacations, enlarging one's home, eating exotic produce). Second, people who work fewer hours have more time available to engage in ecologically beneficial activities that are more time intensive, such as riding one's bike to work, baking one's own bread, and hanging laundry out to dry; indeed, these are some of the very behaviors Kasser and Brown (2003) found people engaged in more when they worked less.

If people are going to switch their conceptions of the good life from an ecologically damaging one based on material affluence to a more ecologically sustainable one based on time affluence, this alternative conception of affluence will need to strongly appeal to individuals. Some evidence suggests that it might. First, at present, many people do indeed report that they want higher levels of time affluence. For instance, a 2003 nationally representative survey of Americans found that a majority feel a pressure to work and would give up a day's pay per week if they could take that day off of work. And in 1998, Danes went on strike for a *sixth* week of vacation! Second, some research suggests that feelings of time affluence may promote higher levels of well-being. For example, Kasser and Sheldon (2009) conducted four studies in which adults and college students reported on both their levels of material affluence (through reports of their income and/or their endorsement of statements such as "I have had enough money to buy what I need to buy") and their levels of time affluence (through reports of hours worked and/or their endorsement of statements such as "I have had enough time to do what I need to do"). Even after controlling for perceived material affluence, time affluence was a significant positive predictor of people's subjective well-being in all four studies. Such findings suggest that people's happiness may increase if their feelings of time affluence also increase, as, of course, sufficient time is the "resource" necessary for the kinds of experiential activities that Lyubomirksy, Sheldon, & Schkade (2005) claim account for nearly 50% of the variance in people's subjective well-being.

There are at least two ways in which attempts to maximize time affluence fit the model of change described in this chapter. First, time affluence might help promote the intrinsic values that stand in opposition to materialistic values. Pursuing one's hobbies (self-acceptance aspirations), loving and caring for others (affiliation aspirations), and volunteering (community feeling aspirations) all take time to do, and being too busy can interfere with all of these kinds of activities. Indeed, Study 4 of Kasser and Sheldon (2009) revealed that adults with higher levels of time affluence reported engaging more frequently in activities consistent with their intrinsic values, which, in turn, partially explained the positive association between time affluence and subjective well-being.

A second important reason to promote time affluence is that doing so may help undermine the dominant social models that prioritize material affluence. Consider, for example, that the United States is one of the very few nations in the world, rich or poor, that has no laws that mandate a minimum paid vacation for all workers or that mandate that mothers receive paid leave from work after they give birth to a child. In contrast, most other nations in the world require that workers receive at least some minimum amount of paid vacation per year (e.g., 4 weeks in the EU, 3 weeks in China) and that new mothers receive adequate paid leave (e.g., the option of 14 weeks of full leave at full wages or of 52 weeks of leave at half wages). If the United States were to pass laws that provided mandatory paid vacation and paid maternal leave, workers would receive a very different message (i.e., time is important) than what they receive now (i.e., work is important). Thus, they would be exposed less to social models encouraging materialistic pursuits, and instead leisure and family would be promoted as more important.

Restrictions on Advertising

Corporations spend millions of dollars yearly to pay researchers (including psychologists) to investigate how to maximize the effectiveness of advertising messages and billions of dollars more to pay for-profit media corporations to deliver these messages to children, adolescents, and adults. Nowadays advertising messages appear in almost every possible media venue, proclaiming that consumption can provide a happy, fun, meaningful life, a sense of self-worth, and the chance for love; through developments in stealth marketing, ads are now even covertly placed in songs, books, and conversations people have with friends and strangers (Schor, 2004; Walker, 2004).

I have already reviewed evidence showing that people place more priority on materialistic values when they watch more television. One study (Good, 2007) has explicitly extended this work into the environmental domain by providing evidence for a mediational model in which television viewing increases people's materialistic values, which in turn accounts for more negative attitudes about the environment. Such correlations are of course consistent with the straightforward social modeling explanation for why people prioritize the types of materialistic values known to undermine positive ecological attitudes.

But watching television is probably only part of the story regarding how advertisements contribute to materialistic values via social modeling. The fact that marketing messages are present in so many arenas of life (i.e., on the Internet, along highways, on buses and subways, in schools) surely helps to establish a set of social norms suggesting that consumption and materialism are acceptable, and perhaps even admirable. Similarly, the omnipresence of advertisements in contemporary culture probably contributes to "the norm of self-interest," i.e., the belief that it is right and good to engage in behaviors that primarily benefit one's self (Miller, 1999). If this is so, the presence of advertising in so many aspects of people's lives may contribute to beliefs such as "high levels of consumption are normal," "everyone purchases a lot," and "good people buy stuff." None of these are beliefs likely to promote ecological sustainability.

Advertisements may also undermine the intrinsic and self-transcendent values that research shows promote more ecologically sustainable behaviors and attitudes. Recall that the value and goal circumplexes presented in Figs. 6.1 and 6.2 reflect both compatibility and conflict between different aims in life. Recent research suggests that when certain values are activated in people's minds, people become more likely to engage in behaviors consistent with compatible values, and less likely to engage in behaviors reflective of values that are in conflict with the value that was activated (see, e.g., Vohs, Mead, & Goode, 2006; Maio et al., 2009). Thus, if encountering advertisements does indeed activate the self-enhancing, materialistic portions of people's value and goal systems, the consequence is likely to be suppression of the self-transcendent and intrinsic portions of people's motivational systems. These are of course the aims in life known to be most consistent with positive ecological attitudes and behaviors.

Another problem with advertisements is that they are likely to contribute to the promotion of materialistic values via the creation of feelings of insecurity (Kasser et al., 2004). The prototypical advertisement narrative, for example, presents people lacking the advertised product as unhappy, unsuccessful, socially outcast, or otherwise insufficient humans, whereas individuals with the product are happy, beautiful, loved, and/or successful. As Richins (1991, 1995) has suggested, such advertisements play on humans' tendency to compare themselves to others and can lead them to wonder whether they too are insufficient. Of course, these advertisements give an easy, and materialistic, solution to such insecurities: imitate those in the advertisement and purchase the product or service.

These arguments suggest that changing society toward greater ecological sustainability is likely to require dethroning advertising from the current place it enjoys in contemporary Western cultures. Quite a number of directions are available toward these ends. Individuals, of course, can choose to stop watching commercial television and cancel their subscriptions to magazines laden with advertisements. Given the extent to which commercial marketing suffuses contemporary culture, however, this will probably be insufficient as an approach. Broader efforts could follow the lead of some localities that have removed all outdoor advertisements (including billboards on highways and business signs over a certain size) and all advertising in public spaces (including subways, buses, and schools); by doing so, people would no longer be forced to view advertising as they went about their daily lives and thus they would be less likely to be exposed to social models promoting materialism and consumerism. Banning all forms of marketing to children under the age of 12 would also be a particularly forceful policy to pursue, as it would end advertisers' ability to prey on youth whose cognitive development makes it difficult for them to understand persuasive intent and whose identities are still in the process of formation. Another important policy would be to tax all expenses that businesses spend on marketing and advertising; in the United States, these expenses are currently tax deductions, and therefore represent huge subsidies to corporations, marketing firms, and for-profit media corporations. If advertising were taxed, businesses would have less incentive and more of a disincentive to advertise. Further, a fundamentally different social norm would be established about the worth of ads. That is, the current norm suggests that ads are essentially equivalent to charitable donations (which are also deductible), whereas taxing advertisements would help create a social norm that views advertisements more akin to a form of materialistic pollution. Imagine for a moment further that revenues from a tax on advertisements were used to fund educational projects that promote intrinsically oriented values, ecologically sustainable activities, and a materially simpler lifestyle.

Changing the Economic System

Imagine next the reactions of governmental officials, corporate leaders, and perhaps a good number of citizens to the proposals described above to encourage a Voluntarily Simple and time-affluent lifestyle and to restrict and/or heavily tax advertising. It seems likely that many people might respond to such proposals with the rejoinder that corporate profits and economic growth would be dampened. They may be right, but whenever proposals to help the environment are met with statements such as "it might create higher prices for consumers," "it might diminish corporate profits," or "it might interfere with economic growth," these counter arguments must be recognized for what they are: counter arguments based in the self-enhancing, materialistic values that are required for the maintenance of an economic system that strives to maximize levels of consumption, corporate profit, and economic growth.

This economic system is, of course, capitalism. As with any other system composing a society, the smooth functioning of the capitalist economic system requires that the people living under it hold certain beliefs, act in certain ways, and support certain institutions (Kasser, Cohn, Kanner, & Ryan, 2007). That is, just as a religion needs its followers to believe in its tenets, to engage in the practices it prescribes, to attend its places of worship, and to listen to its ministers and priests, a capitalistic economic system needs its followers to believe its tenets (i.e., economic growth, free market competition, and high levels of consumption are important), to engage in its practices (i.e., work long hours and consume a lot), to attend its places of worship (i.e., the mall and the couch in front of the television), and to listen to its leaders (i.e., the CEOs and politicians whose job it is to create economic growth and things to buy).

The two pathways toward materialistic values described earlier in this chapter help explain how corporate capitalism has been so successful in integrating itself into the fabric of American life (Kasser et al., 2004). First, self-interested, materialistic values have been encouraged through multiple social models, including, for example, tax laws that create incentives to advertise, policies that allow for-profit companies to own most of the media airways (McChesney, 1997), laws that have given corporations rights associated with personhood (Kelly, 2003; Korten, 1995), international laws that elevate a corporation's right to make a profit over the laws of a particular nation (Cavanagh, Welch, & Retallack, 2001; Cavanagh & Mander, 2004), and government policies that emphasize economic growth at most every turn.

American corporate capitalism also has features that work to create the feelings of insecurity known to enhance people's concern for materialistic values. For example, under American corporate capitalism, the extended social networks from which many people derive support have been in decline, levels of inequality around the world have increased, and a competitive mentality in which a few "winners" profit at the expense of a larger group of "losers" has become common (Kanner & Soule, 2004; Kasser et al., 2004). On top of these, add the fears that common citizens experience about potentially losing their job during corporate takeovers or layoffs, losing their retirement savings in stock market downturns, and losing their habitat to global climate disruption.

Kasser et al. (2007) suggested that one consequence of the privileging of self-enhancing, materialistic values in the US economy is that self-transcendent, intrinsic values are likely to be suppressed. Schwartz (2007) tested this claim by examining how citizens' values in 20 wealthy capitalistic nations were associated with how much the institutions in those nations were oriented in a more cooperative, strategic fashion, (e.g., Germany and Austria) versus a more liberal market fashion (e.g., the United States and the UK; Hall & Gingerich, 2004). Consistent with predictions, the more that nations had liberal market economic organizations (vs. cooperative organizations), the more their citizens valued self-enhancing aims (particularly achievement) and the less they cared about self-transcendent aims (particularly universalism). These, of course, are the very aims that are differentially associated with ecological outcomes, including CO_2 emissions (Kasser, in press).

Thus, it seems that ecological sustainability may only be possible if the juggernaut of capitalism is directly confronted (see also Speth, 2008). Although many directions and approaches could be discussed, I will only discuss one popular approach here, which is to revise national indicators of progress.

In most nations today, national progress and success are predominantly measured by how the stock market is doing, where consumer confidence is this month, and, primarily, the size of their Gross National Product (i.e., the overall amount of economic activity in the nation). Such measures obviously privilege materialistic values. Consider, for example, a case in which a company finds that it achieves higher profits (and thus contributes more to GNP increases) if it manufactures a product in a way that pollutes a nearby river than if it uses ecologically sustainable methods. If the pollution poisons the water in the river, further increases in overall GNP may result when people in the community get sick from drinking that water (i.e., hospital costs) and even if they die (i.e., funeral costs). If community members decide to hire lawyers to sue the company, GNP increases more. And if the company loses the suit and is forced to hire an environmental engineer to clean up the river, GNP goes up further still. People who determine their nation's health on the basis of GNP are thus using an entirely materialistic metric, and one that actually discounts the benefits of health, sustainability, and the like.

Because of these and other problems with GNP, several organizations have proposed a variety of alternative indicators for nations to use. These include Redefining Progress' Genuine Progress Indicator, the nation of Bhutan's Gross National Happiness measures, and the new economic foundation's Happy Planet Index. Others have suggested supplementing GNP measures with direct assessments of citizens' subjective well-being (Diener & Seligman, 2004; Layard, 2005). While each of these indicators has its own idiosyncratic computational formulas and assumptions, common to them all is that the privilege GNP accords to materialistic aims is revoked, and other values (typically self-transcendent, intrinsic ones) are injected into the calculations.

If nations were to adopt such alternative indicators alongside, or even instead of GNP, and if these alternative indicators received nearly as much attention from politicians, the media, and citizens as the Dow Jones Index and the GNP currently receive, then social models of what is important would shift substantially: rather than being told what matters most is economic activity, citizens would be encouraged to think about the self-transcendent, intrinsic values embodied in these alternative indices. What's more, as citizens begin to recognize that increases in GNP do not generally improve national well-being (at least in economically developed nations) and are generally associated with greater ecological damage (Jackson, 2009), they might begin to insist that government officials develop policies and laws aimed at promoting the aspects of these alternative indicators that reflect intrinsic, self-transcendent aims (e.g., caring for others, leisure time, etc.,).

Conclusion

In this chapter I have tried to demonstrate the problematic ecological outcomes associated with strongly valuing self-enhancing, materialistic values and to present an empirically supported, two-pronged model for social change based on (a) understanding and eliminating the causes of materialistic values; and (b) understanding and encouraging the values that stand in opposition to materialistic values. My focus in this chapter on materialistic values should not be taken as suggesting that these values are the only aspect of human functioning that contribute to ecological degradation. The recent American Psychological Association Task Force report on global climate change reviews a variety of other features of human functioning that influence people's ecological attitudes, thinking, and behavior (Swim et al., 2009). And Crompton and Kasser (2009) have shown that the ways humans define themselves relative to non-human nature and the ways that they cope with threats (including environmental threats) bear important associations with ecological outcomes.

The basic philosophy of the two-pronged model presented here might be fruitfully applied to these other environmentally problematic aspects of human behavior as well. Indeed, Crompton and Kasser (2009) identified and made suggestions about how to eliminate the causes of ecologically damaging self-definitions and coping strategies, and identified and made suggestions about how to encourage the kinds of alternative self-definitions and coping strategies that promote ecological sustainability. My hope is that psychologists interested in social change can apply the two-pronged strategy that I've exemplified here with materialistic values to the variety of other aspects of human functioning that threaten future generations and non-human species' chances of living in a healthy habitat here on Earth.

References

Ahuvia, A. C., & Wong, N. Y. (2002). Personality and values based materialism: Their relationship and origins. *Journal of Consumer Psychology, 12*, 389–402.
Andrews, C. (1998). *The circle of simplicity.* New York: Harper Collins.
Banerjee, R., & Dittmar, H. (2008). Individual differences in children's materialism: The role of peer relationships. *Personality and Social Psychology Bulletin, 34*, 17–31.
Brand, J. E., & Greenberg, B. S. (1994). Commercials in the classroom: The impact of Channel One advertising. *Journal of Advertising, 34*, 18–21.
Briers, B., Pandelaere, M., Dewitte, S., & Warlop, L. (2006). Hungry for money: On the exchangeability of financial and caloric resources. *Psychological Science, 17*, 939–943.
Brown, K. W., & Kasser, T. (2005). Are psychological and ecological well-being compatible? The role of values, mindfulness, and lifestyle. *Social Indicators Research, 74*, 349–368.
Cavanagh, J., & Mander, J. (Co-Chairs). (2004). *Alternatives to economic globalization (A better world is possible)* (2nd ed.). San Francisco: Berrett-Koehler.
Cavanagh, J., Welch, C., & Retallack, S. (2001). The IMF formula: Prescription for poverty. *International Forum on Globalization (IFG): Special Poverty Report, 1*(3), 8–10.
Chang, L., & Arkin, R. M. (2002). Materialism as an attempt to cope with uncertainty. *Psychology and Marketing, 19*, 389–406.
Cheung, C., & Chan, C. (1996). Television viewing and mean world value in Hong Kong's adolescents. *Social Behavior and Personality, 24*, 351–364.

Cohen, P., & Cohen, J. (1996). *Life values and adolescent mental health.* Mahwah, NJ: Erlbaum.

Crompton, T., & Kasser, T. (2009). *Meeting environmental challenges: The role of human identity.* Godalming: WWF-UK/Green Books.

Dechesne, M., Pyszczynski, T., Arndt, J., Ransom, S., Sheldon, K. M., van Knippenberg, A., et al. (2003). Literal and symbolic immortality: The effect of evidence of literal immortality on self-esteem striving in response to mortality salience. *Journal of Personality and Social Psychology, 84,* 722–737.

deGraaf, J. (Ed.). (2003). *Take back your time: Fighting overwork and time poverty in America.* San Francisco: Berrett-Koehler.

Diener, E., & Seligman, M. E. P. (2004). Beyond money: Toward an economy of well-being. *Psychological Science in the Public Interest, 5,* 1–31.

Ehrlich, P. R., & Holdren, J. P. (1971). Impact of population growth. *Science, 171,* 1212–1217.

Elgin, D. (1993). *Voluntary simplicity* (Rev. ed.). New York: Morrow.

Gatersleben, B., Meadows, J., Abrahamse, W., & Jackson, T. (2008). *Materialistic and environmental values of young people.* Unpublished manuscript, University of Surrey, UK.

Good, J. (2007). Shop 'til we drop? Television, materialism and attitudes about the natural environment. *Mass Communication and Society, 10,* 365–383.

Grouzet, F. M. E., Kasser, T., Ahuvia, A., Fernandez-Dols, J. M., Kim, Y., Lau, S., et al. (2005). The structure of goal contents across 15 cultures. *Journal of Personality and Social Psychology, 89,* 800–816.

Hall, P. A., & Gingerich, D. W. (2004). *Varieties of capitalism and institutional complementarities in the macroeconomy: An empirical analysis* (MPIfG Discussion Paper 04/5). Cologne: Max Planck Institute for the Study of Societies.

Hayden, A., & Shandra, J. (2009). Hours of work and the ecological footprints of nations: An exploratory analysis. *Local Environment, 14,* 575–600.

Holst, C. (Ed.). (2007). *Get satisfied: How twenty people like you found the satisfaction of enough.* Westport, CT: Easton Studio Press.

Jackson, T. (2009). *Prosperity without growth: Economics for a finite planet.* London: Earthscan.

Kanner, A. D., & Soule, R. G. (2004). Globalization, corporate culture, and freedom. In T. Kasser & A. D. Kanner (Eds.), *Psychology and consumer culture: The struggle for a good life in a materialistic world* (pp. 49–67), Washington, DC: American Psychological Association.

Kasser, T. (2002). *The high price of materialism.* Cambridge, MA: MIT Press.

Kasser, T. (2005). Frugality, generosity, and materialism in children and adolescents. In K. A. Moore & L. H. Lippman (Eds.), *What do children need to flourish? Conceptualizing and measuring indicators of positive development* (pp. 357–373), New York: Springer Science.

Kasser, T. (in press). Cultural values and the well-being of future generations: A cross-national study. *Journal of Cross-Cultural Psychology.*

Kasser, T., & Brown, K. W. (2003). On time, happiness, and ecological footprints. In J. deGraaf (Ed.), *Take back your time: Fighting overwork and time poverty in America* (pp. 107–112). San Francisco: Berrett-Koehler.

Kasser, T., Cohn, S., Kanner, A. D., & Ryan, R. M. (2007). Some costs of American corporate capitalism: A psychological exploration of value and goal conflicts. *Psychological Inquiry, 18,* 1–22.

Kasser, T., & Ryan, R. M. (1996). Further examining the American dream: Differential correlates of intrinsic and extrinsic goals. *Personality and Social Psychology Bulletin, 22,* 280–287.

Kasser, T., & Ryan, R. M. (2001). Be careful what you wish for: Optimal functioning and the relative attainment of intrinsic and extrinsic goals. In P. Schmuck & K. M. Sheldon (Eds.), *Life goals and well-being: Towards a positive psychology of human striving* (pp. 116–131), Goettingen: Hogrefe and Huber Publishers.

Kasser, T., Ryan, R. M., Couchman, C. E., & Sheldon, K. M. (2004). Materialistic values: Their causes and consequences. In T. Kasser & A. D. Kanner (Eds.), *Psychology and consumer culture: The struggle for a good life in a materialistic world* (pp. 11–28), Washington, DC: American Psychological Association.

Kasser, T., Ryan, R. M., Zax, M., & Sameroff, A. J. (1995). The relations of maternal and social environments to late adolescents' materialistic and prosocial values. *Developmental Psychology, 31*, 907–914.

Kasser, T., & Sheldon, K. M. (2000). Of wealth and death: Materialism, mortality salience, and consumption behavior. *Psychological Science, 11*, 352–355.

Kasser, T., & Sheldon, K. M. (2008). Psychological threat and extrinsic goal striving. *Motivation and Emotion, 32*, 37–45.

Kasser, T., & Sheldon, K. M. (2009). Time affluence as a path towards personal happiness and ethical business practice: Empirical evidence from four studies. *Journal of Business Ethics, 84*, 243–255.

Kellert, S., & Wilson, E. O. (1993). *The biophilia hypothesis*. Washington, DC: Island Press.

Kelly, M. (2003). *The divine right of capital: Dethroning the corporate aristocracy*. San Francisco: Berrett-Koehler.

Korten, D. C. (1995). *When corporations rule the world*. West Hartford, CT: Berrett-Koehler.

Layard, R. (2005). *Happiness: Lessons from a new science*. New York: Penguin.

Lyubomirksy, S., Sheldon, K. M., & Schkade, J. (2005). Pursuing happiness: The architecture of sustainable change. *Review of General Psychology, 9*, 111–131.

Maio, G. R., Pakizeh, A., Cheung, W.-Y., & Rees, K. J. (2009). Changing, priming, and acting on values: Effects via motivational relations in a circular model. *Journal of Personality and Social Psychology, 97*, 699–715.

McChesney, R. W. (1997). *Corporate media and the threat to democracy*. New York: Seven Stories Press.

Miller, D. T. (1999). The norm of self-interest. *American Psychologist, 54*, 1053–1060.

Pierce, L. B. (2000). *Choosing simplicity: Real people finding peace and fulfillment in a complex world*. Carmel, CA: Gallagher Press.

Rahtz, D. R., Sirgy, M. J., & Meadow, H. L. (1989). The elderly audience: Correlates of television orientation. *Journal of Advertising, 18*, 9–20.

Ray, P. H. (1997). The emerging culture. *American Demographics, 19*, 28–34.

Richins, M. L. (1991). Social comparison and the idealized images of advertising. *Journal of Consumer Research, 18*, 71–83.

Richins, M. L. (1995). Social comparison, advertising, and consumer discontent. *American Behavioral Scientist, 38*, 593–607.

Richins, M. L., & Dawson, S. (1992). A consumer values orientation for materialism and its measurement: Scale development and validation. *Journal of Consumer Research, 19*, 303–316.

Rindfleisch, A., Burroughs, J. E., & Denton, F. (1997). Family structure, materialism, and compulsive consumption. *Journal of Consumer Research, 23*, 312–325.

Rokeach, M. (1973). *The nature of human values*. New York: Free Press.

Rosnick, D., & Weisbrot, M. (2006). *Are shorter work hours good for the environment? A comparison of U.S. and European energy consumption*. Washington, DC: Center for Economic and Policy Research.

Ryan, R. M., Chirkov, V. I., Little, T. D., Sheldon, K. M., Timoshina, E., & Deci, E. L. (1999). The American dream in Russia: Extrinsic aspirations and well-being in two cultures. *Personality and Social Psychology Bulletin, 25*, 1509–1524.

Saunders, S., & Munro, D. (2000). The construction and validation of a consumer orientation questionnaire (SCOI) designed to measure Fromm's (1955) 'marketing character' in Australia. *Social Behavior and Personality, 28*, 219–240.

Schmuck, P., Kasser, T., & Ryan, R. M. (2000). Intrinsic and extrinsic goals: Their structure and relationship to well-being in German and U.S. college students. *Social Indicators Research, 50*, 225–241.

Schor, J. B. (2004). *Born to buy: The commercialized child and the new consumer culture*. New York: Scribner.

Schor, J. B. (2010). *Plenitude: The new economics of true wealth*. New York: Penguin Press.

Schultz, P. W., Gouveia, V. V., Cameron, L. D., Tankha, G., Schmuck, P., & Franek, M. (2005). Values and their relationship to environmental concern and conservation behavior. *Journal of Cross-Cultural Psychology, 36*, 457–475.

Schwartz, S. H. (1992). Universals in the content and structure of values: Theory and empirical tests in 20 countries. In M. Zanna, (Ed.), *Advances in experimental social psychology* (Vol. 25, pp. 1–65). New York: Academic Press.

Schwartz, S. H. (2006). Les valeurs de base de la personne: théorie, mesures et applications. *Revue Française de Sociologie, 47*(4), 929–968.

Schwartz, S. H. (2007). Cultural and individual value correlates of capitalism: A comparative analysis. *Psychological Inquiry, 18*, 52–57.

Sheldon, K. M., & McGregor, H. (2000). Extrinsic value orientation and the tragedy of the commons. *Journal of Personality, 68*, 383–411.

Shi, D. (1985). *The simple life*. New York: Oxford University Press.

Speth, J. G. (2008). *The bridge at the edge of the world: Capitalism, the environment, and crossing from crisis to sustainability*. New Haven, CT: Yale University Press.

Swim, J., Clayton, S., Doherty, T., Gifford, R., Howard, G., Reser, J., et al. (2009). *Psychology and global climate change: Addressing a multi-faceted phenomenon and set of challenges*. A report by the American Psychological Association's Task Force on the Interface between Psychology and Global Climate Change. Washington, DC: American Psychological Association.

Thogerson, J. B., & Crompton, T. (2009). Simple and painless? The limitations of spillover in environmental campaigning. *Journal of Consumer Policy, 32*, 141–163.

Twenge, J. M., Baumeister, R. F., DeWall, C. N., Ciarocco, N. J., & Bartels, J. M. (2007). Social exclusion decreases prosocial behavior. *Journal of Personality and Social Psychology, 92*, 56–66.

Twenge, J. M., Gentile, B., DeWall, C. N., Ma, D., Lacefield, K., & Schurtz, D. R. (2010). Birth cohort increases in psychopathology among young Americans, 1938–2007: A cross-temporal meta-analysis of the MMPI. *Clinical Psychology Review, 30*, 145–154.

Vohs, K. D., Mead, N. L., & Goode, M. R. (2006). The psychological consequences of money. *Science, 314*, 1154–1156.

Walker, R. (2004, December 5). The hidden (in plain sight) persuaders. *New York Times Magazine*, 69.

Williams, G. C., Cox, E. M., Hedberg, V. A., & Deci, E. L. (2000). Extrinsic life goals and health risk behaviors in adolescents. *Journal of Applied Social Psychology, 30*, 1756–1771.

Chapter 7
Positive Psychology and Public Health

Dora Guðrún Guðmundsdóttir

Public health has been defined as "The science and art of preventing disease, prolonging life and promoting health through the organised efforts of society." (Acheson, 1988). Within the field of public health, health promotion is an area which focuses more on health than diseases. The ideology of mental health promotion is in many ways comparable to the one of positive psychology. Furthermore the development of health promotion, particularly *mental* health promotion within the field of public health, has a lot in common with the development of positive psychology. The aim of this chapter is to highlight the similarities between the ideology of mental health promotion and positive psychology, which both emphasize the positive aspects of health and human beings. A special focus will be on positive mental health and how it can be measured. At the end of the chapter a reflection will be made on how the field of mental health promotion and positive psychology can support each other and lead to social change.

In retrospect, one can say that the consequences of World War II play an important, although different, role for both public health and positive psychology. After the war, the need for a global community highlighting human rights was strong and in the area of public health, the World Health Organisation (WHO) was founded to meet that need in 1948. The constitution of WHO contained a new definition of health, with a strong emphasis on positive health:

> Health is a state of complete physical, mental and social well-being and not merely the absence of disease or infirmity (WHO, 1948).

It is interesting to consider the fact that more than a half century ago health was defined in this way. It is noteworthy that this definition includes the clear statement that health is *not merely the absence of disease*. This declaration broadened the definition of health from strictly a medical concept towards the subjective well-being of the population. Despite this emphasis on positive well-being, health is still seen as a dichotomy between health and disease and health care systems around the world seem to have had their main focus on diseases for decades.

D.G. Guðmundsdóttir (✉)
Public Health Institute of Iceland, Reykjavík, Iceland
e-mail: dora@publichealth.is

R. Biswas-Diener (ed.), *Positive Psychology as Social Change*,
DOI 10.1007/978-90-481-9938-9_7, © Springer Science+Business Media B.V. 2011

While the area of public health did focus on the positive aspects of health after World War II, the field of psychology seems to have been blinded by the negative mental health consequences of the war. During the last decades, psychology has been focusing on mental illness and has done fairly well with it. After World War II, two events changed the face of psychology. In 1946 the Veterans Administration was founded and thousands of psychologists were able to make a living treating mental illness. In 1947, the National Institute of Mental Health (NIMH) was founded and grant options opened for academics studying mental health problems (Seligman, 2002; Seligman & Csikszentmihalyi, 2000). This arrangement has been beneficial for the mission of curing mental illnesses. There has been a great progress in the understanding of and treatment for mental illness in the last decades. At least 14 mental disorders can now be diagnosed and hopefully cured or considerably relieved (Seligman, 2007).

It seems that by relieving the conditions that make life miserable, building the conditions that make life worth living has become less of a priority. People want more than just to correct weaknesses. They want lives filled with meaning and not just to be restless until they die (Seligman, 2002). The positive psychology movement is an attempt to urge psychologists to adopt a more open and appreciative perspective regarding human potentials, motives, and capacities. It is important that the therapeutic environment and clinical interactions focus equally on the client's strengths and skills (Ahmed & Boisvert, 2006).

The Concept of Mental Health

According to WHO's definition of health, mental health is one of the traits of the overall well-being that defines health. This definition is not very descriptive and it can be hard to get a detailed description of mental health since it can be culturally dependent. In the field of public health, societal standards contribute to the meaning of mental health, which many derived from contemporary Western society, as well as standards proposed by the medical profession regarding mental illness. Within the medical model, mental health is often seen merely as the absence of mental illness.

Mental Health, Subjective Well-Being and Psychological Well-Being

Despite the fact that mental health is the subject of both mental health promotion and positive psychology, how it is defined and measured can differ between the fields. The term mental health is normally used in the field of public health, while other related terms are also used in psychology, like psychological well-being (Ryff, 1989) and subjective well-being, which in less formal terms is sometimes labelled "happiness" (Diener, 2000).

Table 7.1 Measurements of mental health (source: adapted from Compton, Smith, Cornish, & Qualls, 1996)

Measurements	SWB (Factor loading)
Happiness (Fordyce, 1977)	0.84
Satisfaction with life (Diener, Emmons, Larsen, & Griffin, 1985)	0.83
Sense of coherence (Antonovsky, 1987)	0.78
Affect balance (Bradburn, 1969)	0.74
Quality of life (Flanagan, 1979)	0.69
Optimism (Scheier & Carver, 1985)	0.69
Psychological well-being (Ryff, 1989)	0.60
Self-esteem (Rosenberg, 1965)	0.51

Even though it can be useful to have many different psychological measures, it can also be confusing. Therefore, it is important to have information on how these measures are related. Compton et al., (1996) investigated the factor structure of numerous mental health questionnaires and obtained a clear first factor (of three factors) that was labelled subjective well-being (see Table 7.1).

As can be seen in Table 7.1, Fordyce's (1977) "Happiness Measure" had the highest loading on the subjective well-being factor, followed by Diener's "Satisfaction with Life Scale" (Diener et al., 1985); Bradburn's (1969) "Affect Balance" (positive affect minus negative affect). These are all well-known and widely used measures. For subjective well-being, the highest correlation was with a general measure on happiness and the second with satisfaction with life. Antonovsky's (1987) "Sense of coherence" also had high loading on the subjective well-being factor as did Flanagan's (1979) "Quality of life" and Scheier and Carver's (1985) Optimism scale. Rosenberg's self-esteem scale loaded 0.51 but it may be a surprise that Ryff's (1989) psychological well-being scale had as high loading on the subjective well-being factor as 0.60. This indicates that subjective well-being and psychological well-being are strongly related.

In her book, *Current concepts of positive mental health*, Jahoda (1958) presents a positive approach to mental health, generated to replace definitions of well-being as the absence of illness where she also offers extensive descriptions of what it means to be in good psychological health. Great similarities are found between Jahoda's definition on positive mental health and psychological well-being defined by Ryff (1989) (see Table 7.2).

Ryff (1989) has developed the psychological well-being scale on the existing literature on positive mental health and psychological well-being. "The psychological well-being scale" consists of six subscales on self-acceptance, personal growth, positive relations with others, autonomy, purpose in life, and environmental mastery. Each subscale has 14 questions which amount to a total of 84 questions.

Ryff and Keyes (1995) argue that there is more to well-being than happiness and satisfaction with life. Comparison of their theory-based indicators of well-being, the

Table 7.2 Comparison of Jahoda's positive mental health and Ryff's PWB

Positive mental health (Jahoda, 1958)		Psychological well-being (Ryff, 1989)	
Attitudes towards the self	(a) adequate self-awareness, (b) accurate self-concept, (c) self-acceptance, and (d) a positive globally caring view of the self	Self-acceptance	(a) positive self-evaluation (b) the ability to acknowledge multiple aspects of self, and (c) the ability to accept both positive and negative qualities into a balanced picture of one's abilities
Growth, development and self-actualization	(a) the ability to accept challenges and tension in the present in the interest of future goals and investment in living or an extension of the self through involvement in different pursuits, (b) a concern for other people, and a desire to help others and be of service	Personal growth	(a) capacity to grow and develop potential, (b) personal changes over time that reflect growing self-knowledge and effectiveness, and (c) openness to new experiences
An integrated personality	(a) desires, impulses, and needs are balanced with rationality, responsibility, and social concerns; (b) a unifying philosophy of life or a sense of meaning and purpose is present (c) the person exhibits anxiety tolerance, frustration tolerance, and the ability to delay gratification	Purpose in life	(a) a sense of purpose and meaning to life and (b) a sense of direction and goals in life
Autonomy	(a) regulation of behaviour from within and (b) independent behaviour. This element speaks of the ability to act independently of environmental reassures	Autonomy	(a) independent and self-determined, (b) ability to resist social pressures, and (c) ability to regulate behaviour from within

Table 7.2 (continued)

Positive mental health (Jahoda, 1958)		Psychological well-being (Ryff, 1989)	
Perception of reality	(a) the ability to see self and others without one's own needs distorting perception of other people or situations (b) empathy and social sensitivity	Positive relations with other	(a) close, warm, and intimate relationships with others, (b) a concern about the welfare of others, and (c) empathy and affection for other people
Environmental mastery	(a) the ability to love, (b) ability to work and play, (c) good interpersonal relations, (d) ability to meet the demands of situations with a sense of mastery and self-efficacy, (e) ability to balance efforts to change the external world with efforts to change one's own psychological world. (f) ability to use adequate problem-solving strategies	Environmental mastery	(a) a sense of mastery and competence and (b) the ability to choose situations and environments that are conducive to meeting goals

Table 7.3 Psychological well-being scales correlations with SWB and depression (source: adapted from Ryff & Keyes, 1995)

SWB	Psychological well-being scales					
	SA	PR	PL	PG	AU	EM
Happiness	0.54*	0.38*	0.41*	0.16*	0.31*	0.51*
Life satisfaction	0.64*	0.40*	0.55*	0.21*	0.30*	0.61*
Depression (CES-D)	−0.70*	−0.46*	−0.56*	−0.22*	−0.48*	−0.68*

* $p<0.05$.
SA, self-acceptance; PR, positive relations with others; PL, purpose in life; PG, personal growth; AU, autonomy; EM, environmental mastery.

psychological well-being scale, with other frequently used measures on subjective well-being and depression can be found in Table 7.3. In the comparison, happiness was measured with the question, "All things considered, how happy are you?" Life satisfaction was measured with the question: "Thinking about your life as a whole, how satisfied are you?" And Depression was measured with CES-D scale (Center for Epidemiological Study Depression Scale).

Moderate to strong associations between two of the subscales (self-acceptance and environmental mastery) were found with the single and multi-item scales of happiness, life satisfaction, and depression (see Table 7.3). However, the remaining four dimensions of psychological well-being (positive relations with others, purpose in life, personal growth, and autonomy) showed mixed or medium relationships with these prior indicators.

As can be seen in Table 7.3 happiness, life satisfaction, and depression had comparable strength of their correlation with the subscales of psychological well-being, except for personal growth. The main difference was that depression had a negative correlation while the others correlated positively with the subscales.

Most people would agree that happiness and depression do not go hand in hand. If a person is happy he or she is not depressed at the same time, and vice versa. Furthermore, one can argue that happiness and depression cannot be opposites on the same dimension since elimination of depression from people does not necessarily make them happy. Many studies have shown a strong negative relation between depression and measures of happiness and life satisfaction (Veenhoven, 1994). Heady and Wearing (1992) found that life satisfaction and happiness had a negative correlation with depression measured with Beck Depression Inventory (BDI) and anxiety, measured with Spielberger scale (see Table 7.4).

Table 7.4 Subjective well-being correlation with depression and anxiety (source: adapted from Heady & Wearing, 1992)

Subjective well-being	Depression	Anxiety
Life satisfaction	−0.59	−0.39
Happiness	−0.35	−0.23

Several studies have demonstrated results that imply that the relationship between happiness and depression seem to be more complicated than just being two opposites on one dimension. In their study of care giving and bereavement in the context of HIV-AIDS, Folkman and Moskowitz (2003) discovered that bereaved partners reported high levels of depressed mood, which is what one would expect. However, they also reported positive emotions at a frequency that was comparable to their reports of negative emotions throughout their care giving and bereavement. According to these results it seems that depressive mood and positive emotions are at least partly independent. These results support the idea that happiness and mental health are something else than just absence of depression or other mental disorders.

These results violate the old assumption that positive and negative emotions are simply opposite and balanced ends of an emotional continuum. After negative emotions are gone, what remains for many people is a neutral state of emotionality, neither positive nor negative. Other actions might therefore be needed to move from a neutral position to more positive emotions, than from a negative to a neutral one (Fredrickson, 2002).

Argyle (2001) noted that the probability of experiencing negative emotionality can be predicted by several factors, such as, unemployment, high stress and low economic status. Eliminating the perceived negative factors by getting a job, reducing stress levels and getting an average income can make a person feel better (the a-process, from Fig. 7.1), but does not automatically provide positive emotions like happiness and psychological well-being to that person (the b-process from Fig. 7.1). The b-process of enhancing well-being is emphasized by both the fields of mental health promotion and positive psychology. To be able to define actions that enable a person to move from a neutral state to a more positive one, it is important to study positive emotions, subjective well-being and positive mental health.

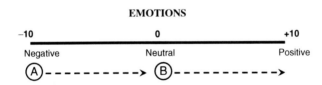

Fig. 7.1 A process from negative state to neutral and from neutral to a positive state

The relationship between happiness and depression might have some similarities with the relationship between health and sickness in general.

Figure 7.2 illustrates how health and sickness overlap, since they are not entirely separate concepts with more complicated relationships than just being opposites. If you are not dead that does not mean that you are in optimal wellness. There are degrees of wellness and of illness. Medical sociologist Aaron Antonovsky (1979, 1987) proposed that we revise our focus, focusing our attention on what enables people to stay well than on what causes people to become ill. Figure 7.2 presents a diagram of an illness-wellness continuum, with death at one end and optimal wellness at the other.

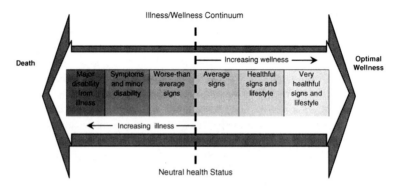

Fig. 7.2 Illness/wellness continuum (source: adapted from Antonovsky, 1987)

The illness-wellness variety represents people's differing health status. Starting at the centre (neutral level) of the diagram, a person's health status is shown as progressively worse to the left and progressively healthier to the right. The segments in the central band describe dominant features that usually characterize different health status. Medical treatment typically begins at the health status to the left of the neutral level and intensifies as the physical condition worsens. Medical treatment can bring the person's health status back to the mid range of the continuum, but to get beyond the mid range, other procedures are needed. Increasing wellness beyond the mid range can be achieved through health promotion where the focus is on the positive aspects of health, with knowledge on optimal wellness (Antonovsky, 1987).

This diagram is in many ways comparable to the emotion dimension in Fig. 7.1 where the b-process is comparable to the increasing wellness beyond the mid range. The ideology of wellness enhancement can therefore also apply for enhancement of positive emotions.

Health Promotion

Health promotion is quite a new ideology. In health promotion, the focus is on the positive aspects of health and to identify effective ways to enhance it. Health promotion was first defined by the World Health Organisation in Ottawa, 1986 as "the process of enabling people to increase control over, and to improve their health" (WHO, 1986). Eriksson and Lindström (2008) argue that the thoughts and the ideas behind Antonovsky's salutogenic model for health have influenced the development of health promotion.

Health promotion can be described as the science and art of helping people to change their lifestyle to move towards a state of optimal health. Optimal health is the balance of physical, mental and social well-being. Lifestyle change can be facilitated through a combination of efforts to enhance awareness, change behaviour and create an environment that supports good health practices (O'Donnell, 1989). The health promotion view of health is that health is created in the context of everyday life where people live, love, work and play (WHO, 1986). This is in conjunction with the ideology of positive psychology which has been described as a science that strives to promote flourishing and fulfilment of each aspect of the individual, group and social levels with a focus on what makes life worth living.

Crossing Point Between Prevention and Promotion

As shown in Fig. 7.3, the fundamental distinction between prevention and promotion lies in their focus. While prevention has its focus on the disease, promotion focuses on health. Prevention action is concerned with avoiding disease while mental health promotion is intended to improve mental health and well-being. By identifying the positive aspects of mental health, one can highlight or target the areas to promote and the goals to be attained. Therefore, it is important to target the positive aspects of mental health together with targeting the illness.

Action:	PROMOTION	PREVENTION	EARLY INTERVENTION	INTERVENTION	REHABILITATION
Focus:	of health	of disease	Screening for disease	Treating disease	after disease

Fig. 7.3   Five stages of health care and their focus (source: adapted from VicHealth, 2000)

The different stages of health care have often been illustrated as a river, for example by Eriksson and Lindström (2008) who developed the illustration *Health in the River of Life* (see Fig. 7.4). It is not enough to promote health by avoiding stress or

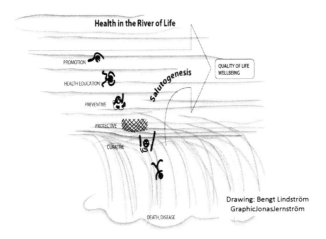

Fig. 7.4   Health in the river of life (source: Eriksson & Lindström, 2008)

by building bridges to keep people from falling into the river; people have to learn to swim (Antonovsky, 1987). Furthermore, it is not enough to teach people to swim if something in the environment prevents them from swimming. The river of life is a simple way to demonstrate the characteristics of medicine (intervention and rehabilitation) and public health (prevention and promotion) shifting the perspective and the focus from medicine to public health and health promotion towards population health.

The difference between the public health actions of prevention and promotion is also crucial. Even though the same action can both prevent an illness and promote health at the same time, the fundamental difference lies in the focus. Positive mental health is the desired outcome of health promotion interventions. Strategies for mental health promotion are related to improving the quality of life and potential for health rather than amelioration of symptoms and deficits. These should be recognized, not as strategies for prevention but as mental health promotion in its most positive sense (Secker, 1998). Nevertheless, it has been argued that policies and interventions which impact the mental health of the population as a whole could be the most effective way to reduce the prevalence of mental illness (Rose, 1989; Stewart-Brown, 2002).

The fundamental difference between prevention and promotion is well recognized within the field of positive psychology. The advocates of positive psychology intend to rationalize that one can study positive aspects of human experience as a specific phenomena, not just as a tool for prevention, coping, health, or some other desirable outcome. They believe that as long as hope, courage, optimism and joy are viewed simply as useful in reducing pathology, it will be impossible to go beyond the homeostatic point of repose and begin to understand those qualities that make life worth living (Seligman & Csikszentmihalyi, 2000; Csikszentmihalyi, 2003).

Positive Psychology

Seligman and Peterson (2003) argue that by working by the medical model and solely looking for the salves to heal the wounds, psychologists misplace much of their science and training. They argue that by embracing the disease model of psychotherapy, psychologists have lost an important aspect of their original profession.

The practice of positive psychology transcends the health care system as it presently exists. Intervention to enhance a client's life may take place within a health care context – for example, by building courage to buffer against social phobia. The growth of the positive traits and subjective well-being, however, is also a matter of child development, of education, of work and of play. Improving the lives of people across all realms of life is psychology's inheritance, and it is time that psychologists pursue that to a further extent (Seligman & Peterson, 2003).

During his time as president of the American Psychological Association (APA) in 1998, Seligman emphasized that mental health should be more than the absence of mental illness. It should be parallel to a vibrant and muscular fitness of the human mind and spirit. Seligman urged psychologists to keep in mind psychology's forgotten mission, that psychology is not just the study of weakness and damage but also the study of strength and virtue. Furthermore, that treatment is not just fixing what is broken but also nurturing what is best within us. He further encouraged psychologists to explore the region beyond zero, to look at what actively made people feel fulfilled, engaged and meaningfully happy (Seligman & Csikszentmihalyi, 2000).

Individuals are seen as decision makers, with choices and preferences, and with the possibility of becoming masterful and efficacious or, in malignant circumstances, helpless and hopeless. Science and practice that rely on the positive psychology approach may have the direct effect of preventing much of the major emotional disorders. It may also have a two-sided effect: making the lives of clients physically healthier, given evidence about the effects of mental well-being on the body and reorienting psychology back to its two neglected missions; making normal people stronger and more productive and maximizing human potential (Seligman & Petereson, 2003).

As a scientific enterprise, positive psychology has focused on understanding and explaining happiness and subjective well-being and accurately predicting factors that influence such states. These objectives are in harmony with the aims of mental health promotion, which is targeting the positive aspects of mental health.

The determinants of mental health include factors related to actions by individuals, such as behaviours and lifestyles, coping skills and good interpersonal relationships. Social and environmental factors like income, social status, education, employment, housing and working conditions, access to appropriate health services and good physical health are also important (Herrman, 2001).

Measuring Mental Health

The majority of measurements of mental health are intended to diagnose mental illness, to evaluate if a person is mentally ill or normal. They focus on the aspects of psychiatrists' and clinical psychologists' mental illness of interests; depression, anxiety, psychosis, drug misuse and, in children, conduct disorder (CD) or attention deficit hyperactivity disorder (ADHD). These measurements do not provide information about the level of mental health in "normal" people (Stewart-Brown, 2002).

Many measures, like the Beck Depression Inventory (BDI) (Beck, 1967; Beck & Beck, 1972), focus only on the negative end of the spectrum of symptoms and are therefore good for diagnosing mental disorders. While some, for example the General Health Questionnaire (GHQ) (Goldberg, 1972), include questions about both positive ("been a happy person") and negative ("lost much sleep over worry") aspects of mental health, their principal goal is still to detect people with mental illness (Stewart-Brown, 2002).

Measurements that are developed to diagnose disorders are good for that purpose; their principal goal is to detect people with mental illness. The result of using that kind of measurements is that the subjects get split into categories; they either have the disorder or not. Consequently, those who do not get the diagnoses are all included in the same category and it's not simple to measure any differences among them. In other words, measures that are designed for diagnosing purpose can provide continuously distributed scores, but the resulting distributions tend to be positively skewed, with most people reporting nearly perfect mental health. Psychological measurements developed to measure happiness and life satisfaction also seem to be positively skewed (Gudmundsdottir, 2009). For the reason that they offer little room for improvement in most people's scores (a ceiling effect), they are not well suited to measuring improvement in positive mental health (Stewart-Brown, 2002).

Measurements that are designed to measure mental well-being in general do get better variation among subjects and are therefore more suitable for measuring changes over time. The Warwick-Edinburgh Mental Well-Being Scale (WEMWBS), for instance, was developed to meet demands for instruments to measure mental well-being (Ruth et al., 2007; Stewart-Brown et al., 2009). The scale has been found to be a reliable measurement on mental well-being with almost no floor or ceiling effects (Gudmundsdottir, 2009).

Mental Health Promotion and Positive Psychology for Social Change

Mental well-being, its definition, measurements and determinants, is the subject of both mental health promotion and positive psychology. Collaboration between these two fields is a clear benefit for knowledge creation, policy making and society at large. A common goal for the collaboration of these two fields is therefore to get policy makers and practitioners in the field to rely on evidence-based knowledge on mental well-being in their decision making. Clearly, a broader collaboration will benefit the general public.

Politicians around the world have shown increased interest in using a national well-being index for detecting the well-being of nations. Good reliable measurements, sensitive to changes in society, are a desirable goal for both fields and for the public. Advocates of positive psychology have made some progress in breaking the barriers between different fields in this area (e.g. Diener, 2006), although further work is needed. Public health extends to science, art and politics of preventing illness and promoting health and well-being.

At the 2009 IPPA (International Positive Psychology Association) conference in Philadelphia, a new field called "positive health" was introduced. For those who have been working in the field of health promotion, this ideology was quite recognizable. The first thing that comes to mind is why we need a new field for something that already exists. Is it so difficult to break barriers between different fields? Whose interests does it serve?

Huppert (2009) concludes in her review on psychological well-being that the science of well-being which focuses on what makes people flourish is a new interesting area of research. I totally agree that the advantages in understanding the behavioural, biological and social pathways to well-being will benefit individuals, organizations and society. It is also clear that it is of both economical and scientific benefit to extend the collaboration of two interrelated research fields which both have the same goal – to focus on the positive aspects of public health and find effective ways to enhance it. With a broad collaboration it will be possible to make a *real* social change.

References

Acheson, D. (1988). *Public health in England: The report of the committee of inquiry into the future development of the public health function* ("Acheson Report"). London: HMSO.

Ahmed, M., & Boisvert, C. M. (2006). Using positive psychology with special mental health populations. *American Psychologist, 61*(4), 333–335.

Antonovsky, A. (1979). *Health, stress, and coping: New perspectives on mental and physical well-being.* San Francisco: Jossey-Bass.

Antonovsky, A. (1987). *Unraveling the mystery of health.* San Francisco: Jossey-Bass.

Argyle, M. (2001). *The psychology of happiness* (2nd ed.). London: Routledge.

Beck, A. T. (1967). *Depression: Causes and treatment.* Philadelphia: University of Pennsylvania Press.

Beck, A. T., & Beck, R. W. (1972). Screening depressed patients in family practice: A rapid technique. *Postgraduate Medicine, 52,* 81–85.

Bradburn, N. M. (1969). *The structure of psychological well-being.* Chicago: Aldine.

Compton, W. C., Smith, M. L., Cornish, K. A., & Qualls, D. L. (1996). Factor structure of mental health measures. *Journal of Personality and Social Psychology, 71*(2), 406–413.

Csikszentmihalyi, M. (2003). Legs or wings? A reply to R. S. Lazarus. *Psychological Inquiry, 14,* 113–115.

Diener, E. (2000). Subjective well-being: The science of happiness and a proposal for a national index. *American psychologist, 55*(1), 34–43.

Diener, E. (2006). Guidelines for national indicators of subjective well-being and ill-being. *The Journal of Happiness studies, 55*(1), 34–43.

Diener, E., Emmons, R. A., Larsen, R. J., & Griffin, S. (1985). Satisfaction with life scale. *Journal of Personality Assessment, 49,* 71–75.

Eriksson, M., & Lindström, B. (2008). A salutogenic interpretation of the Ottawa Charter. *Health Promotion International, 23*(2), 190–199.

Flanagan, J. C. (1979). *Identifying opportunities for improving quality of life of older age groups.* Palo Alto, CA: American Institute for Research.

Folkman, S., & Moskowitz, J. T. (2003). Positive psychology from a coping perspective. *Psychological Inquiry, 14*(2), 121–125.

Fordyce, M. W. (1977). Development of a program to increase personal happiness. *Journal of Counseling Psychology, 24,* 511–520.

Fredrickson, B. L. (2002). Positive emotions. In C. R. Snyder & S. J. Lopez (Eds.), *Handbook of positive psychology* (pp. 120–134). New York: Oxford University Press.

Goldberg, D. P. (1972). *The detection of psychiatric illness by questionnaire.* London: Oxford University Press.

Guðmundsdóttir, D. G. (2009, April 1–3). The short Warwick-Edinburgh mental well-being scale (SWEMWBS): Internal validity and the relationship between SWEMWBS, age, gender and other health and well-being measures. Presented at the 2nd Applied Positive Psychology Conference, Warwick.

Heady, B., & Wearing, A. (1992). *Understanding happiness.* Melbourne: Longman Cheshire.

Herrman, H. (2001). The need for mental health promotion. *Australian and New Zealand Journal of Psychiatry, 35,* 709–715.

Huppert, F. A. (2009). Psychological well-being: Evidence regarding its causes and consequences. *Applied Psychology: Health and Well-Being, 1*(2), 137–164.

Jahoda, M. (1958). *Current concepts of positive mental health.* New York: Basic Books.

O'Donnell, M. (1989). Definition of health promotion: Part III: Stressing the impact of culture. *American Journal of Health Promotion, 3*(3), 5.

Rose, G. (1989). The mental health of populations. In: Williams, P., Wilkinson, G., & Rawnsley, K. (Eds.), *Essays in honour of Michael Shepherd* (pp. 77–85). London: Routledge.

Rosenberg, M. (1965). *Society and the adolescent self-image.* Princeton, NJ: Princeton University Press.

Ruth, T., Louise, H., Ruth, F., Stephen, P., Stephen, J., Scott, W., et al. (2007). The Warwick-Edinburgh mental well-being scale (WEMWBS): Development and UK validation. *Health and Quality of Life Outcomes, 5,* 63.

Ryff, C. D. (1989). Happiness is everything, or is it? Explorations on the meaning of psychological well-being. *Journal of Personality and Social Psychology, 57,* 1069–1081.

Ryff, C. D., & Keyes, C. L. M. (1995). The structure of psychological well-being revisited. *Journal of Personality and Social Psychology, 69*(4), 719–727.

Scheier, M., & Carver, C. (1985). Optimism, coping and health: Assessment and implications of generalized outcome expectancies. *Health Psychology, 4,* 219–247.

Secker, J. (1998). Current conceptualizations of mental health and mental health promotion. *Health Education Research, 13,* 57–66.

Seligman, M. E. P. (2002). *Authentic happiness: Using the new positive psychology to realize your potential for lasting fulfillment.* New York: Free Press.

Seligman, M. E. P. (2007). *What you can change & what you can't* (2nd ed.). New York: Vintage Books.

Seligman, M. E. P., & Csikszentmihalyi, M. (2000). Positive psychology: An introduction. *American Psychologist, 55*(1), 5–14.

Seligman, M. E. P., & Peterson, C. (2003). Positive clinical psychology. In L. G. Aspinwall & U. M. Staudinger(Eds.), *A psychology of human strengths: Fundamental questions and future directions for a positive psychology,* Washington, DC: American Psychological Association.

Stewart-Brown, S. (2002). Measuring the parts most measures do not reach: A necessity for evaluation in mental health promotion. *Journal of Mental Health Promotion, 1*(2), 4–9.

Stewart-Brown, S., Tennant, A., Tennant, R., Platt, S., Parkinson, J., & Weich, S. (2009). Internal construct validity of the Warwick Edinburgh mental well-being scale (WEMWBS): A Rasch analysis using data from the Scottish Health Education Population survey. *Health and Quality of Life Outcomes, 7,* 15.

Veenhoven, R. (1994). *Correlates of happiness* (3 vols.). Rotterdam: RISBO, Center for Socio-Cultural Transformation.

VicHealth. (2000). *Promoting mental health.* Carlton: Victorian Health Promotion Foundation.

WHO. (1948). *Official records of the World Health Organization* (Vol. 2). Geneva: World Health Organization.

WHO. (1986). *Ottawa Charter for health promotion.* Geneva: World Health Organization.

Part III
Positive Psychology and Poverty

Chapter 8
Positive Psychology and Poverty

Robert Biswas-Diener and Lindsey Patterson

As economic growth slows dramatically across the world—as has been the trend in the last couple years—it is estimated that individuals already living in poverty will be hardest hit (World Bank, 2009). Current projections suggest that between 20 and 27% of the world's working poor are living on less than $1.25 per day (World Bank, 2009). Percentages of people living in extreme poverty (less than $1.25 per day) are the highest in Sub-Sahara Africa and South Asia (60–40%, respectively; World Bank, 2009), and many of the countries within Sub-Sahara Africa and South Asia are considered to have low human development ($M = 57.3\%$ living in extreme poverty; United Nations Human Development Programme, 2008). Representing a quarter or more of the world's overall population, the very poor represent one of the most urgent humanitarian crises imaginable.

There is little question that poverty is a pressing material and social concern. Studies of homeless individuals reveal that dire economic circumstances are associated with a variety of negative outcomes ranging from higher rates of anger and depression (Marshall, Burnam, Koegel, Sullivan & Benjamin, 1996) to the deleterious effects of social stigmatization (Lankenau, 1999). On this last point, unpublished pilot survey data of residents of Fresno, California, showed that they dramatically overestimated drug addiction and underestimated physical and mental disability as a cause of homelessness, and reported a negative, untrusting view of the homeless (Biswas-Diener, 2000). While it makes sense to focus on health, social, and other problems related to poverty, Gough and McGregor (2007) caution that people living in poverty should not be "completely defined by their poverty, nor can they be fully understood in its terms alone" (p. 3). Instead, it makes sense to focus on what is "going right" as well as what is "going wrong" in the lives of the poor. From a research, policy, and intervention point of view, we should set an agenda to better understand what makes life bearable for the world's poorest citizens and use this knowledge to help those in poverty gain access to resources and tools that will help them to empower themselves.

R. Biswas-Diener (✉)
Centre for Applied Positive Psychology, Coventry, UK; Portland State University, Portland, OR, USA
e-mail: jayajedi@comcast.net

There is no universally accepted definition for poverty; however, low income, lack of human development, social exclusion, ill-being, poor daily functioning, vulnerability, unsustainable livelihood, unfulfilled basic needs, and relative deprivation are common terms used in the conceptualization of poverty (Maxwell, 1999). Although it might initially seem incongruous, well-being (e.g., happiness, life satisfaction, self-esteem, self-efficacy and related variables), or lack thereof, can also be considered an essential component in defining poverty. In fact, the Millennium Development Goals (MDGs) emphasize the importance of subjective well-being in the "3-D model of individual well-being" (McGregor & Sumner, 2010). In this chapter, we understand poverty principally in economic terms but acknowledge that material deprivation is strongly associated with a wide range of social, emotional and psychological ills. We further assume that a complete understanding of the lives of those living in poverty must also include well-being, successes and other aspects of positive functioning.

This is consistent with the positive psychology approach to understanding human psychological and social phenomena. Positive Psychology is a relatively new branch of psychology that seeks to explore human flourishing and positive functioning as an intellectual counterpoint to psychological maladies. In their introduction to the field, Seligman and Csikszentmihalyi (2000) argue that, in the decades since World War II, psychology

> concentrates on repairing damage within a disease model of human functioning. This almost exclusive attention to pathology neglects the fulfilled individual and the thriving community. The aim of positive psychology is to begin to catalyze a change in the focus of psychology from preoccupation only with repairing the worst things in life to also building positive qualities (p. 5).

From a positive psychology perspective, poverty can best be understood as a unique set of material circumstances that exposes people to violence and social stigma and presents obstacles to fulfilling basic needs but which also fosters resilience, engenders compassion, and presents opportunities for happiness.

Before going further it makes sense to ask "should positive psychologists focus on poverty?" One possible objection to a poverty focus is that poverty, by its very definition, represents a deficit and, therefore, may not be squarely aligned with the positive psychology focus of "optimal functioning." Another possible concern is the fact that addressing poverty can be a political, rather than scientific, undertaking and might therefore be outside the purview of positive psychology. Both of these are sensible cautions and we recommend that each individual positive psychologist reflect on them based on their own values and professional objectives. That said, we also offer counterarguments here: we believe addressing poverty is a moral imperative for all citizens and especially so for those with expert knowledge in researching and improving quality of life. To the point that poverty is a negative rather than positive focus, we argue that positive psychology is, in part, about reaching individual potential, and to the extent that poverty acts as an obstacle to achieving personal potential, it is a positive psychology concern. Further, individuals living within poverty possess strengths, hopes, motivation, happiness, and many other psychological phenomena that are the direct concern of positive psychology research. To the idea that addressing poverty is primarily a political undertaking we argue that science is an important informer of policy and that positive psychology is an applied, rather than a basic science. As such, positive psychologists are in possession of assessment and intervention tools that can be directly used to improve the quality of life of the poor.

This chapter addresses poverty-related issues through a positive psychology perspective. Specifically, this chapter highlights relevant positive psychology research on the relationship between poverty and subjective well-being and examines potential protective factors and agents of change for those living in poverty in seven parts: (1) positive psychology outcomes of happiness; (2) the emotional quality of life of the poor; (3) a positive psychology agenda for poverty; (4) microfinance as a tool to initiate women's empowerment; (5) a microfinance case study; (6) positive psychology interventions for both individuals and groups; and (7) recommendations and conclusions.

Positive Psychology Outcomes, Not Just for the Rich

Among the most interesting research topics in positive psychology and has received much recent attention is the function of positive emotion. Although it has long been assumed that negative emotions, such as fear and anger, serve the evolutionary function of protecting individuals by motivating them toward "fight and flight" behaviors a similar understanding of positive emotions was neglected until relatively recently. Isen (1970) and Isen and her colleagues (1972, 1987) conducted early research on the outcomes related to experiencing positive emotion. Across studies Isen and her colleagues found that feeling good was associated with increased helping behaviors and creativity. Using Isen's research as a foundation, Fredrickson (2000) advanced the "Broaden and Build" theory of positive emotion. According to Fredrickson, positive emotions serve to broaden and build our thought–action repertoires. Follow-up research has supported this theory by showing that positive emotion predicts interest in new activities (Fredrickson & Joiner 2002), creative problem solving (Fredrickson & Joiner, 2002), and health outcomes such as cardiovascular functioning (Fredrickson & Levenson, 1998).

Further support for the benefits of positive affect can be found in a meta-analysis by Lyubomirsky and colleagues (2005). The researchers examined correlational, experimental, and cross-sectional studies, and found that the experience of frequent positive affect was associated, both as a cause and as an effect, with a wide range of desirable outcomes. These include, but are not limited to, better work safety records, lower turnover at work, better immune functioning, fewer hospitalizations, lower rates of drug and alcohol consumption, enhanced creativity, and better social relationships. Although none of the studies included in this meta-analysis employed samples of impoverished individuals there is little reason to think that positive affect would not confer similar tonic effects to the poor.

From a positive psychology perspective, it is worthwhile to understand the happiness of poor individuals. One study of homeless men and women, for example, reveals that even people living in dire poverty experience relatively frequent episodes of affection, joy, and pride (Biswas-Diener & Diener, 2006). Although the people in this study also reported alarming levels of worry, sadness, and anger, it would be a mistake to minimize the importance of their more pleasant emotional experiences. Positive affect has, for instance, been linked to meaning in life (King, Hicks, Krull, & Del Gaiso, 2006; King & Hickes, 2009). Notably, King and colleagues found that positive affect was causally associated with vigilance for meaning relevant stimuli. To the extent that positive emotions serve to enhance meaning and basic areas of functioning, it is important to be aware of when and why poor individuals experience happiness. It could be, for example, that experienced happiness helps buffer people from the dire psychological effects of poverty. Interventions with impoverished societies can be enhanced by understanding the emotional high points of members of the community as well as through the traditional focus on problems and needs assessments.

The Emotional Quality of Life of the Poor

Results from research in psychology have consistently pointed to the association between elements of poverty (i.e., income) and subjective well-being (Diener & Biswas-Diener, 2002). Although factors such as life circumstances (e.g., marital status), wealth of a society, and income satisfaction influence this relationship (Hagerty, 2000; Veenhoven, 1991, 1995), research generally reveals a significant, positive association between income and subjective well-being (Diener, Sandvik, Seidlitz, & Diener, 1993; Hagerty, 2000). In international surveys, for instance, respondents from wealthy nations, such as those in Scandinavia, rank among the happiest in the world (Inglehart & Klingemann, 2000; Veenhoven, 1995). This is especially noticeable in studies using the Gallup World Poll data, which includes representative samples from more than 100 nations (Diener, Helliwell, & Kahneman, 2010; Ng, Diener, Harter, & Arora, 2009). Further, research with a sample of very wealthy people shows that they reported more happiness than did a geographically matched sample of middle-class individuals (Diener, Horowitz, & Emmons, 1985).

Despite the fact that there is such strong evidence linking income—both at the individual and national level—to subjective well-being, there are also a handful of studies specifically focusing on the quality of life of people living in materially deprived circumstances. For example, in a recent study one of us (RBD) used Gallup World Poll data to compare the poorest Americans with the poorest people in Denmark. Two interesting results emerge when looking at the negative and positive affect of the poorest citizens of these two countries (shown in Figs. 8.1 and 8.2, respectively). First, the Danish poor appeared to experience far less negative affect than did their American counterparts. This suggests that there is something about Danish society that protects its poorest citizens against the psychological effects of

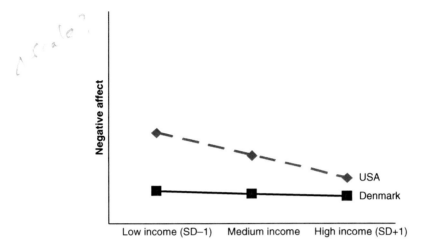

Fig. 8.1 Negative affect of low and high income Americans and Danes

low socioeconomic status. Second, while the poorer citizens of both nations reported slightly less positive emotion than did the richest respondents it should be noted that the poor people in both countries experienced relatively high positive affect. This is consistent with past research showing that "most people are happy" (Diener & Diener, 1995), including those who live in economic hardship (Biswas-Diener & Diener, 2001).

A more detailed look at the well-being of the very poor comes from a study of homeless people living in India and the United States of America. Biswas-Diener and Diener (2006) measured the life satisfaction of three groups of homeless people: (1) people living on sidewalks in Kolkata (Calcutta), India; (2) people residing in an

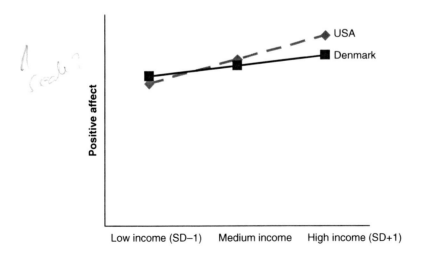

Fig. 8.2 Positive affect of low and high income Americans and Danes

organized tent camp in Portland, Oregon; and (3) people living on the streets and homeless shelters of Fresno, California. Results across the three samples yield interesting patterns of well-being. Members of all three groups, for instance, reported high satisfaction with themselves, including satisfaction with their own morality, physical appearance, and intelligence. This finding alone presents an interesting scientific counterpoint to the common view of the homeless as being socially downtrodden and spiritually defeated. The homeless men and women in the study, in essence, thought highly of themselves, and this could be a potential launching point for intervention because it suggests a degree of investment in the self and assumes some knowledge of personal or psychological assets. In addition, analyses of significant differences between these three groups showed that the homeless in India reported higher satisfaction with their social life and their family relationships as well as higher overall life satisfaction. It could be that the experience of stronger family ties and a more satisfying social life in Kolkata act in a bottom-up way to promote higher life satisfaction among India's poor relative to their American counterparts. Although further research is needed, the existing evidence is encouraging in that it points to several potentially fruitful areas for positive psychological intervention with homeless people: building on a foundation of self-satisfaction and developing programs that strengthen social ties.

This last point—that social relations are crucial to well-being (Diener & Seligman, 2002)—has interesting ramifications for homeless people. Many homeless interventions and social services are aimed either at providing the most basic services, such as food and shelter, or equipping individuals with job, social, and other skills that will help reintegrate them into mainstream society. Sometimes absent from these types of services is an emphasis on group level, rather than individual, well-being. This could be the practical result of the fact that homeless populations tend to be heterogeneous and often do not have an identifiable community center, either social or physical. Even so, positive psychology-oriented programs for homeless and poor individuals should include some emphasis on forming social bonds and helping others.

To illustrate the idea of a poverty program that focuses both on individual and collective well-being, we would like to introduce a case study in positive intervention related to poverty: *Dignity Village*. Dignity Village is an organized tent camp at the outskirts of Portland, Oregon, a metropolitan area of about 1.8 million people. Dignity Village is unusual in that it is a self-organized, self-governing tent camp with 501 (c) (3) charitable tax exempt status. Dignity Village is a drug- and alcohol-free community that is home to approximately 60 people who would otherwise be "houseless." This community includes toilet and shower facilities, wind-powered energy, access to the internet, a community garden and annual fundraisers including their own calendar, bazaar, and plant sale. The camp has a formal governance structure, with an elected committee of policymakers and a communal meeting hall. Make no mistake; however, the citizens of Dignity Village experience many of the problems typical to other homeless people. They report, for example, high rates of disability and previous incarceration, chronic difficulties with long-term employment and a high incidence of being estranged from their families.

Qualitative information collected at Dignity Village suggests that the people who dwell there enjoy many protections from some of the dangers typically associated with homelessness as well as a variety of social and economic opportunities largely unavailable to "average" homeless people (Biswas-Diener & Diener, 2006). Because of their status as a model village, the Dignity Village residents benefit from community volunteer support, positive media coverage, and municipal services that are rare for homeless people. Quantitative data on the well-being of the Dignity Villagers suggest that these social and infrastructure benefits translate directly into psychological dividends. They report experiencing, for example, significantly lower rates of sadness than homeless comparison groups in Kolkata and California. In addition, when compared with a "typical" sample of homeless people from California, the residents of Dignity Village reported higher absolute satisfaction with their social lives, romantic relationships, and friends. Although these differences were not significant, they were larger for the residents of Dignity Village compared to a sample of homeless people in California and might become significant with a larger sample. This is evidenced by the fact that the residents of Dignity Village reported significantly higher affection than did the homeless in California (Biswas-Diener & Diener, 2006).

Although Dignity Village was initiated by the homeless themselves, and not by positive psychologists, it is emblematic of positive psychology principles. It is a program that assumes people are whole, motivated, and capable, and one that creates structures to enable people to reach their potential. Further, it is, fundamentally, a social change program. While Dignity Village offers support and opportunities to individuals, it emphasizes social harmony, working together on super ordinate goals, offering support in relationships and other aspects of collective welfare.

A Positive Psychology Agenda for Poverty

Like all programs that focus on poverty reduction or alleviation, positive psychology must look at systemic as well as individual success. Positive psychologists, in particular, are able to address this complex issue from both the basic research and application/intervention point of view. First, researchers are well poised to look at positive deviance—those individuals who experience success despite impoverished circumstances—and to use these individuals as instructive instances of overcoming life obstacles (Barker, 2000). Positive psychology researchers are potentially able to identify the factors that lead to individual success in adverse circumstances and, more importantly, assess how transferable these individual decisions, behaviors, and thoughts are to other people in similar circumstances. For example, it would be considered an important finding to discover that a low-income person high in optimism is more likely to persevere and experience positive outcomes in job searches. It is even more valuable to know to what extent this type of optimism can be taught and who are the best candidates for this type of "positive psychology transfer." In addition, positive psychology researchers are able to examine whether these case studies represent "top-down" or "bottom-up" influences. It could be, for example, that improving life for an individual within a community will bene-fit the community as a whole to the extent that the individual can then better serve others. Alternately, it could be that creating positive community structures could serve a top-down influence on the well-being of individuals within that commu-nity. These types of influences have been examined in the frame work of happiness (e.g., Diener, 1984) but could be more strategically evaluated by positive psychology researchers interested in poverty. Second, positive psychology practitioners—those educators, coaches, therapists, and consultants who are heavily influenced by this theoretical and research perspective—can create new interventions that help poor individuals gain resilience, employ their strengths and otherwise flourish relative to their circumstances. While a number of happiness increasing interventions have been reported within positive psychology research (Lyubomirsky, 2008), there are relatively fewer group-level interventions.

One way of bridging the gap between individual and collective positive psy-chology interventions is to expand the scope of the outcome variables that are commonly used in this type of research. Traditionally, positive psychologists have used individual happiness as the predominant outcome variable for interventions (see Chapter 8 by Biswas-Diener, this volume). Expanding the nature of well-being to include social dimensions of life, as Ryff (1989) advocates, can lay the foundation for creating interventions that both raise happiness and improve connections. Diener and Biswas-Diener (2008) propose a model of "complete happiness" —called *psy-chological wealth*—that extends beyond one's affective state to include material circumstances, spiritual development, health, social relationships, and mental state. This more complete approach to a person's quality of life, both psychological and otherwise, allows for a more straightforward connection between individual and group-level well-being. One example of intervention programs that directly influence an individual's psychological wealth while also potentially affecting com-munity welfare is empowerment programs. We will discuss these more in-depth in the following section.

Microfinance as a Tool to Initiate Women's Empowerment

International aid and development work related to addressing poverty often focuses on the issue of empowerment. Empowerment is most commonly thought of in economic and political terms. The World Bank (2002), for example, defines empow-erment as "the expansion of assets and capabilities of poor people to participate in, negotiate with, influence, control and hold accountable institutions that affect their lives" (p. 14). Although not explicitly listed, it is easy to see that empower-ment, as defined here, would necessarily have positive psychological consequences related to self-efficacy, dignity, and other aspects of mental health. Interestingly, empowerment is an issue that is already talked about within the framework of indi-vidual and collective welfare. The World Bank (2002) reports "There is a reciprocal relationship between individual assets and capabilities and the capability to act collectively....Poor people who are healthy, educated and secure can contribute more effectively to collective action; at the same time, collective action can improve poor people's access to quality schools or health clinics" (p. 15). Despite the fact that empowerment programs undoubtedly have psychological benefits, they are most often framed in economic terms and presented as economic interventions. This is, perhaps, the reason that there has not been more attention to such programs within positive psychology itself.

Since the 1980s, the economic tool of microfinance has been used to combat poverty in some of the poorest countries in the world. Microfinance programs provide poor women, and occasionally men, across the world with small loans to use toward life betterment including business startup or improvement, home improvement, or other family matters. When implemented appropriately, microfinance programs have seen success in financial as well as social and psychological aspects of women's lives. In fact, some microfinance programs have helped women become more empowered in their household and community. Theoretically, empowerment has the potential to impact individuals in three ways: (1) *power to*; (2) *power over*; and (3) *power within*. Microfinance programs have been found to impact all three of these categories for women in economically developing countries (Kim et al., 2007).

Power to is a personal sense of efficacy or influence and can be used to understand the psychological benefits of the empowerment process including autonomy, self-confidence, and self-esteem. Microfinance programs in Bangladesh, India, Nepal, and South Africa have been found to increase these characteristic components of psychological empowerment for women living in poverty (Amin, Becker & Bayes, 1998; Holvoet, 2005; Kim et al., 2007; Mahmud, 2003; Sharma, 2007). For example, a study by Sharma (2007) found that Nepalese women reported increased self-confidence, autonomy, and awareness of social issues after participating in a microfinance program. Similarly, another study found that women participating in a microfinance program in South Africa reported higher levels of self-confidence, financial confidence, and more progressive attitudes toward gender norms and relations compared to South African women that did not participate (Kim et al., 2007).

Microfinance programs have also been associated with increases in the *power over* component of empowerment. *Power over* is an individual's ability to make personally or socially impactful actions. Studies have associated women's participation in microfinance programs with women's increased reports of decision-making, bargaining power, and communication with their husbands as well as improvements in spousal relationships and appreciation for women's work in the household (Amin et al., 1998; Holvoet, 2005; Kim et al., 2007; Mahmud, 2003; Sharma, 2007).

Finally, it has been suggested that microfinance programs positively impact women's sense of *power within* or an individual's ability to participate in organizations and agencies in her own community. Women who participate in microfinance programs across the world have reported to be more active in social organizations as well as seek out more community activity and collective action (Kim et al., 2007; Mahmud, 2003; Sharma, 2007). Research shows that participation in microfinance programs serves to help women gain access to resources and increase mobility which provide a stepping stone for women to enter social and political arenas (Mahmud, 2003).

Microfinance programs have been criticized for a number of failures negatively impacting women's financial, social, and psychological well-being, and many critiques recognize that microfinance opportunities do not immediately alleviate poverty or empower women simply by program implementation or participation (Kabeer, 2001; Leach & Sitaram, 2002; Rogaly, 1996). However, it is important to recognize that, when implemented appropriately, microfinance programs can be successful and positively impact many aspects of women's lives. Taking into account women's needs, community needs and resources and societal norms and values (e.g., gender relations), microfinance programs can be tailored to fit a specific group of women. By doing so, organizations and communities increase the chances of the program's success and enhance the potential to help women overcome poverty and find ways to empower themselves.

A Microfinance Case Study

India is home to many of the microfinance programs where various forms of micro-lending (e.g., Grameen model and Self-Help Group model) have been implemented and evaluated. The following case study of an Indian microfinance program was originally presented by Anand (2002) and serves as an exemplary model for women's empowerment through microfinance.

The successful microfinance program, called the Bhoodan Vikas Mandal (BVM), that Anand (2002) studied lies in the State of Kerala, India. Kerala is, in many ways, a test state for social programs. In 1957, for instance, the citizens of Kerala elected a communist government to power that created sweeping land and educational reforms. By 1986, Kerala had a higher literacy rate and life expectancy and lower infant mortality relative to the Indian average rates (Franke & Chasin, 1989). While economic and political tides have shifted over the decades since, the emphasis on grassroots social programs has not.

The BVM is a non-governmental organization that was established in 1996. It is relatively small, supporting microfinance self-help groups (SHG) for women in three towns (Edakkara, Chungathara, and Kurumbalangode). The primary goal of the BVM is to eliminate poverty in rural families. The BVM serves 57 SHGs consisting of, at most, 20 women each. Women meet weekly and discuss loan proposals, loan use, and repayments. Some features of BVM SHGs include byelaws for each group, evaluation and monitoring from the BVM office, and independent group decision making.

The BVM has seen both success and struggles within small SHGs in the last 13 years. The BVM has helped Indian women save significant amounts of money and contribute to, on average, 35% of their family income. Beyond financial success, the BVM has helped women gain necessary tools of empowerment. Research suggests that women participating in the BVM were more involved in social organizations and increased their political participation (i.e., voting) as well as increased their mobility, self-esteem, self-confidence, and communication skills. Despite these successes, however, the BVM also discovered a few barriers during the development and implementation processes as well as during daily functioning. One of the major concerns for SHGs in the BVM was that each group's growth and success heavily depended on the group's leader, where some leaders were more active than others. Since many of the leaders were the most educated or were the most skilled at business and finance within their group, many of the SHGs maintained the same leaders over many years. For some groups, leadership by one or a few women became problematic because many of the leadership, business, and financials skills were not always passed down to all members of the SHG. Other problems that some of the SHGs in the BVM encountered were a lack of group clarity of group goals and a lack of understanding of microfinance basics due the rush in the formation of some groups. Finally, most of the BVM SHGs were successful at micro-lending to individuals within the group; however, very few groups ventured to obtain loans for the group as whole, which was only problematic if the group wanted to begin a larger scale business or an individual required a loan larger than the group could give.

The BVM model of microfinance, consisting of many small SHGs, is similar to other SHG models that have experienced both success and failure across the world. Women in programs that have seen success often report the same benefits that the women in the BVM model experienced, including increased financial skills, increased confidence and self-esteem, better communication skills, and increased mobility and social participation. It is important to recognize that the BVM model, like many other SHG models, developed over time. In fact, it took many groups 2 or 3 years to develop a consistent group of women and solidify the byelaws and goals of the group. Furthermore, it is not sufficient to simply give women the economic resources to achieve their goals. The women who participated in the BVM model of SHGs were most successful when they were also provided with educational, emotional, and social support from the organization as well as from other women within their group. Through the examination of the BVM, it is apparent that, with much planning and commitment from both participating women and the supporting organization, poor women can benefit financially, socially, and psychologically from small self-help microfinance groups.

Positive Psychology Interventions for Both Individuals and Groups

Microfinance and related empowerment programs are, of course, only a single instance of positive psychology relevant interventions. Rojas (2009) argues that the basic assumption of such programs—that increasing economic prosperity will translate to greater well-being—may be wrong. Specifically, Rojas uses an annual national survey from Costa Rica to demonstrate that income deprivation is not a perfect corollary to well-being deprivation, and policies aimed at one do not necessarily affect the other in a one-to-one relationship. Although Rojas' comments are aimed particularly at public policy initiatives, they serve as an important cautionary note for psychological intervention strategies as well. With these comments in mind, we suggest a wider range of potential positive psychology applications and interventions for poverty:

1. *Measurement and policy*: There are currently a variety of initiatives to measure well-being along with traditional economic indicators of quality of life. Diener and colleagues (2009) make a case for using well-being variables to inform public policy and provide specific suggestions for doing so (see also Chapter 4 by Diener and Diener, this volume). In their book, Diener and colleagues (2009) specifically address the idea that well-being—the preeminent positive psychology variable—is directly relevant to the "good society" as well as the "good life." They write:

   > We suggest that even if well-being measures cannot completely resolve disputes about the nature of the good society, they yield an additional perspective on these debates. For example, are people happier in regions where the arts flourish, or is well-being equally high where these forms of entertainment are much less common? After all, if the arts are important enough to deserve government support, they should produce positive and measurable outcomes. At an even broader level, the well-being measures can shed light on whether more authoritarian or more libertarian societies experience the highest well-being. And of course, if these effects depend on cultural values, well-being measures should be able to reveal this too. (p. 61)

   This approach is consistent with the basic research side of positive psychology because it is principally about measurement of positive aspects of human psychology and functioning. Further, these types of measures can be used to inform policies and interventions related to empowering the poor, psychologically and otherwise.

2. *Strengths:* One of the conceptual "pillars" of positive psychology is a focus on strengths (Seligman, 2002). Strengths represents a major focus of theory (e.g., Linley, 2008), assessment (Peterson & Seligman, 2004), and intervention (Seligman, Steen, Park, & Peterson, 2005). Strengths are preexisting capacities that are authentic and energizing which lead to optimal functioning when they are employed (Linley, 2008). Strengths have been found to be universal phenomena, including cultures and societies where people live without material luxuries or modern conveniences (Biswas-Diener, 2006). To the extent this is true, strengths represent a set of personal resources that individuals and groups living in poverty can use to enhance their personal and collective well-being. Strengths-based programs are already being piloted in impoverished communities (see Chapter 10 by Linley, this volume).

3. *A focus on what works*: Finally, positive psychology is, by definition, about what works. By looking at established individual and collective successes, we can identify factors related to success and establish methods for transferring social, situational, and personal benefactors to those who might best use them. There are already two examples of how this is done, both tangentially associated with positive psychology. The first is *positive deviance*. Positive deviance is the process by which paragons of success are systematically identified and used to create interventions by which their success-relevant behaviors are transferred to others. This technique has been used effectively with impoverished groups (Lapping et al., 2002). The second is *appreciative inquiry*. Appreciative inquiry is, in short, a method of increasing group cohesiveness and effectiveness by raising positive emotion through a facilitated process of focusing on group assets and how these might be leveraged for future success (Cooperrider, Whitney, Stavros, & Fry, 2008). Appreciative inquiry is commonly used in organizations and has also been advanced as a topic relevant to social change (Cooperrider & Pasmore, 1991). Both *Positive Deviance* and *Appreciative Inquiry* are conceptually tied to positive psychology in their focus on successes rather than failures and strengths over weaknesses. Further, these approaches represent an established model of intervention for positive psychologists who want to address poverty.

Recommendations and Conclusions

In the end, positive psychology is best served by transitioning from a focus on individual well-being to a wider focus on collective success and welfare. By adding a scientific exploration of the good society to the current research on the good life, positive psychologists can positively impact the lives of those living in poverty as well as more affluent individuals. There are, however, several noteworthy obstacles to doing so. First, applied positive psychologists—those delivering interventions and services rooted in positive psychology research—will naturally gravitate, as a practical concern, toward the better financed areas of practice. Currently, these include organizational consultation, coaching, and other private-sector opportunities. It should be noted that this is true even outside of positive psychology: there tends to be more money in private sector and free enterprise undertakings than in non-profit, humanitarian, and poverty intervention services. Increasing funds for poverty intervention through research grants, government programs and non-profits services will be an important prerequisite to attracting scholars and practitioners to this field. In addition, positive psychologists are hampered in their ability to help the poor achieve a better quality of life by the simplicity of our interventions and the lack of knowledge of top-down and bottom-up influences on well-being. In the future, we will need to create more sophisticated group-level interventions that are both culturally appropriate and effective. Whether these are government policies, community aid or targeted empowerment programs, the science of positive psychology has much to offer those living in poverty, and it has the moral obligation to do so.

References

Amin, R., Becker, S., & Bayes, A. (1998). NGO-promoted microcredit programs and women's empowerment in rural Bangladesh: Quantitative and qualitative evidence. *Journal of Developing Areas, 32*(2), 221–236.

Anand, J. S. (2002). *Self-help groups in empowering women: Case study of selected SHGs and NHGs*. Kerala Research Programme on Local Level Development, Center for Development Studies. Retrieved January 18, 2010, from http://krpcds.org/w38.pdf

Barker, G. (2000). Gender equitable boys in a gender inequitable world: Reflections from qualitative research and program development with young men in Rio de Janeiro, Brazil. *Sexual and Relationship Therapy, 15*, 263–282.

Biswas-Diener, R. (2000). *Perceptions of homelessness*. Unpublished pilot data collected September through December, 2000 in Fresno, California.

Biswas-Diener, R., & Diener, E. (2001). Making the best of a bad situation: Satisfaction in the slums of Calcutta. *Social Indicators Research, 55*, 329–352.

Biswas-Diener, R., & Diener, E. (2006). Subjective well-being of the homeless, and related lessons for happiness. *Social Indicators Research, 76*, 185–205.

Cooperrider, D., & Pasmore, W. A. (1991). The organization dimension of global change. *Human Relations, 44*, 763–787.

Cooperrider, D., Whitney, D., Stavros, J. M., & Fry, R. (2008). *Appreciative inquiry handbook: For leader of change*. San Francisco: Berrett-Koehler Publishers.

Diener, E. (1984). Subjective well-being. *Psychological Bulletin, 95*, 542–575.

Diener, E., & Biswas-Diener, R. (2002). Will money increase subjective well-being? A literature review and guide to needed research. *Social Indicators Research, 57*, 119–169.

Diener, E., & Biswas-Diener, R. (2008). *Happiness: Unlocking the mysteries of psychological wealth*. Boston: Blackwell.

Diener, E., & Diener, C. (1995). The wealth of nations revisited: Income and quality of life. *Social Indicators Research, 36*, 275–286.

Diener, E., Helliwell, J. F., & Kahneman, D. (Eds.). (2010). *International differences in well-being*. New York: Oxford University Press.

Diener, E., Horowitz, J., & Emmons, R. (1985). Happiness of the very wealthy. *Journal of Personality Assessment, 49*, pp. 71–75.

Diener, E., Lucas, R., Schimmack, U., & Helliwell, J. (2009). *Well-being for public policy*. Oxford: Oxford University Press.

Diener, E., Sandvik, E., Seidlitz, L., & Diener, M. (1993). The relationship between income and subjective well-being: Relative or absolute? *Social Indicators Research, 28*, 195–223.

Diener, E., & Seligman, M. E. P. (2002). Very happy people. *Psychological Science, 13*, 80–83.

Franke, R. W., & Chasin, B. H. (1989). *Kerala: Radical reform as development in an Indian state*. San Francisco: Food First Books.

Fredrickson, B. L. (2000). Cultivating positive emotions to optimize health and well-being. Target article in *Prevention and Treatment, 3*. Available from http://journals.apa.org/prevention

Fredrickson, B. L., & Joiner, T. (2002). Positive emotions trigger upward spirals toward emotional well-being. *Psychological Science, 13*, 172–175.

Fredrickson, B., & Levenson, W. (1998). Positive emotions speed recovery from the cardiovascular sequelae of negative emotions. *Cognition & Emotion, 12*, 191–220.

Gough, I., & McGregor, J. A. (2007). *Wellbeing in developing countries: From theory to research*. Cambridge: Cambridge University Press.

Hagerty, M. R. (2000). Social comparisons of income in one's community: Evidence from national surveys of income and happiness. *Journal of Personality and Social Psychology, 78*(4), 764–771.

Holvoet, N. (2005). The impact of microfinance on decision-making agency: Evidence from South India. *Development and Change, 36*(1), 75–102.

Inglehart, R., & Klingemann, H.-D. (2000). Genes, culture, democracy, and happiness. In E. Diener & E. M. Suh (Eds.), *Culture and subjective well-being* (pp. 165–183). Cambridge, MA: MIT Press.

Isen, A. M. (1970). Success, failure, attention, and reactions to others: The warm glow of success. *Journal of Personality and Social Psychology, 15*, 294–301.

Isen, A. M., Daubman, K. A., & Nowicki, G. P. (1987). Positive affect facilitates creative problem solving. *Journal of Personality and Social Psychology, 52*, 1122–1131.

Isen, A. M., & Levin, P. F. (1972). The effect of feeling good on helping: Cookies and kindness. *Journal of Personality and Social Psychology, 21*, 384–388.

Kabeer, N. (2001). *The power to choose: Bangladeshi women and labour market decisions in London*. New York: Verso.

Kim, J. C., Watts, C. H., Hargreaves, J. R., Ndhlovu, L. X., Phetia, G., Morison, L. A., et al. (2007). Understanding the impact of a microfinance-based intervention on women's empowerment and the reduction of intimate partner violence in South Africa. *American Journal of Public Health, 97*(10), 1794–1802.

King, L. A., & Hicks, J. A. (2009). The detection and construction of meaning in life events. *Journal of Positive Psychology, 4*, 317–330.

King, L. A., Hicks, J. A., Krull, J., & Del Gaiso, A. K. (2006). Positive affect and the experience of meaning in life. *Journal of Personality and Social Psychology, 90*, 179–196.

Lankenau, S. E. (1999). Stronger than dirt: Public humiliation and status enhancement among panhandlers. *Journal of Contemporary Ethnography, 28*, pp. 288–318.

Lapping, K., Marsh, D. R., Rosenbaum, J., Swedberg, E., Sternin, J., Sternin, M., & Schroeder, D. G. (2002). The positive deviance approach: Challenges and opportunities for the future. *Food and Nutrition Bulletin, 23*, 128–135.

Leach, F., & Sitaram, S. (2002). Microfinance and women's empowerment: A lesson from India. *Development in Practice, 12*(5), 575–588.

Linley, P. A. (2008). *Average to A+*. Coventry: CAPP Press.

Lyubomirsky, S. (2008). *The how of happiness: A scientific approach to getting the life you want*. New York: Penguin Press.

Lyubomirsky, S., King, L. A., & Diener, E. (2005). The benefits of frequent positive affect. *Psychological Bulletin, 131*, 803–855.

Mahmud, S. (2003). Actually how empowering is microcredit? *Development and Change, 34*(4), 577–605.

Marshall, G. N., Burnam, M. A., Koegel, P., Sullivan, G., & Benjamin, B. (1996). Objective life circumstances and life satisfaction: Results from the course of homelessness study. *Journal of Health & Behavior, 37*, 44–58.

Maxwell, S. (1999). The meaning and measurement of poverty. *Overseas Development Institute: Poverty Briefing, 3*, 1–4.

McGregor, A., & Sumner, A. (2010). What might 3-D wellbeing contribute to MDG momentum? In A. Sumner & C. Melamed (Eds.), *The MDGs and beyond: Pro-poor policy in a changing world* (pp. 26–27). Brasilia: International Policy Centre for Inclusive Growth, United Nations Development Programme.

Ng, W., Diener, E., Harter, J., & Arora, R. (2009). Affluence, feelings of stress, and well-being. *Social Indicators Research, 94*, 257–271.

Peterson, C., & Seligman, M. E. P. (2004). *Character strengths and virtues*. Oxford and Washington, DC: Ocford University Press and American Psychological Association.

Rogaly, B. (1996). Micro-finance evangelism, 'destitute women', and the hard selling of a new anti-poverty formula. *Development in Practice, 6*(2), 100–112.

Rojas, M. (2009). Enhancing poverty-abatement programs: A subjective well-being contribution. *Applied Research in Quality of Life, 4*, 179–199.

Ryff, C. D. (1989). Happiness is everything, or is it? Explorations on the meaning of psychological well-being. *Journal of Personality and Social Psychology, 57*, 1069–1081.

Seligman, M. E. P. (2002). *Authentic happiness: Using the new science of positive psychology to realize your potential for lasting fulfillment.* New York: Free Press.

Seligman, M., & Csikszentmihalyi, M. (2000). Positive psychology: An introduction. *American Psychologist, 55*, 5–14.

Seligman, M. E. P., Steen, T., Park, N., & Peterson, C. (2005). Positive psychology progress: Empirical validation of interventions. *American Psychologist, 60*(5), 410–421.

Sharma, P. R. (2007). Micro-finance and women empowerment. *The Journal of Nepalese Business Studies, 4*(1), 16–27.

United Nations Development Programme. (2008). *Human development indices: A statistical update 2008.* Retrieved January 4, 2010, from http://hdr.undp.org/en/media/HDI_2008_EN_Tables.pdf

Veenhoven, R. (1991). Is happiness relative? *Social Indicators Research, 24*, 1–34.

Veenhoven, R. (1995). The cross-national pattern of happiness: Test of predictions implied in three theories of happiness. *Social Indicators Research, 34*, 33–68.

World Bank. (2002). *Empowerment and poverty reduction: A sourcebook.* Washington, DC: The World Bank.

World Bank. (2009). *World development indicators.* Retrieved January 8, 2010, from http://go.worldbank.org/U0FSM7AQ40

Chapter 9
Strengthening Underprivileged Communities: Strengths-Based Approaches as a Force for Positive Social Change in Community Development

P. Alex Linley, Avirupa Bhaduri, Debasish Sen Sharma, and Reena Govindji

Positive psychology came about to redress the perceived imbalance in the focus of the psychology endeavour, which was perceived to be unduly weighted towards the negative side of human experience, with insufficient experience being paid to the positive. This nascent discipline was originally conceptualised as having three pillars of focus, namely, positive subjective experience (e.g. happiness), positive personal characteristics (e.g. strengths) and positive institutions (e.g. schools, organisations, communities that in some way applied the principles of positive psychology (Seligman & Csikszentmihalyi, 2000). Perhaps unsurprisingly, given the discipline's status as a psychological science, the predominant focus of positive psychology research and practice has been at the level of the individual, particularly subjective experience and characteristics (Linley, Joseph, Harrington, & Wood, 2006). Historically, over the first decade of positive psychology's life, less attention has been paid to the organisational, community and social applications of the work – although this is now changing, as is well attested by the arrival of the current volume.

Notwithstanding this more recent shift, positive psychology has been subject to criticisms that it may *appear*, at least, as the preserve of the white, middle-class intellectual, and has been charged with the same (Constantine & Sue, 2006). Given the predominant make-up of psychology faculties, this may not be an unreasonable observation, nor is it unrealistic to see why, since as social psychology has well-established, all of us have a natural tendency to see the world through our own lenses, biases and even prejudices. Notwithstanding this, efforts are increasingly being made to bring more of a culturally informed lens to our understanding of positive psychology topics, such as subjective well-being (Suh & Diener, 2000) and character strengths, including international surveys (Park, Peterson, & Seligman, 2006), and in innovative fashion for the discipline, qualitative field research with culturally diverse communities in situ (Biswas-Diener, 2006; Biswas-Diener & Diener, 2001).

P.A. Linley (✉)
Centre of Applied Positive Psychology, Coventry, UK
e-mail: Alex.linley@cappeu.com

R. Biswas-Diener (ed.), *Positive Psychology as Social Change*,
DOI 10.1007/978-90-481-9938-9_9, © Springer Science+Business Media B.V. 2011

In the field of positive psychology and social change however, which is itself in the very early days of emergence, there is very little that has as yet been done to take positive psychology out of the "ivory tower" of academic research labs, and into the potentially less salubrious environs of underprivileged communities where social change could not be needed more desperately.

In this chapter, therefore, our intention is to introduce the reader to how we and others have been doing exactly that, by using positive psychology and strengths-based approaches in community development. We showcase three examples of this work, drawing from the ABCD Institute and LASA Development, together with focusing on our work with the Shiriti slum community in Kolkata, India, in support of which we describe the work of The Strengths Project, including how and why it was established, and the guiding principles by which it operates. The chapter concludes by looking forward at some of the challenges and opportunities faced by strengths-based approaches to social change. Before we examine specific examples of strengths-based approaches to community development, however, we set the broader context for our work in two ways: first, by reviewing the evidence that strengths matter and that strengths-based approaches specifically make a difference; second, by reviewing extant work from other fields that have attempted to take strengths-based approaches into the arena of social policy formation and delivery.

What Is the Evidence That Strengths Make a Difference?

Much of our work in the applications of positive psychology is concerned with how we can take strengths approaches into practice. To this end, we are also constantly engaged in our own strengths research, as well as keeping abreast of developments in the field. Rather than present an exhaustive literature review that would probably be over-the-top for the focus of this chapter, let us give you a bullet point summary of the evidence that strengths approaches make a difference:

- In a study of 19,187 employees from 34 organisations across seven industries and 29 countries, the Corporate Leadership Council (2002) found that when managers emphasised performance strengths, performance was 36.4% higher, and when they emphasised personality strengths, performance was 21.3% higher. In contrast, emphasising weaknesses led to a 26.8% decline for performance weaknesses and a 5.5% decline for personality weaknesses;
- Strengths use was associated with higher levels of happiness, fulfilment, vitality, self-esteem and self-efficacy in a study of 214 college students (Govindji & Linley, 2007). In regression analyses controlling for other variables, strengths use remained a significant predictor of these outcomes, together with self-esteem;
- Strengths use was significantly associated with subjective well-being, self-esteem, self-efficacy, and physical and mental health in a sample of 135 college

students. It was also a significant predictor of subjective well-being together with self-esteem (Proctor, Maltby, & Linley, 2009);

- Using character strengths in pursuit of goals makes us more likely to achieve those goals, as demonstrated in a repeated-measures longitudinal design over a 3-month period by Linley and colleagues (2010a). Goal attainment, in turn, was associated with need satisfaction and in turn with greater happiness and well-being;
- The opportunity to do what one does best each day, that is, using our strengths, is a core predictor of workplace engagement, which, in turn, is a core predictor of a range of business outcomes (Harter, Schmidt, & Keyes, 2002);
- Greater endorsement of character strengths is associated with higher levels of life satisfaction, particularly for so-called "strengths of the heart" (Park, Peterson, & Seligman, 2004);
- People instructed to use their top five character strengths in a new and different way each day for 1 week reported higher levels of well-being and lower levels of depression, even up to 6 months later, with this being moderated by continued practice of the activity (Seligman, Steen, Park, & Peterson, 2005);
- When focusing on self-development, people improve faster on areas where they are already strong, than they do in areas where they are weak, contrary to some popular perceptions that focusing on weakness development brings the greatest return (Sheldon, Kasser, Smith, & Share, 2002);
- Developing realised or unrealised strengths over a 4-week period led to increases in self-esteem, happiness and well-being, and lower levels of stress in a sample of university administrators (Minhas, 2010).

Based on a combination of empirical, theoretical, experiential and anecdotal work, Linley (2008) has suggested that realising strengths in ourselves and others may be the "smallest thing to make the biggest difference". He also sets out the three pillars of responsibility of the strengths approach: first, a personal responsibility to use and develop our strengths; second, a collective responsibility to create the conditions that enable the strengths of others; and third, a social responsibility to harness strengths for the benefit of wider society (Linley, 2008, Chap. 8).

Our organisational consulting through CAPP allows us to reach large numbers of people through strengthening individuals and strengthening organisations. We do so as a strengths-based organisation ourselves, and therefore are focused on delivering against the first and second pillars of personal and collective responsibility. Our work through The Strengths Project, as we go on to discuss below, has as an explicit aim to strengthen underprivileged communities who would not otherwise have access to this work, and so help us in discharging something of the third pillar, our social responsibility to harness strengths for the wider benefit of society. Before moving on to look specifically at our work through The Strengths Project, we first turn our attention to how strengths approaches have been used to effect social change to date.

Strengths-Based Approaches to Effect Social Change: The Practice of American Social Work

The strongest evidence for the use of strengths approaches to effect social change is to be found through the activities of American social work. Consider, for example, the following extracts from the National Association of Social Workers Code of Ethics (2008):

> The primary mission of the social work profession is *to enhance human well-being* and help meet the basic human needs of all people, with particular attention to the needs and empowerment of people who are vulnerable, oppressed, and living in poverty. *A historic and defining feature of social work is the profession's focus on individual well-being in a social context and the well-being of society* ... Social workers promote social justice and social change with and on behalf of clients .... *Social workers seek to enhance the capacity of people to address their own needs.* Social workers also seek to promote the responsiveness of organizations, communities, and other social institutions to individuals' needs and social problems. [Italics added]

Here is a body that holds the enhancement of human well-being at its core, and which is focused on helping people to enhance their own capacity and ability to address their own needs. In practice, this has led to the development of strengths-based social work practice as being a core social work model and approach (e.g. Rapp & Goscha, 2006; Saleebey, 2006).

Notably, however, there are core similarities but also differences in how social work views the strengths approach and how it is understood by psychologists. This difference is not surprising, given the differing levels of analysis and interpretation that typically guide each discipline in broad terms, namely, the level of the individual and group (psychology) and the level of the community and society (social work). As such, the two approaches tend to share core philosophical assumptions of the strengths approach, but implement those assumptions are differing levels of specificity in practice. Importantly, these differing levels of specificity are in no way mutually exclusive, but in contrast could be synergistically reinforcing – an opportunity to which we return below.

In practice for the strengths approach, this plays out that in social work, the strengths approach is taken to be focused philosophically on the assets, talents, capabilities, capacities, skills, abilities, resources and aspirations that exist within people and communities, and which can be tapped into as a means of creating the social change they desire. In psychology, the strengths approach holds this same philosophical assumption, but is focused more specifically at the level of the individual and individual characteristics, in the form of specific character strengths or psychological strengths, or the generic use of strengths (notwithstanding more recent work on the development of strengths-based organisations; e.g. Garcea, Harrington, & Linley, 2010; Chapter 10 by Garcea and Linley, this volume).

The strengths approach in social work practice has been and continues to be applied across a wide range of settings and populations, including family work, youth work, chronic illness, substance, misuse, poverty and community development, to name but a few (Saleebey, 2006).

In specific terms of strengths-based *policy development*, however, the approach is emergent (Hill, 2008). Most policy development tends to be led top-down by politicians whose re-election rests, they believe, on the amelioration or improvement of social or economic problems. As such, their focus is naturally on problems, and their approaches tend to be problem-led, rather than solution-focused or strengths-based. Through the efforts of the American Psychological Association Division 27/37 Task Force on Strengths-based Research and Policy, however, specific attention is being given to how policy development may be better informed from a strengths perspective, and work is being undertaken to review and revisit policy development that builds on inherent strengths, rather than focusing exclusively on the presenting problems (Maton, Schellenbach, Leadbeater, & Solarz, 2004).

As examples of how this "policy approach" can and is actually being used in practice, we turn our attention now to exploring three examples of strengths-based community development and positive social change, from the Asset-Based Community Development Institute in the United States, LASA Development working in Nepal and our own work through The Strengths Project in Kolkata, India.

The Asset-Based Community Development Institute

As a specific example of the strengths approach in practice in community development, the work of the Asset-Based Community Development Institute (www.abcdinstitute.org) is instructive. The ABCD Institute was founded by John McKnight and Jody Kretzmann, and is based at the School of Education and Social Policy at Northwestern University. It is engaged in four primary community-building activities:

(i) building community capacity through engaging directly with community groups to support their asset-based community development activities;
(ii) conducting research through partnering with community residents and other local entities so as to inform the development of community objectives;
(iii) working directly with students and others to help build the next generation of community and civic leaders; and
(iv) producing community-building publications and other resources to support practitioners in the field and build the evidence base for the role of asset-based community development in strengthening communities (see http://www.abcdinstitute.org/about/).

The ABCD Institute considers the local assets of communities as the primary building blocks of sustainable community development, and define these as:

- the skills of local residents;
- the power of local associations;
- the resources of public, private and non-profit institutions;
- the physical infrastructure and space in a community;

- the economic resources and potential of local places; and
- the local history and culture of a neighbourhood.

Building on the skills of local residents, the power of local associations, and the supportive functions of local institutions, asset-based community development draws upon existing community strengths to build stronger, more sustainable communities for the future.

A key focus of the ABCD Institute approach to community-building is through the asset-mapping of the current strengths and resources of the community with which they are working. It is this focus on the positives that are already in existence for a community, rather than a focus on lamenting what it lacks, that truly defines their approach as strengths-based. As the founders of the ABCD Institute describe it:

> Each community boasts a unique combination of assets on which to build its future. A thorough map of those assets would begin with an inventory of the gifts, skills, and capacities of the community's residents. Household by household, building by building, block by block, the capacity mapmakers will discover a vast and often surprising array of individual talents and productive skills, few of which are being mobilized for community-building purposes. (Kretzmann & McKnight, 1993)

As such, the focus of the work of the ABCD Institute is on how the existing assets of a community can be harnessed to create the future that the residents of that community want to enjoy, as the Mercado Central case illustrates.

A Case Study in the United States: The Mercado Central Minneapolis, Minnesota – ABCD Institute

In Minneapolis, Minnesota, asset-based community development principles were merged with traditional community organising in a process of connecting the talent and energy of the community around issues such as building a church and working on immigration issues. These organising efforts had primed the community to be ready for change, and the Mercado Central is the economic engine for change they decided to create.

The Mercado Central is a retail business cooperative that was developed by the Latino immigrant community in Minneapolis, Minnesota. It is the result of the creativity and hard work of members of this community, who joined forces with a faith-based organising group and numerous community organisations to build a traditional marketplace in their inner-city neighbourhood. In doing so, the Mercado Central has transformed the lives of people in this community by recognising their capacity to build their own local economy in a manner that reflected their traditions. It is home to 44 businesses and represents unfaltering commitment to leadership development, as well as being a signal example about how the power of community working together can overcome individual limitations when people strive to overcome the challenges they face alone.

As a result of this initiative, these are some of the outcomes that they achieved:

- The community purchase and renovation of three dilapidated buildings; $2.4 million invested;
- Over US $277,000 in small business loans made to new Latino businesses;
- Forty-four businesses established and/or expanded in the local community;
- First-year sales of over US $2 million at Mercado businesses, benefiting both owners – many of whom are local residents – and the neighbourhood itself;
- Increased local employment opportunities at Mercado Central businesses, with more than 70 new jobs created, employing mostly local people;
- Increased city and state revenues – over US $80,000 in sales tax paid out by Mercado Central merchants in the first year of operation.

LASA Development

Another example of a community-building organisation that operates from strengths-based principles is LASA Development. Founded by Patricia Lustig in 1990, LASA Development is a service organisation that has implicitly developed a strengths-based approach both to the way in which they work as an organisation and the contribution that they make to the developing world. LASA is successful as a result of utilising synergies with other organisations, either in partnership or as joint ventures based on their experience in leadership, coaching, creativity and organisational change. LASA has conducted projects in both Nepal and the United Kingdom, and we include an example of one of their projects in Nepal here.

A Case Study in Nepal: Discover Dream Design and Delivery in Phakel – LASA Development

In one of LASA's projects in 1998, they were interested in using the strengths-based principles of Appreciative Inquiry in working with villagers in Nepal. The project was led by Mac Odell who had adapted Appreciative Inquiry to work with villagers. At the outset of the project, drawing from Appreciative Inquiry (Cooperrider & Srivastva, 1987), LASA ran a mini-4D cycle (Discovery, Dream, Design and Delivery) in 2 h, which was all the time the subsistence-level farmers had to give them, in Phakhel, Nepal.

Throughout the project, they held meetings every few months and visited the villagers about three times a year to support the process. They separated the men, women and children into different groups and came together to share information and go through the 4D cycle as follows:

- *Discovery* – asking villagers to tell a story about something that had gone well in the village, which they had done together. They had them draw on flip chart paper because most of them were illiterate. Extra time was necessary in the beginning to get the women to even pick up a pen!

- *Dreaming* – asking the groups what kind of a village they would like for their children and grandchildren, again getting them to draw their dreams for the future;
- *Design* – asking the villagers to plan – they discovered that people who could not read did not seem to have developed the logical sides of their brains enough and did not know how to plan, so this had to be taught! To teach how to plan, LASA Development worked with things they were already doing (like when to plant their crops and the steps they needed to take) and built upon that – a classic example of building on the strengths that already existed within the people;
- *Delivery* – when the villagers came back to report on the Design, they all stood up and went straight into who committed to do what. In this way, they were committing to each other the steps that they would each take, individually and collectively, in order to make the delivery of their design a reality. They then debriefed to see what they had learned throughout the process. Finally, the people danced and sang to celebrate their achievements, and to leave them with a fun memory of the work they have done.

Through this Appreciative Inquiry as a means of community-building, note the outcomes that have been achieved:

- The villagers raised ₹ 34,000 (an incredible amount for a community of 88 families where the average income for a family of six is about ₹ 10,000 per year) and had sunk the school foundations when LASA Development visited them in May 2000. They then built upon the foundations subsequently, once these had stabilised during the monsoon season;
- The village received a grant for ₹ 2.2 million from PLAN International to build the first model secondary school. The school has 14 classrooms on two floors;
- The villagers had raised in excess of ₹ 162,000 themselves. This money was put towards the registration fee, because secondary schools are not provided by the government, which requires a fee of ₹ 50,000 for a secondary school to be registered with them. The registration fee was paid, and additional funds were used for paying the teachers' salaries and buying equipment and books, as the government does not support secondary schools in any way. Teachers earn on average between ₹ 4,000 and 8,000 per month;
- The village has moved from strength to strength with these outcomes. The project reflected strong community organisation, led by an unmarried lady in her forties, a 70-year-old grandfather and another gentleman in his forties who does have children, now attending secondary school far away from home in Kathmandu.

This has become a truly sustainable project based on the foundations of building upon community strengths and positive psychology, as illustrated by this quote from a man, who, during the 4D sessions, got up to say:

> This really brings it home to me. We've been bloody lazy! For the past 40 years we have been holding our hands out for aid from the government and what do we get? We fight, we

can't agree on anything and we don't feel good about ourselves. 40 years ago, we did a lot together because there was no one else to help us and you know what? We were proud of what we did! We were proud of our village. Are any of you proud now? No? Well, let's do this together and be proud again!

This quote powerfully illustrates the potential of strengths approaches to help people, groups, organisations and communities, to develop themselves and build a better future by realising the best of what they already have within themselves. This is a theme that resonates throughout our work with The Strengths Project, which we go on to describe next.

The Strengths Project: Background, Establishment and Objectives

For the vast majority of us, the only experience or exposure that we are likely to have had to the an Indian slum community way of life is through the Danny Boyle-directed film, *Slumdog Millionaire*, itself based on the original novel *Q & A* by Vikas Swarup (2005), or any of the numerous documentary spin-offs that seem to have followed the box office success of *Slumdog*, such as Kevin McCloud's *Slumming It*, which was recently broadcast on Channel 4 in the UK.

This cannot be said of our colleague Robert Biswas-Diener, whose field work conducting qualitative interviews and collecting survey data with sex workers and slum dwellers in Kolkata has proved seminal for the field (Biswas-Diener & Diener, 2001). Nor can it be said of the two native Indian authors of this chapter, Bhaduri and Sen Sharma, who both spend a significant proportion of their time working with slum dwellers in their role as Community Workers for The Strengths Project. And for Linley and Govindji, our first-hand experience of working with slum communities in Kolkata comes from our first visit there of February 2008, during which we were able to spend several days visiting a number of different slum communities in Kolkata, but particularly the Shiriti community with whom we are now working through The Strengths Project. For those less fortunate than us who do not have this opportunity, we strongly recommend *Calcutta: The Human Face of Poverty*, by Frederic C. Thomas (1999), which provides one of the best descriptions of life as it is lived in Kolkata that we have ever read.

Initial Experiences of the Shiriti Kalabagan Slum Community

To help you picture the scene, consider the following, all of which we experienced first-hand on visiting the slum:

- The floor is compacted dirt, since there is no tarmac or paving stones;
- The homes are constructed of corrugated iron, advertising hoardings, large concrete pipes, wooden boards, tree trunks and anything else available that can be put to good use;

- There is a toxic lake off to one side, where we are told a young boy from the slum drowned a couple of years previously. The lake is littered with rubbish and there are no barriers of any description to prevent the children from reaching it;
- There is one toilet that serves the community of c. 2,500 people. It is a corrugated iron construction of about two square metres in area, which sits over a hole in the ground, since there are of course no sewage works in place;
- There is one tap with cold running water that serves this same community of 800 people. It is only on at certain times of the day, so outside of these times people have to go without or make do with water they have put by from earlier;
- Where people have electricity, it is often provided through a maze of over-ground cables that have illegally tapped into the municipal lamppost or similar.
  And yet, note also the following:
- The children are typically happy – even very happy – appearing carefree and having fun with whatever they are doing and whatever is available;
- The women work hard to maintain a real sense of pride in their homes, polishing their display ornaments and cooking meals to provide nourishment to the best of their abilities;
- The men go out to find work, whether as factory hands, farm labourers, or more typically, auto-rickshaw drivers or rickshaw pullers;
- People talk to each other wherever they go, everybody seems to know everybody else and there is an intricate web of social interactions at every moment of the day;
- There is a real sense of community – never have I (PAL) felt such an outsider when I first entered the slum, to then feel the safest and most connected I have ever felt as part of a community when I was accepted into the slum community.

It is of course a cliché, and yet we still do not see people queuing up to trade places with them, but there is clearly much that we can learn from these communal networks of social integration and interdependency. They are *communities* in the truest sense of the word, something which we in the "developed" Western world seem to have done much to lose (e.g. Putnam, 2001), but hopefully may yet regain (Putnam & Feldstein, 2005).

Our visits to Shiriti and other slum communities in Kolkata were for a specific purpose. Through the establishment of The Strengths Project, we wanted to take positive psychology and strengths approaches out to communities who would not otherwise have access to these resources. It is a travesty of the social order against which many of us labour, but the natural law seems to dictate that those who need things least find it the easiest to get them, whereas those who need them the most find it the hardest – whether it is food or finance, or, in the case of The Strengths Project, access to the individual, group and community-building knowledge, technologies and resources of strengths and positive psychology.

Having conducted our field visits, together with Robert Biswas-Diener and under the guidance and language translation of our co-authors, Avirupa Bhaduri and Debasish Sen Sharma, we set about working out how we could take The Strengths Project forward into practice through working with a slum community in Kolkata.

We identified the Shiriti slum as our primary focus, on the basis that it was more of a permanent structure, and more organised, than other slum communities we had visited, and so had some of the community infrastructure that was necessary for our work. Avirupa Bhaduri was appointed as a full-time Community Worker for the project, and Debasish Sen Sharma provided additional support on a part-time basis.

A Case Study in India: Strengthening the Shiriti Kalabagan Slum Community in Kolkata – The Strengths Project

Our first work was focused on exploring the strengths that existed within this slum community. We did so through using an approach adapted from the Individual Strengths Assessments which were developed by CAPP as a means of identifying, exploring and developing strengths in individual people (Linley, 2008, Chap. 4). At this time, we were unaware of the work of the ABCD Institute, and particularly their seminal work on community asset mapping (Kretzmann & McKnight, 1993), to which we would strongly recommend any interested reader.

Notwithstanding this, the interviews conducted with the Shiriti slum dwellers by Avirupa Bhaduri provided rich data to inform our future work with the community. For reference, the interview schedule used is included at Appendix 1. Avirupa Bhaduri describes some of the outcomes and experiences that came through this first phase of the project:

In March 2008 we had first thought of mapping the strengths in Shiriti, a slum in south Kolkata, which is home of about 500 families, each comprising of 5 members on an average. This was a pioneering idea. The objective was to learn how positive psychology could effectively be applied to bring in social change. We did an initial survey, the outcome was inspiring. We found that most people, even in the face of poverty and hardship, led a thriving family and community life. The women were especially strong, and retained many core strengths. We conducted a specially designed ISA with them and realized that there was a clear prospect of improving their lives, based on their own strengths. Unlike most charitable organizations, we decided not to donate money. Instead we held a meeting with the women. In that meeting two clear facts emerged. They need extra income and most of them were keen to learn sewing as they felt there's a demand for sewing jobs which they can do in their free time sitting in the comfort of their home.

We decided to start by forming a sewing group. The women were asked to sign up for an 8–10 months course of sewing. Within the next couple of weeks there was a huge response. A total of 60 women from all age group signed up. Then the hunt for a teacher began. We found the perfect teacher in Sutapa Paul. Being a struggler herself she understood the group very well. Then on the inaugural day four sewing machines were donated from Robert [Biswas-Diener] and a women's sewing group [in Portland, Oregon].

The women gave a hearty welcome to the machines. A puja was conducted; the machines were decorated with garlands. The tiny room of the local club was filled with laughter and shouts of joy. The enthusiasm was infectious. The class started on 14th March in that small room. The local boys happily agreed to let the women use their room during noon, when it usually remained unused. After a month some left the group but most stuck on. However the women who left, kept in touch and insisted that they wanted to be a part of the group in other ways. Some expressed desire to buy material and fabrics at the best rate; some said they were good at keeping the books. Others claimed that they have contacts with local tailors and will try and get orders for the group. So all of us decided to form a co-operative which will be run by the group, where everyone will do what they liked best.

Some very enthusiastic women, among them Seema, Tulsi, Orpita, Jyotsna, Hena, came together on a fine March afternoon, for their first lesson in sewing at Nabadiganta club, located just on the fringes of Shiriti Kalabagan slum. It's a pioneering effort whereby initially the women group was given support like, buying four sewing machines, supplying them with raw materials, (fabric, needles, thread and so on), also arranging a trainer for them till such time they are skilled. The aim is to eventually form a co-operative where the jobs will be aligned according to their strengths.

The class starts at 2 p.m., 3 days a week, with approximately 25 people in each batch. They gather much before that, and each day they take turns to clean the room and assemble the class. As soon as Sutapa Paul, the teacher arrives, the class begins. The group by now has learnt quite a lot. They have already made petticoats, baby frocks, and is now learning to make salwar kameez. Few are quick learners, but all of them are very enthusiastic. Our next target is to arrange for an exhibition of the wares at an alternative city art gallery, so that the co-op will have a confidence boost that will surge our endeavour forward!!F During the Bengali New Year the group will showcase the various items that they have made during their course in a stall in the same club premise. We are now making preparations and finalizing the ideas for the stall decoration, fixing the price etc. All of us are excited and are determined to make it a success."

In Conclusion: Challenges and Possibilities for Strengths as a Means of Social Change

A cynical question would be to ask whether we could possibly make any substantive difference in a city of 9 million like Kolkata when we work with only a single community of 2,500 people; this, especially in the larger context of a billion people in our world who are below the poverty line (Collier, 2007; Sachs, 2005). Our response is simple. Like the boy walking along the beach littered with starfish that had been washed up by the tide, challenged by his father that he could make no difference as he picked them up one at a time and threw them back into the sea, he replied, "Well, I made a difference to that one ... and that one ... and that one ...".

All we can do is our best, trying to make a difference when and where we can. Not even to try is the greatest quitting of all, doing something that changes even one life for the better is something worth doing. If we all took this philosophy into practice, the world could well be a very different and more positive place.

As but two inspirational examples, consider the original US $27 that Muhammad Yunus ultimately turned into the billion-dollar people-owned Grameen Bank (Yunus, 1998), and for which he and Grameen were awarded the Nobel Peace Prize, or BRAC, regarded as the largest and most successful NGO in the world, which started in Bangladesh and is now spreading its methodology of grassroots activities and community involvement to overcome poverty around the world (Smillie, 2009). For other examples, see the inspirational stories of social change agents and social entrepreneurs included in Baderman and Law (2006), Bornstein (2007), and Elkington and Hartigan (2008).

Further, as the experiences reported by the ABCD Institute and LASA Development show, and also in our work with The Strengths Project, we have found that adopting and applying strengths-based approaches to community development can be a powerful and transformative force for positive social change. By building on the strengths (however broadly defined) of the individuals, families, groups that make up these community populations, as well as those of their wider social networks, it is possible to harness an intrinsic motivation for change that was always there, but latent, and in doing so, to inspire people with a passion for their own potential, a belief in their own capabilities and what they can achieve through them.

For us, this is the real payoff through using strengths as a force for positive social change, because we are enabling people to use their strengths to strengthen themselves and also to strengthen others, in doing so strengthening their communities and opportunities for future growth, development, fulfilment and flourishing. In doing so, we are proud to be meeting each of the three pillars of responsibility of the strengths approach that were laid out by Linley (2008): first, a personal responsibility to use and develop our strengths; second, a collective responsibility to create the conditions that enable the strengths of others; and third, a social responsibility to harness strengths for the benefit of wider society (Linley, 2008, Chap. 8). For our own work, both in practice and in dissemination, such as through this chapter, it is one of the key ways in which we deliver against CAPP's mission of *Strengthening the World*. We hope that in doing so we have been able to inspire you to use your strengths to strengthen others as well.

Acknowledgements We each wish to acknowledge our deep gratitude and profound respect for the work of our friend and colleague, Dr. Robert Biswas-Diener, the volume editor, whose work on positive psychology and poverty, including his field visits to Kolkata, provided the foundation on which The Strengths Project was established, and hence the basis on which this chapter was able to be written. Thank you, Robert, for your advocacy of the poor and underprivileged through positive psychology, and for your work as a Founding Trustee of The Strengths Project. We also acknowledge and thank our colleague Linda Woolston, who also serves with us as a Trustee of The Strengths Project. Finally, we wish to recognise the resilience and positivity of all those underprivileged communities with whom we have worked, and who continue to inspire us every day.

Appendix: Shiriti Kalabagan Strengths Mapping Interview Schedule

1. Tell me about your daily routine. What activities do you typically do?
2. Which of these activities do you enjoy/enjoy most?
3. What is it you like best about these activities?
4. What other work-related activities do you enjoy?
5. How about recreational activities? How do you like to spend your free time?
6. What do you like about this activity/these activities?

7. Are there activities you do not have the opportunity to do as much as you would like? What might those be?
8. When your friends or family members give you compliments what do they typically say?
9. Think back to a specific day or time that you are especially proud of.... Tell me about that day.
10. What made that day so special?
11. What did you do to contribute to making that day special?
12. What accomplishment are you most proud of in life?
13. What have you contributed, specifically, that makes you proud of this?
14. Tell me when you feel the most energised and happy? What are you typically doing?
15. What is so energising about that activity?
16. If you could choose a vision of the future to aim for, what would it be?
17. Why would you choose that vision rather than others?
18. In this future vision, what personal contributions do you see yourself making?
19. What do you feel your strengths are? That is, what are you best at?
20. How often do you have the opportunity to use these strengths?
21. When you compare Shiritri, to what you know of other bustees, what do you think makes it different?
22. What do you think Shiritri has going for it that makes it as successful as it is (or, more successful than other bustees)?
23. When do you have the opportunity to do what you do best?
24. Do you have someone who supports and encourages you?
25. When you think back to yesterday, did you have the opportunity to learn something new yesterday? What?

References

Baderman, J., & Law, J. (2006). *Everyday legends: The stories of 20 great UK social entrepreneurs.* York: WW Publishing.

Biswas-Diener, R. (2006). From the equator to the North Pole: A study of character strengths. *Journal of Happiness Studies, 7,* 293–310.

Biswas-Diener, R., & Diener, E. (2001). Making the best of a bad situation: Satisfaction in the slums of Calcutta. *Social Indicators Research, 55,* 329–352.

Bornstein, D. (2007). *How to change the world: Social entrepreneurs and the power of new ideas.* Oxford: Oxford University Press.

Collier, P. (2007). *The bottom billion: Why the poorest countries are failing and what can be done about it.* Oxford: Oxford University Press.

Constantine, M. G., & Sue, D. W. (2006). Factors contributing to optimal human functioning in people of color in the United States. *The Counseling Psychologist, 34,* 228–244.

Cooperrider, D. L., & Srivastva, S. (1987). Appreciative inquiry in organizational life. In R. W. Woodman & W. A. Pasmore (Eds.), *Research in organizational change and development* (Vol. 1, pp. 129–169). Greenwich, CT: JAI Press.

Corporate Leadership Council. (2002). *Performance management survey.* Washington, DC: Author.

Elkington, J., & Hartigan, P. (2008). *The power of unreasonable people: How social entrepreneurs create markets that change the world*. Boston: Harvard Business Press.

Garcea, N., Harrington, S., & Linley, P. A. (Eds.). (2010). *Oxford handbook of positive psychology and work*. New York: Oxford University Press.

Govindji, R., & Linley, P. A. (2007). Strengths use, self-concordance and well-being: Implications for strengths coaching and coaching psychologists. *International Coaching Psychology Review*, 2(2), 143–153.

Harter, J. K., Schmidt, F. L., & Hayes, T. L. (2002). Business-unit-level relationship between employee satisfaction, employee engagement, and business outcomes: A meta-analysis. *Journal of Applied Psychology*, 87, 268–279.

Hill, K. (2008). A strengths-based framework for social policy: Barriers and possibilities. *Journal of Policy Practice*, 7(2–3), 106–121.

Kretzman, J., & McKnight, J. L. (1993). *Building communities from the inside out: Centre for Urban Affairs and Policy Research*. Chicago: ACTA Publications.

Linley, A. (2008). *Average to A: Realising strengths in yourself and others*. Coventry: CAPP Press.

Linley, P. A., Joseph, S., Harrington, S., & Wood, A. M. (2006). Positive psychology: Past, present, and (possible) future. *Journal of Positive Psychology*, 1, 3–16.

Linley, P. A., Nielsen, K. M., Wood, A. M., Gillett, R., & Biswas-Diener, R. (2010a). Using signature strengths in pursuit of goals: Effects on goal progress, need satisfaction, and well-being, and implications for coaching psychologists. *International Coaching Psychology Review*, 5(1), 6–15.

Linley, A., Willars, J., & Biswas-Diener, R. (2010b). *The strengths book: Be confident, be successful, and enjoy better relationships by realising the best of you*. Coventry: CAPP Press.

Maton, K. I., Schellenbach, C. J., Leadbeater, B. J., & Solarz, A. L. (Eds.). (2004). *Investing in children, youth, families, and communities: Strengths-based research and policy*. Washington, DC: American Psychological Association.

Minhas, G. (2010). Developing realised and unrealised strengths: Implications for engagement, self-esteem, life satisfaction and well-being. *Assessment and Development Matters*, 2, 12–16.

National Association of Social Workers. (2008). *Code of ethics of the National Association of Social Workers*. Retrieved February 13, 2010, from http://www.socialworkers.org/pubs/code/code.asp

Park, N., Peterson, C., & Seligman, M. E. P. (2004). Strengths of character and well-being. *Journal of Social and Clinical Psychology*, 23, 603–619.

Park, N., Peterson, C., & Seligman, M. E. P. (2006). Character strengths in fifty-four nations and the fifty US states. *Journal of Positive Psychology*, 1, 118–129.

Proctor, C., Maltby, J., & Linley, P. A. (2009). Strengths use as a predictor of well-being and health-related quality of life. *Journal of Happiness Studies*, 10, 583–630.

Putnam, R. D. (2001). *Bowling alone: The collapse and revival of American community*. New York: Simon & Schuster.

Putnam, R. D., & Feldstein, L. M. (2005). *Better together: Restoring the American community*. New York: Simon & Schuster.

Rapp, C. A., & Goscha, R. J. (Eds.). (2006). *The strengths model: Case management with people with psychiatric difficulties*. New York: Oxford University Press.

Sachs, J. (2005). *The end of poverty: How we can make it happen in our lifetime*. Harmondsworth: Penguin.

Saleebey, D. (Ed.). (2006). *The strengths perspective in social work practice* (4th ed.). Boston: Allyn & Bacon.

Seligman, M. E. P., & Csikszentmihalyi, M. (2000). Positive psychology: An introduction. *American Psychologist*, 55, 5–14.

Seligman, M. E. P., Steen, T. A., Park, N., & Peterson, C. (2005). Positive psychology progress: Empirical validation of interventions. *American Psychologist, 60,* 410–421.

Sheldon, K. M., Kasser, T., Smith, K., & Share, T. (2002). Personal goals and psychological growth: Testing an intervention to enhance goal-attainment and personality integration. *Journal of Personality, 70,* 5–31.

Smillie, I. (2009). *Freedom from want: The remarkable success story of BRAC, the global grassroots organization that's winning the fight against poverty.* Sterling, VA: Kumarian Press.

Suh, E. M., & Diener, E. (Eds.). (2000). *Culture and subjective well-being.* Cambridge, MA: MIT Press.

Swarup, V. (2005). *Q & A.* New York: Scribner Book Company.

Thomas, F. C. (1999). *Calcutta: The human face of poverty.* Calcutta: Penguin Books.

Yunus, M. (1998). *Banker to the poor: The story of Grameen Bank.* London: Aurum Press.

Chapter 10
Creating Positive Social Change Through Building Positive Organizations: Four Levels of Intervention

Nicky Garcea and P. Alex Linley

Positive psychology is both reflective and enabling of wider cultural trends – the zeitgeist of our times
(Linley, Joseph, Harrington, & Wood, 2006).

There is no doubt that in the last decade applications of positive psychology in the workplace have provided organizations with "another way" of doing business and managing people. The term "positive organization" shares its origins with Seligman's (2002) third pillar of authentic happiness as being "positive institutions." While the first pillar of positive emotion, and the second pillar of positive characteristics have been examined in detail, the third pillar of positive institutions has received less attention – which is probably symptomatic of psychology's typically predominant focus on the individual or interpersonal level of interaction, as distinct from the level of the institution, community, or social system (of course with exceptions – please allow us to speak in general terms here). In practice, however, the concept of the positive institution has captured the attention of many organizations that are increasingly grappling with questions of their own identity, purpose, and sustainability in the context of our changing economic, social, technological, and environmental world order.

These organizations often start off with the broad questions of "What would a positive organization look like?" or "How do we build a positive organization?" The answer to this question lies in how we conceptualize organizations in the first instance. The accepted conceptualization of organizations can be traced back to the early influence of people like Max Weber (bureaucratic structures) and Frederick Winslow Taylor (time and motion studies; the demarcation of labor), both of whom have had immeasurable impact on organizational design that continues to this day – often unappreciated by those who unwittingly and unconsciously apply their precepts, simply on the basis that "this is the way things are," rather than asking themselves the more challenging but worthwhile question of "How ought organizations to be?"

N. Garcea (✉)
Centre of Applied Positive Psychology, Coventry, UK
e-mail: Nicky.garcea@cappeu.com

R. Biswas-Diener (ed.), *Positive Psychology as Social Change*,
DOI 10.1007/978-90-481-9938-9_10, © Springer Science+Business Media B.V. 2011

Leading management and organizational thinkers have recently begun to turn their attention to these questions, and early views of alternative models for organization are beginning to emerge. For example, Dave Ulrich writes on the "abundant organization" (Ulrich, 2009) and Gary Hamel considers the future of management through greater management innovation. So, while we acknowledge the progress that is being made, we recognize that nonetheless, for many people in many organizations, the institutions in which they work remain constructed on the basis of mental models of how things should be done that date back to the nineteenth century – notwithstanding the fact that we're now in the twenty-first!

In this chapter, we will introduce our work on helping organizations to re-imagine and reinvent themselves as positive organizations. In doing so, our focus on this occasion is not to attend to organizations themselves as agents of positive social change through their outputs per se (see Garcea, Harrington, & Linley, 2009, for some of our thoughts on this), and which has been the subject of much sustained interest in recent years. Instead, we focus our attention on the steps through which organizations may evolve to become more "positive organizations" and we do so through attending to the difference that can be made to their employees' experience of work as a result. It is our aim that this chapter will heighten practitioners' awareness of the potential impact that their interventions can have on the entire organizational system, thereby developing individuals, teams, and organizations to find meaning and fulfillment in their "great work."

Developing Positive Organizations

Positive organizations are developed by the actions of the people, groups, and leaders working within them, the fabric of the system. Developing positive organization for many is an organizational development process. Essentially, it is when we apply positive psychology principles in the design of our interventions, with the aim of creating organizations that are more performance-enhancing, life-affirming, and fulfillment-giving. In the business world context that is following the trauma of the global recession, and as many organizations look to rebuild organizational life with the mandate of "doing more with less," positive psychology interventions have much to offer and much that is needed. The key question, which we are asked and face so often, is where to begin?

There was a time that we thought there was actually an answer to this question – that if we knew enough, read more, collected enough experiences – then we would be able to say, "Yes, you begin to build positive organizations by doing ..." and then go on to lay out a tried and trusted roadmap of the steps that need to be taken. Two things happened. One: the world has changed, and it's not changing back. The speed of change means that fixed models of organizational change are more broken than they ever were before. Two: we got wise (or at least wiser) – we hope. In true social constructionist fashion, we've come to see that there is not, and could never be, one single answer to this question that is always the right answer (despite what the leading management consultants might tell you). Instead, there is (to paraphrase Aristotle and the golden mean), the right answer for that organization, in that context, at that point in time.

In different ways, with different organizations, in different contexts, at different points in time, we have tried different approaches to building positive organization. All of them have succeeded in some ways and failed in others, leading us ever more to conclude that there is no single right answer. We have started at the top of the organization, working exclusively with the senior management team on the basis that if they "got it" then the roll out would be smooth and supported from the top-down. It probably would have been – had the roll out ever happened. Instead, time and circumstances moved on, and the bigger opportunity was lost, although a truly positive impact was achieved with the members of the senior management team as individuals, an impact, which also cascaded to an extent and was noticed through their "leadership shadow."

We have also started at the bottom of the organization, recruiting people for their positive characteristics in an attempt to shift the culture from the ground up. It works, at least to an extent. The infusion of positivity helps to shift the culture, but then comes up against the more powerful force of the existing culture. Without leadership support for its infusion, the new culture can be subsumed into the old. So top-down can work, to an extent and bottom-up can work, to an extent. Putting them both together, you might think they would meet in the middle – but the reality is they rarely do without more specific interventions to enable it.

In contrast, we can effect change in the same way that nature effects change. Through social contagion, through dialog, through creating movements that draw everyone together and move them in the same direction. This is the focus of many emerging approaches to organizational change, which draw on biological metaphors and chaos theory principles of nonlinear dynamics, to create viral approaches to change (e.g., Christakis & Fowler, 2010; Herrero, 2008).

So, there might be three broad approaches to organizational change and building positive organizations, but how do you ever know what that answer is and which approach to take? This is where judgment comes into play, and it's that more often than not we are actually getting paid for as consultants. So, while we can't give you the perennial roadmap for building positive organizations, we can share with you examples of some of the questions that we might typically ask in constructing our judgment on how best to go forward with that organization, in that context, at that point in time.

- What is the strategic imperative and fit for this work?
- What are the compelling challenges in your business environment? How can building a positive organization help you to deal with these challenges?
- Is there an existing change initiative, being driven by business imperatives, which could be supported more effectively through adopting positive approaches?
- Is there an under-performing business unit where you could experiment with the approach and see if it makes a difference?

- Who holds the power in the organization and what payoff will they get through building a more positive organization?
- Who are the shadow stakeholders who might benefit from subverting the process?

Ultimately, as should be clear from the above, our work in practice is pragmatic rather than ideological. We do what we do because we believe in it, but we also construct the business case for doing it by focusing on the business benefits and deliverables. To effect change we need to speak in the language of those whom we seek to change, since change only rarely happens from the outside in, but far more often from the inside out. Change also happens through *dialog*. The word *dialog* comes from the ancient Greek routes of *dia* (through) and *logos* (meaning), which together can be understood as "meaning flowing through." Understood in this way, it's easy to see why dialog can be at the heart of any change initiative, because change only happens when meanings are shared and "flowing through" the different people who are both impacted by and enacting the change. This being so, we go on to explore with you the four levels at which our interventions may typically be designed to impact: the intrapersonal, the interpersonal, the group, and the organization. We provide examples of interventions that we have had first-hand experience of implementing through our consultancy and research practice at CAPP, describing both our successes and our struggles.

Intrapersonal Interventions

The biggest challenge we face in shifting the intrapersonal landscape – people's perception of and dialog with themselves – is our inherent negativity bias. We say inherent deliberately, since there is good evidence to suggest that this negativity bias is an evolutionary outcome that has stayed with us throughout our evolutionary adaptation – and for good reason: it works (Baumeister, 2001; Rozin & Royzman, 2001). Quite simply, if we don't pay attention to danger, threats, or problems, we're far more likely to end up dead. It's for this reason that the weakness focused takes root in us so deeply, because its tentacles reach deep into our archetypal psyche which is geared up to pay attention to what's wrong, what's broken, what isn't working, what's threatening. Yet, we also know that if we focus exclusively on the negative, we not only suffer, we also miss out on so much more that could be better. The right way to handle this is to recognize that our negativity bias is like a volume control: we can turn it up or turn it down as much as we want to. We don't have to turn it off, but we can choose how much, or how little, we allow it to dominate our perceptions and our lives.

These two simple things, first, understanding that we have an inherent negativity bias, and second, recognizing that we can choose to turn it up or turn it down, like a volume control, have revolutionized the perspective of many people with whom we have worked. Suddenly, they feel like they are in control of their own lives much more again. From this more solidly positive foundation, their attention then turns to what they are attending to if they are not attending to the negative all the time. In doing so, it quickly becomes apparent that they have a far poorer vocabulary for what they are good at, what they enjoy doing, what they do well.

This is where our seeding of the language of strengths comes into play. This again illustrates the power of dialog as a force for change, since by changing the language and vocabulary that people use, we are able to change the social constructions on which they focus, and in turn the ways that they respond and behave.

"Seeding" a language of strengths is often the first foundation to building a positive organizations (Page & Carter, 2008). At CAPP we developed Realise2, our online strengths assessment and development tool and model, to help individuals accurately identify their strengths, whether realized or unrealized, their weaknesses, and their learned behaviors. In our experience, individuals often have clarity when describing their weaknesses (there goes the negativity bias again), but they are less specific when describing their strengths. For this reason, seeding a language of strengths, and so changing the nature of people's dialog, at first with themselves, can be the foundation stone of intrapersonal change.

Our work at the intrapersonal level of change tends to include interventions for an individual to complete alone, since they are designed to encourage self-reflection with the intention that this intrapersonal work will stimulate shifts in thinking and behavior. As any sports professional will tell you, this work on mindset and mental preparation takes time and an equal amount, if not more practiced, than cognitive skill development. The positive psychology literature has provided a rich source of research at the intrapersonal level of interventions, including, for example, gratitude visits (Seligman, Steen, Park, & Peterson, 2005), positivity portfolios (Fredrickson, 2009), and counting your blessings (Sheldon & Lyubomirsky, 2006). Many of these interventions were reviewed by Sin and Lyubomirsky (2009), who were interested in their impact on depression and happiness.

Intrapersonal interventions can also be a critical precursor to interpersonal interventions. At CAPP, we will often ask participants who are going to take part in a team intervention to spend time on an intrapersonal activity in preparation as a way of raising their self-awareness. In our work, this is often about helping people to identify and build on their strengths more, so we ask them to complete the Realise2 online strengths assessment and reflect on their own results. Having done so, people are then well-placed to look at how their strengths can be best deployed through their relationships with others, which takes us on to the interpersonal level of intervention.

Interpersonal Interventions

In the field of organizational development, the term "using self as instrument for change" is used in relation to the organizational development practitioner's role in initiating and sustaining change processes. By using themselves as instruments for change, practitioners can position themselves in a unique role to give feedback to the system and to catalyze change. In this way, we believe individuals who are working on developing their "best selves" are likely to be the most informed and observant practitioners, leaders, and employees. It is the collection of this individual action aligned to collective outcomes that can serve the wider building of the positive organizational system.

Through shifting the nature of people's dialogs, through enabling them to have a shared language and understanding of their own strengths and the strengths of the people with whom they work, we are able to generate a more positive work culture from the outset (Minhas, 2010). The nature of people's conversations and interactions changes, and they are able to look at themselves in different and more positive ways.

The Realise2 online strengths assessment examines 60 different attributes according to the three dimensions of energy, performance, and use. It provides users with a comprehensive profile report that details there as follows:

- *Realized strengths* – the things that energize you and you do well;
- *Unrealized strengths* – the things that energize you and you do well, but maybe don't get sufficient opportunity to use as much;
- *Learned behaviors* – the things you do well but are not energized by;
- *Weaknesses* – the things you don't do well and which drain you (Fig. 10.1).

As this model reveals, through using this tool as an individual intervention we are placing substantial emphasis on unrealized strengths being our greatest areas for development. In our experience, few people know how to use their strengths more, and are not always equipped with the expertise to recognize or grow strengths

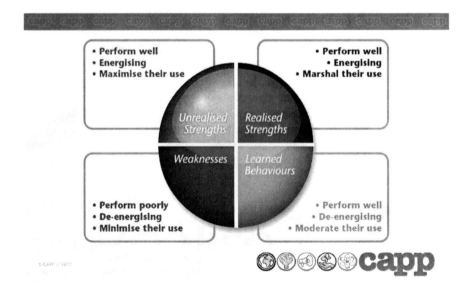

Fig. 10.1 Capp's Realise2 strengths development model

in themselves. Once individuals increase their awareness of their strengths, learned behaviors, and weaknesses we work with them to take action, using the CAPP 4 M model, which encourages individuals to:

1. *Marshal realized strengths* – dial back the use of a realized strength so as not to overuse it, or use it in a new and different situation that will be stretching and performance-enhancing.
2. *Maximize unrealized strengths* – share unrealized strengths with others, aligning them to goals, conducting upward strength social comparisons, and identifying role models who use this strengths well.
3. *Moderate learned behaviors* – Stand back and assess their impact, try to limit your reliance on them, use them alongside an unrealized strength, and most of all try to reverse your reputation if you are known only for your use of your learned behaviors.
4. *Minimize weaknesses* – if your area of weakness is not performance critical then do not focus on minimizing its impact; if it is, then consider working with a complementary partner, adjusting your role or taking action to bring the weakness up to an acceptable level.

As people understand and integrate the 4 M model into their work and development, they come to see how they can draw effectively from others through complementary partnerships or strengths-based team working. In essence, both of these involve identifying what you as an individual do best and love to do, and crafting your work to find more opportunities to do so. In parallel, it is about working with others to share out and allocate those tasks between people that can be done better by someone else in the partnership or on the team. The key question with which we leave people in this regard is "Am I the best person to be doing this task?" By learning to ask themselves this consistently, we help people to shift their behavior so that they are more consistently working to the strengths of both themselves and the people around them.

A key success factor for any interventions is that it can be sustained by the individual post-intervention. Essentially, it is our mission that at the individual level, we are providing individuals with lasting intrapersonal resources that they can sustain and nurture over time. This means that we are placing a greater emphasis on individuals taking responsibility for their own personal development. The discipline of personal responsibility is a critical success factor in individual interventions, since we are looking to people to take responsibility for their own growth and development, and to pursue this and take it in the direction that is right for them.

An additional lesson that we have also learnt at this level is that some of the simplest interventions evoke deep emotional responses. Recently, a coachee that we were working with experienced an immediate emotional reaction when she realized that her recent great work was not being demonstrated outside of work. Similarly, we have coached employees who have realized that they have continually sought roles and promotions that were aligned to their learned behaviors. For practitioners in this field it is important to reflect not only on the levels of the system, which we are designing for interventions, but also by the levels of depth which our interventions may touch. We have observed activities using pictures, movement, and simple questions evoke deep unconscious reactions, hitting participants at the "covert" level, touching their values and beliefs. What is critical to remember is that if it is change that we are seeking to evoke then it will be essential that as practitioners we are prepared to work at these deeper levels. This is a topic to which we will return in exploring designing interventions at the group level.

Group Interventions

With all group interventions it is important to distinguish between the content (or the *what*) of the group's work versus the process (or the *how*) of it (Minahan, 2006). When we are looking at the content of group activities, we are considering the tasks that they complete and the goals they are working on. In contrast, when we are considering group processes, we are focusing on how members join the group, how leadership occurs, how the group communicates and delegates work. For the positive psychology practitioner, we are able to offer significant interventions that support teams to increase their performance and delivery of tasks by intervening in ways that affect the group process, the "how" they work together.

Positive psychology interventions that can be designed to affect group processes include the following:

- Observing positive and negative ratios;
- Positive group 360 feedback;
- Strengths-based goal setting and delegation;
- Strengths-based team management.

In Section "Organizational System Interventions" we will focus on two of the above-group interventions, observing positive and negative emotions and strengths-based goal setting.

Through the pioneering work of Barbara Fredrickson over the last 20 years, our understanding of the role of positive emotion in teams has significantly increased (Fredrickson, 2009). Fredrickson's work highlights how achieving optimal levels of positive emotion can be a critical element in the success of teams and workgroups, especially where creativity, strategic thinking, cohesion, co-operation, and resilience are required. Her "Broaden and Build" research shows how experiencing positive emotions, such as joy, enthusiasm, interest, gratitude, and serenity can have significant repercussions at the group level. Fredrickson's work highlights how experiencing enhanced and authentic emotion can broaden people's mindsets, encouraging them to discover novel lines of thought or action; they fuel resilience and undo the lingering after-effects of negative emotions; and they can generate an upward spiral that promotes optimal functioning. In the business context, teams with higher levels of expressed positivity among group members have been linked not only to greater behavioral variability within moment-to-moment interactions, but also to long-range indicators of business success (Losada & Heaphy, 2004).

In working to improve team effectiveness, we have found that increasing the experience of positive emotion is a powerful (and enjoyable) intervention. Introducing simple exercises to enhance mood, promote (appropriate) humor, and encourage appreciation have a noticeable effect on team climate and productivity. One exercise, which we have found quickly, promotes group positive emotion and individual insight is to ask one member of the group to take it in turns to receive positive, affirmative, strengths-based feedback. Other activities that promote team rituals and savoring have also proved to increase the mood of groups. At Aviva, this practice has been embedded with their call center staff by introducing "huddles" at the start of a shift. Huddle topics can vary from sharing positive news, to letting people know when they last used a new strength. What is noticeable in the interventions we have both designed and observed in this area is that they are each simple, short, and easily integrated in to the day-to-day work of the group.

It is critical to recognize, however, that this focusing on the positive is in no way an excuse for a "happy-clappy love in," as some detractors of positive psychology in organizations would claim. As evidence shows, interventions should be balanced (Fredrickson & Losada, 2005). For teams to function effectively, team interactions and discussions need an emotional atmosphere that balances positive and appropriate negative aspects. In individual flourishing, at least three positive emotions are needed for every negative emotion – but no more than 11:1, otherwise we get stuck in a positive, ineffective feedback loop. In teams, at least six positive interventions (such as providing support, expressing encouragement, offering humor, acknowledging others perspectives, building on others ideas and showing appreciation) are required to counteract the effect of every negative statement (e.g., disapproval, sarcasm, or cynicism). High performing teams maintain or exceed this ratio and also achieve a balance between inquiry (genuine questioning to explore issues) and advocacy (arguing in favor of one's own position). Low-performing teams are characterized by a lower ratio of positive to negative interventions. The negativity leads to the loss of behavioral flexibility and the ability to question; these teams tend to get stuck in an endless loop of self-absorbed advocacy, with members focused on promoting their own views, at the expense of listening and constructive engagement.

At CAPP we also address these fundamental issues of balance at the design stage, in all of our interventions. This is one of the core reasons why Realise2 includes weaknesses; it is also why, when constructing group training material, we build in space and time to address criticisms of approaches and challenges. Indeed, there have been times when we have not done so – and groups have gone into revolt because they have not had enough time to get things off their chest. It's worth noting that most of the time, this resistance comes from misunderstanding or misinformation, rather than any fundamental disagreement – and as such, providing the time and space for these concerns to be aired and dealt with can reap rich dividends in terms of ensuring buy-in and commitment for moving forward.

Further, when setting up group interventions, this time to address the "elephant in the room" can be critical. We use two broad methods to support groups in sharing the challenges that they have on their mind. These include asking people to draw what is *on their table*, for example, what people know I feel, think, and do, as distinct from what is *under their table*, for example, what people don't know I feel, think, and do (Marshak, 2006). The second is an exercise which Edgar Schein writes about in his book *Helping* (Schein, 2009). Schein highlights the usefulness of "camp fire conversations," an activity where members of the group can speak about the challenges that they are facing, sitting in the group they can speak to the center of the circle, namely "the camp fire." This is a ritual that Schein encourages practitioners to carry out with teams at the start of off-site group interventions. In designing positive group interventions, ensuring this time and space is provided for groups to off-load is key to interventions gaining traction and the group being able to move to a desired future state.

With the resistance and blockers put on the table and dealt with, we then move more specifically to looking at how to build on the strengths of those in the group. To quote Peter Drucker, "To achieve results, one has to use all the available strengths ... These strengths are the true opportunities. The unique purpose of organization is to make strength productive." (Drucker, 1967, p. 75).

In our experience, one of the key ways in which organizations can make strengths productive is to support teams to operate by playing to the combined strengths of their team members, at the same time as making their individual weaknesses irrelevant. There are five ways in which we typically might support teams to work in this way.

1. *Ensure team and goal alignment:* Identify the goals and purpose of the team: what has it been put together to achieve? Lack of goal clarity leads different people to pull in different directions for different reasons. Ensuring team and goal alignment is the critical first step on which everything else rests.
2. *Identify the team activities that will deliver success:* What are the key activities the team needs to deliver in order to be successful? Break these down into their constituent parts, so that the flexibility of who does what can be increased. Breaking team goals down into key activities means that those activities can be divided up differently and allocated to the people who will deliver the best results.
3. *Align individual strengths to team activities:* From team members' Realise2 reports, identify which strengths can best deliver which activities, then allocate and align those activities according to the strengths of people on the team. Avoid requiring people to work from their weaknesses by using complementary partnering, swaps, and trade-offs – "I can do this for you if you can do that for me." Use learned behaviors only when activities cannot be allocated according to team member's strengths. Developmental assignments can be used to help team members to explore and develop their unrealized strengths.
4. *Deal with the "no-takers" activities:* There may well be those activities that nobody seems to want to do. Deal with them in one of the following ways: Allocate it to the team member who has a learned behavior aligned to the

activity – they might not want to do it all the time, but at least they can do it well. Rotate the activity, so that people take turns to do it. Offer special recognition to whoever does the activity, so as to take the edge off doing it. Sandwich the activity between other things that are working from people's strengths – that way they can re-charge and re-energize either side of doing the thing that drains them, but that nonetheless needs to be done.

5. *Re-evaluate periodically:* Nothing lasts forever. Team deliverables change, people's aspirations change, working relationships change. Keep check on the energy you see in the team and re-allocate and re-align responsibilities to keep people fresh, energized, and engaged. Variety can be the spice of life, just so long as it's not based on having people spending all their time on trying to master the things that drain them and that they will never perform well.

To evoke change successfully at the group level, there are some fundamental factors that also impact on the effectiveness of introducing positive psychology and strengths-based interventions. First, much of the research in positive psychology that can be applied to the group is focusing on process and the "how," however, these are often the areas that groups feel least comfortable discussing. Groups will frequently want to revert back to addressing the task and the "what" they do. We have run many strengths building team sessions where groups have found it difficult to consider actions to take forward that relate to emotion or behavior. Understanding the skew of positive psychology interventions toward emotions, and the preferences of groups to avoid working in this space, can support good intervention design and practice from the outset.

Second, as we work less on task and more on process, our focus shifts into the group "maintenance" space. As practitioners working on maintenance we move from the role of facilitator to "group process consultant" or "team coach." This subtle shift requires a different range of skills and capabilities, since it means that our role is not about imparting our knowledge and maneuvering people through our group exercises, but working more as OD or group process consultants "in service of the group," maintaining processes so that, through our presence, the psychological needs of the group can be met. Being in this role means that at times we may decide to share feedback that relates to overt and covert processes, and as so many positive psychological interventions target emotion that we will need to be adept at working at the covert level. Balance, again, is key and we need to be aware that practitioners who plan to work with groups at this deep and intense level, without taking some steps to pay attention to the overt and task level first, may see groups resisting their positive psychology interventions, or indeed that those interventions fail.

Organizational System Interventions

It has only been in the last 30 years that "whole" system level interventions have been used to evoke change. The "system" level interventions that were first implemented in the 1980s were based on theory and practice that can be traced back to the

1950s and 1960s. Studies of British Coal workers in the 1950s by Eric Trist and Fred Emery reported how technology can disrupt system functioning. In 1960, Ronald Lippitt at the University of Michigan was also noticing that his work on problem solving was energy-draining. Over the 20 years that followed, Lippitt looked to taking a solution-focus approach to his consulting, starting to consult with groups in Michigan on "creating a plan for a new future" (Lippitt, 1980). The work of Marvin Weisbord (1987) was considered to be one of the first places in which a clear statement was written about positive whole system approaches. Essentially, Weisbord's book recommended the need to get all of the stakeholders in the room. Possibly, the best-known whole system intervention that is considered to have a link to positive psychology is appreciative inquiry. Next we go on to look at how appreciative inquiry is being used by organizations as an intervention for whole system change.

"Appreciative Inquiry is described as the coevolutionary search for the best in people, their organizations, and the relevant world around them. In its broadest focus, it involves systematic discovery of what gives "life" to a living system when it is most alive, most effective, and most constructively capable in economic, ecological, and human terms" (Cooperrider & Whitney, 2008). In the first phase of appreciative inquiry (AI), the "discovery" phase, participants are asked about their positive experiences in the organization and what they see as the organization's strengths and values. The "Discovery" phase can be carried out in advance, or during an AI Summit meeting. The second phase, the "Dream" phase, uses the whole system or stakeholders from the whole system to plan how to build the positive elements into a vision of the desired future state. At this stage, groups are encouraged to establish a common ground about what they would like more of in the future. At the "Design" phase, participants plan actions to create the future they want. At the "Destiny" phase, participants conclude how they will sustain and evaluate the success of the change. At CAPP, from our experience of running AI events, we will also at times ask a 5th D, about the "Derailers," between Dream and Design. The introduction of this 5th element to our AI processes has been borne out of recognition for the need to work with some aspects of critique and challenge, in order to ensure that energy and creativity are sustained for the other parts of the AI process. By allowing people the opportunity to focus on and deal with the Derailers, we have found that the resistance will then dissipate or can then be better managed, both of which are more conducive to a positive outcome overall.

In the academic world, David Cooperrider and the Center for Business as an Agent of World Benefit, part of the Weatherhead School of Management at Case Western Reserve University (see http://worldbenefit.case.edu) are exemplary. Building on his discovery and development of appreciative inquiry, Cooperrider and his team are now using this characteristic methodology of the abundance approach to turn their attention to how organizations specifically and business generally can be deployed as an agent of world benefit, providing corporations with the tools and techniques to "do well by doing good" (Laszlo, 2008). This is mirrored by the work of people like Dave Ulrich (2009) on the abundant organization, and Kim Cameron and his colleagues in positive organizational scholarship on the difference made by abundance approaches (Cameron & Lavine, 2006).

AI provides us with an intervention that can involve the whole system, but there are also key custodians of the system, which are key to its success: the leaders. Although working with the leaders of an organization may be seen as an individual intervention, working with leaders and talent from across the system can be key in initiating change. It is also important that leaders recognize the impact of their actions on the system. It is becoming increasingly understood that leaders are what Naumann and Bennett (2000) have described as "climate engineers." That is, whether they like it or not, leaders and what they convey through their personality, values, beliefs, preferences, and behaviors, leave an indelible imprint on the character of the organizations they lead (Hogan, 2007). As highlighted by Morris and Garrett (2009), climate engineers do not just determine how the employees that they touch will grow and develop – their shadow will also extend to affect the brand, clients, and customers, together with their reach and perception into their communities and the wider world. Research also shows that consumers are also more driven to purchase from companies and leaders who they consider demonstrate ethics and fairness (Hilton & Gibbons, 2002). So, how can our interventions support leaders to be more consciously a force for social change?

Organizational-Level Interventions for Social Change

Mark Leach (2006), in his work on organizational development as a force for social change, highlights some of the fundamental variables that leaders need to consider if they are to create an organization that promotes social change and good. Leach highlights the need for leaders to be clear on the links between the organization's mission and its activities. It is critical that there is congruence between both what the organization says it does, and the actions that it takes year-on-year.

Research has also shown the benefit of leaders using an Appreciative Inquiry (AI) methodology, in order to co-create a vision-based strategy (Cooperrider & Whitney, 2005). In our work at CAPP, we have supported organizations in developing their strengths-based and positive organization strategy, through combining both the principles of strengths-based development with the key components of AI. We have found that this blended approach helps to build leaders' and organizations' confidence, creativity, and aspirations, together with considering their strategy in the light of their individual and collective strengths. The alignment of their collective strengths to the strategy that they have developed as a team leads to significant commitment and buy-in, goal orientation, and delivery.

In our experience, organizations can also be resistant to working at the "whole system level;" equally for those organizations who can be persuaded to work at this level, it can be where some of our most impactful work in evoking change happens. With the exception of AI, the positive psychology literature has provided less research and insights to working at the whole system level. For positive psychology to be a force for positive change within organizations there should be a greater focus of interventions that extend beyond just AI, and which draw more broadly from the organization development literature and the four levels of intervention that we have described here.

Factors That Influence Success

As well as greater research required at the whole system level, it is also critical that practitioners examine the design of the interventions to ensure change is initiated (Farquhar, 2006). As Farquhar highlights, designing and preparing an intervention strategy requires us to consider the following:

- The purpose(s) of the intervention;
- The environment in which the organization functions;
- The organization's culture including its core leadership, and professional identity;
- The circumstances in which the strategy will be used;
- The appropriate depth of the intervention;
- The likelihood and consequences of collateral effects of the intervention;
- The fit of the strategy within the available time frame and its flow inside the sequence of the intervention;
- The client's response to the proposal for the intervention.

With all of the above in mind, our experience shows that organizations can be more resistant to positive or strengths-based interventions, than they are interventions that come from more traditional practice or are not specifically positioned as overtly positive. This reaction highlights the negativity bias and deficit mindset that is often in play for some clients within organizations. Working with individual mindsets like this requires us as practitioner to be crystal clear from the outset that there is sufficient appetite to engage with and sustain change. For many, this can mean ensuring there are mechanisms in place, which can help to support the change. At CAPP, we often find that while individuals or groups find the discovery of their strengths interesting, post-training or coaching, they can often find the temptation to focus back onto their weaknesses too tempting. In instances like this, the role of the team members, managers, and the setting up of action learning sets can be critical to ensuring that the change is sustained. Again, changing the dialog through the nature of the conversations that people have can be one fundamental way in which we do this, as we started this chapter describing.

Conclusion

It has been our aim in this chapter to highlight how a collection of positive psychology research and activities can be applied to the three different levels of system, which can evoke change. Change cannot be evoked in any system by positive psychology alone. Positive psychology provides a lens for practitioners to examine and judge whether, a positive and strengths-based solution will evoke the desired change.

As practitioners in this emerging field, we have to take care and pride in the design of our interventions, always being mindful of the levels of the organizational system at which we are intervening and the depth we will reach.

In explicitly addressing these four levels of the system we have hoped to show different ways in which positive organizational change can be evoked. Positive psychology has sometimes been criticized for only focusing on the individual level, and practitioners have suggested that in doing this we are not intervening with positive psychology in the most powerful way. We disagree, because as we have described above, the intrapersonal and interpersonal interventions are often a stepping-stone to broader group and organization level interventions. Notwithstanding this, there is no doubt that more research is required at developing and evaluating "whole system" interventions that have been informed by positive psychology.

Overall, though, we hope to have demonstrated to you through this chapter the four levels at which we can intervene to make a positive difference to the lives of employees within organizations, on the basis that in doing so, we can transform the experience of the millions of people in our societies who spend a significant proportion of their waking lives at work in organizations. Our view is that by helping organizations to become more positive places for people to exist, we enable those same organizations to be taking a role as powerful custodians in bringing about positive social change.

References

Baumeister, R. F., Bratslavsky, E., Finkenauer, C., & Vohs, K. D. (2001). Bad is stronger than good. *Review of General Psychology, 5*, 323–370.

Cameron, K., & Lavine, M. (2006). *Making the impossible possible: Leading extraordinary performance: The Rocky Flats story.* San Francisco: Berrett-Koehler.

Christakis, N., & Fowler, J. (2010). *Amazing power of social networks and how they shape our lives.* HarperCollins.

Cooperrider, D., & Whitney, D. (2005). *Appreciative inquiry: A positive revolution in change.* San Francisco: Berrett-Koehler Publishers.

Cooperrider, D., & Whitney, D. (2008). *Appreciative inquiry handbook: For leaders of change.* San Francisco: Berrett-Koehler Publishers.

Drucker, P. F. (1967). *The effective executive.* London: Heinemann.

Emery, F. E., & Trist, E. L. (1960). Socio-technical systems. In C. W. Churchman & M. Verhurst (Eds.), *Management sciences, models and techniques* (Vol. 2, pp. 83–97). London: Pergamon.

Farquhar, K. (2006). Intervention phase. In B. B. Jones & M. Brazzel (Eds.), *The NTL handbook of organizational development and change.* San Francisco: Pfeiffer.

Fredrickson, B. L. (2009). *Positivity: Discover the ratio that tips your life toward flourishing.* New York: Crown Books.

Fredrickson, B. L., & Losada, M. (2005). Positive emotions and the complex dynamics of human flourishing. *American Psychologist, 60*, 678–686.

Garcea, N., Harrington, S., & Linley, P. A. (2009). Building Positive Organizations. In P. A. Linley, S. Harrington & N. Garcea (Eds.), *Oxford Handbook of Positive Psychology and Work.* New York: Oxford University Press.

Govindji, R., & Linley, P. A. (2007). Strengths use, self-concordance and well-being: Implications for strengths coaching and coaching psychologists. *International Coaching Psychology Review, 2*(2), 143–153.

Herrero, L. (2008). *Viral Change: the alternative to slow, painful and unsuccessful management of change in organisation*. Beaconsfield, UK: Meetingminds.

Hilton, S., & Gibbons, G. (2002). *Good business: Your world needs you*. London: Texere.

Hogan, R. (2007). *Personality and the fate of organizations*. Mahwah, NJ: Erlbaum.

Laszlo, C. (2008). *Sustainable value: How the world's leading companies are doing well by doing good*. Sheffield: Greenleaf Publishing.

Leach, M. (2006). Changing organizations and systems from the outside: OD practitioners as agents for social change. In B. B. Jones & M. Brazzel (Eds.), *The NTL handbook of organizational development and change*. San Francisco: Pfeiffer.

Linley, P. A., Joseph, S., Harrington, S., & Wood, A. M. (2006). Positive psychology: Past, present, and (possible) future. *The Journal of Positive Psychology, 1*, 3–16.

Lippitt, R. (1980). *Choosing the future you prefer*. Washington, DC: Development.

Losada, M., & Heaphy, E. (2004). The role of positivity and connectivity in the performance of business teams: A nonlinear dynamics model. *American Behavioral Scientist, 47*(6), 740–765.

Marshak, R. J. (2006). *Covert processes at work: Managing the five hidden dimensions of organizational change*. San Francisco: Berrett-Koehler Publishers.

Minahan, M. (2006). Working with groups in organizations. In B. B. Jones & M. Brazzel (Eds.), *The NTL handbook of organizational development and change*. San Francisco: Pfeiffer.

Minhas, G. (2010). Developing realised and unrealised strengths: Implications for engagement, self-esteem, life satisfaction and well-being. *Assessment and Development Matters, 2*(1), 12–16

Morris, D., & Garrett, J. (2009). Strengths: Your leading edge. In P. A. Linley, S. Harrington, & N. J. Garcea (Eds.), *Oxford handbook of positive psychology and work*. New York: Oxford University Press.

Naumann, S. E., & Bennett, N. (2000). A case for procedural justice climate: Development and test of a multilevel model. *Academy of Management Journal, 43*, 881–889.

Page, N., & Carter, D. (2008). Strengths-based organization. In S. J. Lopez (Ed.), *The encyclopaedia of positive psychology*. Oxford: Blackwell.

Rozin, P., & Royzam, E. (2001). Negativity bias, negativity dominance, and contagion. *Personality and Social Psychology Review, 5*, 296–320.

Schein, E. H. (2009). *Helping: How to offer, give, and receive help*. New York: McGraw Hill.

Seligman, M. E. P. (2002). *Authentic happiness*. New York: Free Press.

Seligman, M. E. P., Steen, T. A., Park, N., & Peterson, C. (2005). Positive psychology progress: Empirical validation of interventions. *American Psychologist, 60*(5), 410–421.

Sheldon, K. M., & Lyubomirsky, S. (2006). How to increase and sustain positive emotion: The effects of expressing gratitude and visualizing best possible selves. *The Journal of Positive Psychology, 1*, 73–82.

Sin, N. L., & Lyubomirsky, S. (2009). Enhancing well-being and alleviating depressive symptoms with positive psychology interventions: A practice-friendly meta-analysis. *Journal of Clinical Psychology: In Session, 65*, 467–487.

Ulrich, D. (2009). The abundant organization [foreword]. In P. A. Linley, S. Harrington, & N. Garcea (Eds.), *Oxford Handbook of Positive Psychology and Work*. New York: Oxford University Press.

Weisbord, M. R. (1987). *Productive workplaces: Organizing and managing for dignity, meaningand community*. San Francisco: Jossey-Basss.

Chapter 11
Organizational Democracy as a Force for Social Change

Traci L. Fenton

Imagine an organization that

- Lets you vote on the CEO's performance.
- Allows you, not your boss, to determine your work projects.
- Uses open e-mail discussion lists to make critical decisions.
- Is fully transparent about the organization's financial health.
- Rotates all leadership roles on a regular basis.

Sound far-fetched? Well, it's not. These innovative examples of organizational democracy are being practiced in companies all over the world of every size – from small to Fortune 500. It's a growing trend that reflects an inescapable fact: organizations that embrace a democratic style are building healthier workplaces and cultures and better bottom lines. In the process, they are also becoming a force for social change in the world, proving that *how* a company operates is just as important as what it does.

Organizational Democracy as a Force for Social Change

This is the dawn of the most entrepreneurial and socially aware era in human history. More individuals than ever before are passionate about corporate social responsibility, a greener environment, and human rights. And we're creating organizations all over the world to advance these noble causes.

But are these organizations operating consistently with the principles of freedom and democracy that enliven their progressive missions? Far too often they are patterned after the same outdated command and control organizational structures that have been stifling individual voice and reserving power for those at the top of the management hierarchy born with the Industrial Age.

T.L. Fenton (✉)
WorldBlu, Inc., Cedar Rapids, Iowa, USA
e-mail: traci@worldblu.com

R. Biswas-Diener (ed.), *Positive Psychology as Social Change*,
DOI 10.1007/978-90-481-9938-9_11, © Springer Science+Business Media B.V. 2011

We are limiting the scope of the social change impact we seek by not consciously designing our organizations to operate in a way that advances human development, peace, and economic prosperity, even as we design products and services that might.

Operating an organization using the principles of organizational democracy can solve this problem and have a ripple-effect in several areas. For example:

Democratic workplaces build more peaceful and prosperous societies. In her recent study of nearly 80 nations, Gretchen Spreitzer, a University of Michigan professor of management and organizations, found that there was significantly less corruption or unrest and more peace in nations where employees have the freedom to make decisions at work and where organizations are managed using a participatory leadership style. Conversely, in countries where employees have to be more compliant in following a manager's decision, there is more unrest. Spreitzer found that democratically run workplaces not only benefit economically from progressive management practices, but also enhance peace in their community by reducing the feeling of powerlessness at work (Spritzer, 2007).

Democratic workplaces are healthier. What about the impact of workplace democracy on an employee's physical health? Gallup reports that 62% of "engaged" employees in the United States believe that being engaged at work has a positive impact on their health, whereas a combined 84% of "not engaged" or "actively disengaged" employees feel that not being engaged has a negative impact on their physical health (Gallup Organization, 2005). In addition to investments in wellness programs and on-site gyms, companies could also consider increasing employee opportunities to fully engage at work as a means of lowering their healthcare costs.

Democratic workplaces create more democratic citizens. In Botswana, a nation working hard to build and sustain its political democracy, organizations are expected and encouraged to operate democratically. In 1993, the Ministry of Education decided to transition all secondary schools from an authoritarian to a democratic management structure. The result? According to the *International Education Journal*, students, administrators, and the country as a whole are benefiting from a more democratic citizenry (Monyatsi, 2005).

Democratic workplaces contribute to human development. Democratically run organizations naturally help employees develop their ability to communicate effectively, manage conflicts, respect different views, listen, compromise, and work in harmony. Employees who feel valued at work also learn to value themselves more, contributing to a growing sense of self-worth. This can then ripple-out to contribute to more positive interactions in the home as well as in civic life.

Choosing to operate a company democratically can make a significant impact on elevating human worth, untapping potential, enhancing communication skills, and cultivating a more engaged and peaceful citizenry.

What Is Organizational Democracy?

We've explored the societal benefits of a company operating democratically, but what is organizational democracy exactly and why is it so relevant today? Most people work in organizations that are far from democratic. Indeed, most organizations aren't democratic at all! Instead, they operate using the military-inspired hierarchical command and control model, which was adopted during the Industrial Age. A recent Zogby International Poll, in conjunction with the Workplace Democracy Association, found that one out of every four Americans believes he works in a dictatorship. And 80% believe that if they had more freedom at work they would do a better job (Zogby, 2008).

Unfortunately, because we've created organizations that often dehumanize the people who work in them, employees do not perform to their full potential. Democratic organizations, however, by the nature of their design, inspire the opposite, and have found a way to successfully answer the following business questions:

1. Why can't employees choose their bosses?
2. Why can't employees hire, fire, or otherwise hold accountable the people on whom they increasingly depend to run the organization?
3. Why can't employees benefit directly from the ideas they come up with that result in higher profits for the organization?
4. Why can't employees set their own goals?
5. Why can't employees have access to financial information that would enhance the quality of their decisions?

Organizational democracy provides a fresh and systemic answer to all of these questions. Simply put, organizational democracy is a system of organizational management that is based on freedom, instead of fear and control. It's a way of designing organizations to amplify the possibilities of human potential – and of the organization as a whole.

The *term* democracy comes from the Greek words *demos*, "the people," and *kratein*, "to rule." The essence of democracy is the concept that people have the power and ability to shape their lives and their future both individually and collectively.

A democratic organization chooses freedom rather than fear, peer-to-peer relationships rather than paternalism, engagement rather than estrangement in its daily operations. Beyond giving employees a vote, democratic organizations give them a real voice in the decisions that impact their job and the organization.

Here's a look at what organizational democracy is – and isn't.

Organizational democracy is not	Organizational democracy is
Politics	Business
Concensus-only	Conversations
Being flat	Decentralized networks
Management	Leadership
American-only ideals	Universal ideals
Size	Strategy
Being slow	Knowing when to be fast AND when to be slow
Giving up control	Giving up the delusion that you're in control
Ignoring profits	Profits and people
Cosmetic office parks	Creating meaningful work
Being a great workplace for everyone	Being a great workplace for those who can thrive in a decentralized and dynamic environment
Analyzing decision-making techniques	Making decisions
Only a triple bottom line	A quadruple bottom line (financial, community, external environment, AND internal environment)
Voting on everything	Ongoing participation in things that matter

Organizational democracy is a way to tap the ingenuity of employees to solve problems by understanding that traditional hierarchical workplace structures that perpetuate disengagement and the delusion of control are a recipe for defeat in today's collaborative world.

Operating a company democratically also helps boost the bottom line: It trims unnecessary layers of management, decreases turnover costs through improved employee morale and satisfaction, and increases innovation by tapping employee creativity. Other benefits include:

- Increases in productivity, profitability, sales, and efficiency.
- Improvements in customer service.
- An increased ability to attract and retain top talent.
- Decreases in turnover and absenteeism.
- Increasing levels of trust and communication.
- Greater levels of innovation.
- Higher employee satisfaction.
- An increased ability to adapt to market changes.

Organizational democracy – decentralizing power and decision-making to employees at every level of a company – is a potent approach to unleashing human capacity and benefiting the bottom line.

The End of the Industrial Age

Organizational democracy, however, is more than just a powerful business strategy – it is an idea whose time has finally come. While various management thinkers and scholars have been heralding the ideal of a democratic organization for years, a convergence of factors are now making this model of organization all the more relevant – and vital.

With the bursting of the dot-com bubble in the late 1990s and now with the global Great Recession upon us at the time of this writing, another bubble has also been slowly losing its air – the Industrial Age bubble. This bubble contained the old economy "air" that we've been breathing for the last century or more. Like a fish in water, until the recent birth of the "new" economy powered by the Internet, we haven't known anything different.

The "old" economy was built in the Industrial Age. With the dawning of industry in the early 1900s came the need to organize large groups of people, which eventually led to the creation of what we know today as the modern corporation. Up to that point, we had been a largely agrarian society with the skills and mind-set to organize and manage only small groups of people. So, we turned for help to the most developed model at that time for how to organize and manage large groups of people – the military model. And that model – with its hierarchy, command and control, and bureaucracy – became the *corporate* model of organization, despite the fact that their purposes and aims were quite different.

In the military, one needs to make what are – literally – life-or-death decisions and there needs to be speed and order in the decision-making chain. In corporations, however, although the decision environment is intense at times, it does not form the hinge between life and death. The stakes – as well as the desired outcome – are different, and therefore the operating model should be as well. However, at the start of the twentieth century, in the absence of another tested model for how to organize large groups of people, the military model prevailed and became the default and eventually the standard for how to structure a company.

The militaristic, command and control model of organization was, for the most part, effective, if you measure effectiveness by economic output and development. But mid-way through the twentieth century, management experts such as Peter Drucker began to question the industrial model of organization in terms of its effects both on workers and productivity. The rebellion started to crescendo when other management and leadership thought-leaders such as Margaret Wheatley, Peter Senge, Dee Hock, Russell Ackoff, Tom Malone, Lynda Gratton, and others started weighing in. Their common mantra: There's a better way to organize and it isn't like this.

Now, at the beginning of the twenty-first century, the prevailing sentiment is that the Industrial Age is officially Jurassic, and not just because the new Internet-driven collaborative economy has come along. Over the last 5 years, the Gallup Organization's annual employee engagement index has shown a marked increase in employee disengagement from 54 to 73% in the United States alone (Gallup Management Journal, 2005). In other words, nearly three-fourths of the

US workforce is disengaged at work, costing the United States over \$300 billion annually. But in a global age, problems aren't just local, and neither is this one. For example, 82% of Australian workers, 88% of Chinese workers, and 91% of Japanese workers are all disengaged at work (Gallup Management Journal, 2005). Workers are increasingly disenfranchised with the command and control system.

Here's a chart that shows some of the characteristics of the old command and control model compared to a democratic model.

Characteristics of a command + control model	Characteristics of a democratic model
Paternalistic relationships	Peer-to-peer relationships
Employees are order-takers	Employees are decision-makers
Layers of management	Decentralized leadership
Ego + greed	Humility + resolve
Secret society	Responsible transparency
Layers of hierarchy	Decentralized networks

© 2010 WorldBlu, Inc.

With the bursting of the Industrial Age bubble and growing disengagement among workers comes new expectations about voice, transparency, collaboration, and working in a way that is meaningful and makes an impact on social advancement. Welcome to the Democratic Age.

Here's a brief look at the eight trends moving organizations into this new age.

Trend One: The Internet and Technology

The Internet, blogging, Twitter, Facebook, podcasts, social media, and online democratization tools are the new technologies for communication and sharing information, usurping traditional lines of communication, and making information that was only available to a few available to almost everyone. The effect of this trend: Expect employees to want to have a voice and influence in decisions that affect them at work.

Trend Two: Generations X and Y Have Arrived

Generations X and Y expect to have a voice at work, to be involved, to make a contribution. I know because I'm a borderline Gen X/Gen Y-er. We want openness. We crave authenticity. Our lifestyle of connectedness and belief in our abilities (as well as our disenfranchisement with how we saw Big Business treat our parents) means we want to work in organizations that value our unique contribution. The effect of this trend: Expect Gen X and Y to demand a more egalitarian workplace.

Trend Three: Wall Street Backlash

People are tired of the greedy model of business encapsulated by the rise and fall of companies like Enron and most recently, the major corporations on Wall Street. Recent corporate scandals and Ponzi schemes churned up strong emotions and led to mounting resolve for a different way of running a corporation – and a global economy. The effect of this trend: New laws and regulations requiring transparency and accountability will reshape the way works gets done.

Trend Four: Political Transitions

In the last 15 years, there has been a large jump in the number of countries embracing political democracy. Two-thirds of the world is now considered politically democratic, according to Freedom House. As more countries become democratic, businesses will be pressed to rethink their command and control structures for an organizational system more compatible with a democratically organized world. The effect of this trend on organizations: Employees who get to vote at the polls may also expect their voice to count at work (Freedom House, 2010).

Trend Five: The Search for Meaning

Futurist Patricia Aburdene identifies the number one megatrend of our time as the search for meaning and spirituality (Aburdene, 2007). People increasingly want their work to not just be work – they want it to matter. They want to feel that the work they do is making a difference in the world, not just lining their bosses' pockets. The effect of this trend: Employees will expect to find meaning in the *way* they work, not just the end product they help produce.

Trend Six: Corporate Social Responsibility

Businesses are increasingly embracing the idea of corporate social responsibility (CSR), conscious capitalism, and the "triple bottom line" – financial, community, and the external environment. Democracy in the workplace aligns closely with this growing trend and adds a fourth dimension – the way employees are treated in the internal environment of the organization. The effect of this trend: Embrace CSR values to attract smart, globally aware employees to your workplace.

Trend Seven: Lifestyle Democracy

Today I checked the headlines on GroundReport.com, a citizen journalism website, listened to Pandora and voted for my favorite music, checked out a course using MIT's "open courseware" project, and voted on a friend's t-shirt design on

Treadless.com. It is the rise of what I call "lifestyle democracy," where everything from media to music, education to fashion is being democratized. The effect of this trend: With everyday life becoming democratized, employees will expect the same at work.

Trend Eight: Feminine Values

There is a growing recognition that masculine qualities alone in the business world won't get us where we need to go, and are often the cause of our economic woes. Increasingly, traditionally identified feminine qualities like collaboration, emotional intelligence, accountability, and integrity in both women *and* men are being heralded as crucial to bringing the world and our economies back into balance. The effect of this trend: Expect to see workplaces that are deliberately being reshaped to value feminine qualities.

These eight trends are rapidly and radically reshaping the business landscape, bringing us into a whole new era and making democratically designed organizations not just a nice idea, but also an *imperative*.

The Birth of Blu

I founded WorldBlu, a global social enterprise committed to championing the growth of democratic organizations worldwide, in 1997 after my first job out of college awakened me to the need for more democracy in the workplace. I had accepted a position as an advertising account executive for a local newspaper owned by a Fortune 500 company. Although I considered the job to be far from ideal, I was nonetheless excited to be a part of a large company and make a positive contribution.

However, my dreams hit reality hard the first day on the job. Day 1 was nothing less than culture shock as the harsh reality of the command and control model greeted me at the door. I entered the office building as a confident, bright-eyed college graduate who had held various leadership positions during college. I left later that day demoralized and deflated, feeling more like a child than an empowered employee.

My first few days were spent being told what I could and could not do, how I was to behave, who was important in the organization – and who was *not*. I was told what my sales goals were and how I was to accomplish those goals. Any questions I had were either shrugged off or ignored. I was assigned to a cubicle with the minimal resources needed to do my job. I was not trained; instead, I was told to just "get out there and figure it out as you go." By the end of the first week I had never felt so low in all my life. I remember thinking, "If this is what I'm supposed to expect from work for the next 40 years of my life, I quit!"

When I did decide to resign 4 months later, my boss said to me, "When I hired you I knew you wouldn't last more than 6 months. You're too smart to let yourself be treated the way we treat people here." Those were the kindest words he'd ever spoken to me.

This scenario of dehumanization is repeated across the United States and around the world each day for countless individuals. In far too many cases, people begin working at an organization only to quickly discover that no one is interested in hearing *their* ideas about how to improve the company. No one is interested in what *their* personal life-goals are and how they might be actualized within the company – benefitting the company along the way. They're expected to be committed, show up on time, and give it their all, but often at the expense of self-respect, meaning, and personal development. Employees soon learn that they are there to serve the company – with little reward or fulfillment beyond a paycheck in return.

Kenneth Cloke and Joan Goldsmith write in their book, *The End of Management and the Rise of Organizational Democracy,* about the results of undemocratic work environments on employees:

> Through years of experience, employees learn that it is safer to suppress their innate capacity to solve problems and wait instead for commands from above. They lose their initiative and ability to see how things can be improved. They learn not to care and to accept things the way they are. They justify making mistakes and are allowed to be irresponsible and pass the blame to others for their mistakes. They become mindlessly obedient, fatalistic, intransigent, and hostile. Yet in spite of the obvious limitations created by these responses, managers continue giving orders rather than helping employees learn for themselves what needs to be done and how and when to do it best (Cloke & Goldsmith, 2002).

Sound familiar? I have told my experience to people from over 100 different countries and consistently see nods of agreement and understanding smiles. We have all been there. We all know what it's like to be treated like a Nobody. The thing is, the era of Nobodies is over. Information has given power to the people – to the average employee – not just to management. Suddenly, everybody can be a *Somebody*, and you don't have to climb a corporate ladder or wait 30 years to get there.

The WorldBlu Organizational Democracy Framework

My experience in Corporate America led me to start WorldBlu and launched a journey to discover the answer to the timely question: What is organizational democracy and how it can be realized in companies? I wanted to understand the *principles* that created a democratic system, rather than just identify commonly assumed democratic *practices*. A principle-based system is more universally understood, applicable, and scalable.

My research into the core principles of organizational democracy took a decade. Throughout the process, I researched what democracy is – and what it isn't. I studied classical democratic thought and as well as leading contemporary thinkers. I traveled throughout democratic and undemocratic countries around the world querying dozens and dozens of practitioners of democracy as well as CEOs of democratically run non- and for-profit organizations.

Overall, I was looking for a core set of *causal principles* that must be present in order to create a democratic system. My premise was that if even one of these core principles were removed, then the system could no longer be considered democratic. I also recognized that the principles had to create a dynamic tension between them, ultimately holding the entire system in balance. With these factors in mind, a list of ten core principles of democracy then emerged. These form the WorldBlu Organizational Democracy Framework^{TM} (Fenton, 2002).

The Ten WorldBlu Principles of Organizational Democracy

1:: *Purpose + Vision*: When an organization and the individual know their reasons for existing and have a sense of intentional direction.
2:: *Transparency:* When ideas flow freely and information is openly and responsibly shared.
3:: *Dialogue + Listening:* When people listen and engage in conversations in a way that brings out new levels of meaning and connection.
4:: *Fairness + Dignity:* When each person is treated justly and regarded impartially.
5:: *Accountability:* When each person and the organization as a whole are responsible to each other and their community for their actions.
6:: *Individual + Collective:* When individuals understand the unique contribution they make toward achieving collective goals.
7:: *Choice:* When each person is encouraged to exercise his or her right to choose between a diversity of possibilities.
8:: *Integrity:* When each person steadfastly adheres to high moral and ethical principles.
9:: *Decentralization:* When power is appropriately shared among people throughout the organization.
10:: *Reflection + Evaluation:* When there is a commitment to continuous feedback and development and a willingness to learn from the past and apply lessons to improve the future.

In short, democratic companies operate on *freedom*, not fear. What makes democratic companies uniquely *democratic* is that they have implemented *all* of the ten principles into the design of the organization, creating a powerful freedom-centered culture as a result.

Organizational Democracy at DaVita

Organizational democracy is not some fad among startups or small companies. It is a growing trend that reflects an inescapable fact: All businesses that embrace a democratic style are building healthier workplaces and better bottom lines while changing the world in the process.

As business leaders consider the prospect of establishing democratic practices, they'll undoubtedly face obstacles – some real, some invented. Size shouldn't be one of them. Think about it. In the spread of political democracy, countries ranging from a few hundred inhabitants to more than a billion people have all embraced it. So, why should corporate giants fear it, especially at a time when the world desperately needs models of large companies operating with integrity, transparency, and accountability?

Since 2007, WorldBlu has recognized the top companies in the world operating democratically. Organizations that have received our award are from both the non-profit and for-profit sectors, range from small to large, and are found in industries as diverse as manufacturing, technology, food service, consulting, healthcare, technology, and consumer goods.

One such company is DaVita. Today, the Denver, Colorado-based company is the largest independent provider of dialysis services in the United States, with more than 33,000 employees and annual sales of over $6 billion.

But back in 1999, the situation was bleak. The company was functionally bankrupt, under investigation by the US Securities and Exchange Commission, being sued by shareholders, and the majority of senior executives had left. Its new CEO, Kent Thiry, understood that changing course meant embracing a fresh, democratic approach. They decided to look at DaVita as a community *first*, and a company second. They committed themselves to creating an environment in which people felt valued, heard, and respected (Pfeffer, 2006).

To that end, they started radically changing things at DaVita to embrace a democratic model, resulting in them being named the first Fortune 500 company to receive the WorldBlu List of Most Democratic Workplaces award, in 2008.

DaVita's democratic approach to leadership and engagement is a far cry from that of the Fortune 500 where I started my career back in 1997. So, what does the application of democracy look like in a large company? Let's take a look at how DaVita practices the ten WorldBlu Principles of Organizational Democracy:

Democratic Companies Have Purpose and Vision

At DaVita, organizational democracy begins with each person thinking of his or herself first as part of a community, and second as part of a company. There is a clear sense of purpose, vision, and values that they call "The DaVita Way," which includes "Caring for Our Patients, Caring for Each Other, and Caring for Our World." DaVita's vision is to become the "Greatest kidney care company the world has ever seen." Employees are called "teammates" because "team" is one of their core values. And like any organized community, there is a top leader. At DaVita, the CEO, Kent Thiry, is called The Mayor – and he even has a Mayor uniform, which he wears from time to time. Recently a marketing firm surveyed DaVita teammates to identify the one word they use to sum up their company. That word was "village," which connotes the spirit of equality and connectivity organizational democracy can engender within a company (Pfeffer, 2006).

Democratic Companies Are Transparent

Each quarter, DaVita teammates are invited to participate in a "Voice of the Village" call with the CEO and senior leadership team. The purpose of the call is to openly share information about the state of the company and to address any areas of concern. At the end of the call, the floor is open to teammates in a question and answer session to ask the CEO or any member of the senior leadership team anything they would like. Leaders also send a weekly e-mail communication to all teammates to give them an "inside look" at the company and keep lines of communication open, and they publish a semi-annual internal magazine as well. Through these open channels, teammates can share their thoughts, questions, and suggestions on a regular basis with senior leadership (Fenton, 2009).

Democratic Companies Encourage Accountability

Every year, each DaVita business department is empowered to set its own goals and be accountable to them, rather than the traditional command and control approach which would have goals set at corporate headquarters and then decreed from "on high." This kind of grassroots accountability engenders a feeling of ownership and teamwork. DaVita then recognizes each department that reaches its goals with a financial reward. This practice of shared and distributed accountability encourages continuous improvement and teamwork and provides momentum for reaching shared goals (Fenton, 2009).

Democratic Companies Provide Choice

Remarkably enough, DaVita regularly invites their teammates to vote on various issues, which is practically unheard of in the business world, particularly among Fortune 500 companies. Instead of simply dictating major decisions to employees, DaVita has historically been know to present their employees with a set of choices and then invite them to vote on what they want. The DaVita leadership team has asked teammates to vote on different program names, logos, and new practices, among other things. The teammates even chose the company's name, DaVita, which means "giving life." During the company's annual meetings, several ballots are often cast to get teammate feedback on new initiatives that DaVita is considering for the upcoming year (Fenton, 2008).

Democratic Companies Have Integrity

Integrity is at the core of organizational democracy, which means making the right moral and ethical decisions that enable a company to prosper. While patients, physicians, teammates, and communities have benefited from the DaVita Community, innovation in healthcare still attracts critics. People question the motives and methods of the healthcare industry, and there are those that even question the value of providing a better quality of life for dialysis patients. The entire concept and approach of the DaVita Community is all about setting an example of integrity and innovation by rethinking the company's role in society and in the healthcare industry as a whole, and they have been broadly recognized for their leadership in this arena (Fenton, 2009).

Democratic Companies Decentralize Power

It would be easy for a large company like DaVita working in the life-or-death healthcare industry to be very command and control with its 1,500 clinics nationwide. However, at DaVita, they've found that providing a set of guiding parameters and then giving each clinic the freedom to be its own boss within those, is the best way to decentralize power. By doing this, a message of trust and respect is communicated to all teammates, innovation is encouraged, and the development of leaders throughout the organization occurs (Fenton, 2008).

Democratic Companies Engage in Dialogue and Listening

DaVita regularly conducts "Town Hall" meetings, ensuring that dialogue – not one way, top-down monologue – occurs throughout the company. The goal is to make sure teammates know what's going on in the DaVita community. At the Town Hall meetings, teammates showcase new programs, managers recognize teammates who have excelled in their respective jobs, and departments share updates. The Town Hall meetings are also an opportunity to have leaders openly answer any questions teammates may have about the company's business practices and where the company is headed. DaVita has more than 100 vice presidents, so the company also guarantees that whenever a vice president visits a local DaVita center or business office, he or she also holds a Town Hall meeting for the local team (Fenton, 2008).

Democratic Companies Treat People with Fairness and Dignity

DaVita strives to treat its teammates with fairness and dignity, and this practice continues beyond the corporate boundary to include DaVita's patients as well. At each DaVita clinic across the United States there is a "Wall of Fame" to honor and dignify every local patient and teammate. Also, DaVita leaders are trained in active listening and how to ask open-ended questions. These techniques encourage mutual respect and openness and minimize the misunderstandings and feelings of isolation that are all too common at many major corporations (Fenton, 2009).

Democratic Companies Embrace Both the Individual and the Collective

As more and more individuals yearn for workplaces where they can find meaning and express their individual talents and gifts, it is important that organizations understand how to embrace the diversity of their individual teammates while communicating how they fit into the collective picture. Often companies expect workers to check their individuality at the door in favor of conformity. But at DaVita, one of the core values is "Fulfillment," which is the company's way of highlighting the importance of being fulfilled on both a personal and professional level. For example, although clinics are staffed during normal office hours, teammates have the flexibility to fulfill their obligations outside of work. Their leaders make several accommodations possible for these personal needs, while still meeting the needs of the patients and the organization. DaVita has also established the KT Community Foundation, which provides grants that allow teammates to contribute time, skills, and energy to transform the communities in which they live (Fenton, 2009).

Democratic Companies Engage in Reflection and Evaluation

One of the most important things democratic companies do is allow space to reflect on their daily practices and share their successes and failures. Sharing successes is easy to do, but sharing mistakes is a lot more challenging. However, the leaders at DaVita understand that sharing failure is one way to encourage people to take risks and learn. Each year, DaVita hosts annual meetings at which the CEO and COO publicly share their personal successes and failures in front of more than 2,000 teammates at the company. Also, DaVita leaders annually complete a mission and values report card, where they evaluate themselves and then report back to the community. The report card is not about business results; it strictly evaluates a leader's ability to practice and uphold the mission and values of the organization throughout the community (Fenton, 2008).

As a result of DaVita's transformation from a command and control to a democratic model, it dramatically reduced its turnover rate, stimulated organic growth above the industry average, and became the industry leader. Net operating revenue grew from $1.45 billion in 1999 to $6.1 billion in 2009 (Fenton, 2009).

DaVita's CEO, Kent Thiry told me, "We feel our approach adds more value to the American health system, not just in savings but also in transparency and accountability. I firmly believe that every company can be a democratic community. And I know it's worth it! "

His statement underscores the potential of organizational democracy to transform not only corporations, but also the millions of lives they affect. That, in turn, raises a pressing question: Do big businesses especially have a responsibility to be organized democratically because of the power they wield and the number of people they employ?

If more Fortune 500 companies operated democratically, it could mean less corporate malfeasance, happier employees, and a noticeably more stable economy. And it would allow a powerful alignment between the political system much of humanity embraces and the places we work in each day.

DaVita serves as a powerful example of what a democratic approach can achieve within an organization. In this new Democratic Age, leaders with the courage and vision to transition from the now defunct command and control model to the freedom-centered, democratic approach will help usher in a new era and a new economy based on transparency and accountability, allowing each one of us to fully realize our potential – and change the world for the better.

References

Aburdene, P. (2007, April 17). *Megatrends 2010: The rise of conscious capitalism.* Newburyport, MA: Hampton Roads Publishing.

Cloke, K., & Goldsmith, J. (2002). *The end of management and the rise of organizational democracy* (p. 10). San Francisco: Jossey-Bass.

Crabtree, S. (2005, January 13). Engagement keeps the doctor away. *Gallup Management Journal.*

Fenton, T. (2002). *The democratic company.* Austin, TX: WorldBlu, Inc.

Fenton, T. (2008, May 6). Even big companies are embracing a democratic style. *The Christian Science Monitor.*

Fenton, T. (2009). Interviews at DaVita, Inc. in El Segundo, California, October 13, 2009 with various employees.

Freedom House. (2008). *Freedom in the World 2010.* http://www.freedomhouse.org/template.cfm?page=505

Monyatsi, P. P. (2005). Transforming schools into democratic organisations: The case of the secondary schools management development project in Botswana. *International Education Journal, 6*(3), 354–366. Shannon Research Press. http://www.iej.cjb.net

Pfeffer, J. (2006, February 23). *Kent Thiry and DaVita: Leadership challenges in building and growing a great company* (pp. 1–2). Stanford, CA: Stanford Graduate School of Business, Stanford University, Case: OB-54.

Spreitzer, G. (2007). Giving peace a chance: Organizational leadership, empowerment, and peace. *Journal of Organizational Behavior, 28,* 1077–1095. Wiley InterScience, Published online August 23, 2007.

Zogby Poll. (2008, June 23). As Independence Day Nears, Workplace Democracy Association Survey Finds One in Four Working Americans Describe Their Employer as a "Dictatorship". www.zogby.com/News/ReadNews.cfm?ID=1520

Part V

Positive Psychology and a Focus on Others

Chapter 12
Better Living Through Perspective Taking

Sara D. Hodges, Brian A.M. Clark, and Michael W. Myers

One of us (SDH) teaches an undergraduate seminar in the University of Oregon's Honors College called "Normal People Behaving Badly." It's all about tendencies that are common (if not universal) among mentally healthy humans – that is, people without any kind of psychopathology – but that nonetheless result in conduct and attitudes that are commonly (perhaps universally) condemned, such as hypocrisy, prejudice, and selfishness. The psychological mechanisms behind these bad behaviors are not inherently "evil" and in fact, they probably persist in the human repertoire because they developed alongside some other useful purpose, such as reducing cognitive effort in processing information or increasing the likelihood of survival.

The seminar has been popular, enrolling as many literature, history, and political science majors as psychology majors. However, at some point into the course, after several weeks of listening to the litany of "bad behaviors" and analysis thereof, students start to show signs of being a little overwhelmed and depressed. Not only does the course cover loathsome behaviors, such as acts of discrimination and slander, and even atrocities like genocide, but also furthermore, because part of the underlying course message is that these acts are related to "normal" human tendencies, the "normal" students enrolled in the class do not have the comfort of being assured that they are above such behaviors. In fact, only unrealistic self-serving biases (something actually covered in the course ...) could really keep a student from thinking he or she was entirely immune. Eventually, the students start to plead for mercy from the seemingly endless barrage of nasty human foibles and plaintively ask, "Can't *something* be done? Is there something *we* can do?" The long answer of course is complicated: Historical wrongs would have to be righted, ingrained prejudices would have to be reversed, and cultural and institutional traditions (some of which serve very positive purposes) would have to be unlearned and dismantled. However, to keep the students' despair at bay, a little ray of sunshine is offered – in the form of perspective taking. Virtually every "bad behavior" covered in the course has appeared in some empirical psychology study alongside

S.D. Hodges (✉)
University of Oregon, Eugene, OR 97403, USA
e-mail: sdhodges@uoregon.edu

R. Biswas-Diener (ed.), *Positive Psychology as Social Change*,
DOI 10.1007/978-90-481-9938-9_12, © Springer Science+Business Media B.V. 2011

a manipulation of perspective taking, and these studies conclude with a common moral: People behave better – more acceptably, more admirably, more prosocially – after perspective taking.

What exactly are the effects of this simple panacea? This is the question we will address in this chapter, but to begin, the simplest answer that encompasses the most territory can be summed up in two parts. First, perspective taking has been consistently found to increase compassionate emotions (commonly called empathy, but the precise label in this case is "empathic concern") toward the person whose perspective has been taken. Second, perspective taking leads people to view and treat other people more like the self, viewing them as possessing more traits in common with the self, and symbolically having "merged," at least partially, with the self in terms of cognitive representations and descriptions of personality and explanations of behavior.

Are these two general outcomes separable? Our answer is only speculative – and requires treading carefully. There has been a spirited debate about *helping* others whose perspective we take and whether this helping is "truly" altruistic or egoistic, given that the recipient of the helping may be linked to the self (see, Batson, Sager, et al., 1997; Cialdini, Brown, Lewis, Luce, & Neuberg, 1997). Interestingly, this debate has focused on the "either/or" question of what mediates helping behavior: Is it EITHER empathic concern OR similarity/merging? One answer is clear: Perspective taking does ultimately lead to more helping behaviors, regardless of which mediators are involved. However, researchers have not generally asked a question that we think is more fundamental: Does perspective taking have separable effects on empathic concern and similarity/merging, or are these two sides of the same construct? We know of only three studies (two published) that have explicitly explored the *simultaneous* effects of perspective taking on empathic concern *and* similarity/merging, and the results do not explicitly answer this question. Maner et al. (2002) found that perspective taking increased empathic concern across the board, and that it also increased one measure of merging (Aron, Aron, & Smollan's 1992 "Inclusion of Other in Self" [IOS] scale), but this latter effect occurred only when no information was provided about how similar the target of perspective taking was to the perspective taker. Batson, Sager, et al. (1997) found that perspective taking increased empathic concern and affected some measures of merging, but not others. Finally, Myers and Hodges (unpublished manuscript) found that perspective taking increased empathic concern, and increased merging on some measures more than others. Without studies that specifically set out to test whether one part mediates perspective taking's effect on the other, an answer may be premature.

In this chapter, although we will present numerous examples of the direct effects of perspective taking on empathic concern and related outcomes, we will not try to tackle the much larger and more diffuse relationship between the broader construct of empathy (or other moral emotions) and the potential for positive social change (for reviews, see Haidt, 2003; Pizarro, 2000; Tangney, Stuewig, & Mashek, 2007). Instead, we will focus specifically on perspective taking, which is sometimes identified as the "cognitive" side of the multidimensional construct of empathy

(Davis,1983; Hodges & Biswas-Diener, 2007). We will further narrow our focus by not attempting to cover the extensive literature on *accuracy* in perspective taking – for example, accurately guessing other people's attitudes, intentions, thoughts, and feelings (for this topic, we refer to the reader to other sources, such as Baron-Cohen, 1997; Hall & Bernieri, 2001; Ickes, 2003; Smith, Ickes, Hall, & Hodges, in press). Instead, we will limit our discussion to the effects of *engaging* in perspective taking, regardless of whether the perspective taken is accurate or not. Even with these limits, there is plenty to say about the potential for perspective taking to lead to positive social change.

Cross-Cultural Caveat

Virtually all of the studies we have referred to so far and those that we will refer to subsequently were conducted using North American samples. Although we would like to believe that the claims we are making about perspective taking are universal, there is good reason to expect that many of the effects we report would be moderated by culture. Particularly, results would be expected to differ between individualist cultures (particularly associated with North America) and collectivist cultures (particularly those associated with Asian countries, like Japan and Taiwan), largely because of different conceptions of the self in these two broad classes of culture. In individualist cultures, the self is viewed largely as independent of others and in fact may even be defined by how the self differs from others. In collectivist cultures, the self is defined in relation to others, and reflects a self that is part of a larger collective whole (Markus & Kitayama, 1991). Thus, the idea of "taking" someone else's perspective might be a more meaningful concept in individualist cultures, where the self and others would be thought to have different perspectives. In a collectivist culture, the embedded self might already have a perspective that reflects the perspective of others (see Brewer & Gardner, 1996; Wu & Keysar, 2007), without having to "take" anything new.

Some intriguing research findings support these ideas. For example, Cohen and Gunz (2002) evoked specific emotions (e.g., fear, shame, or anger) in individualist and collectivist participants by having them recall events in which those specific emotions were predominant. Participants then viewed pictures of faces and were asked to rate the emotions being felt by the people in the pictures. People with individualist cultural backgrounds showed evidence of what the authors called "egocentric projection": They rated the faces as more frightened when they had reported a frightening memory. However, people with collectivist backgrounds showed "relational projection": They saw more of whatever emotion would likely have *prompted* or been felt *in response* to their own emotion. So, for example, when they felt fear, they saw the other faces as angrier; when they felt sad, they saw the other faces as more sympathetic; when they felt contempt, they saw the other faces as more shameful.

People with collectivist cultural backgrounds are also relatively more likely to recall memories from a third-person perspective – one that could be shared by others – and relatively less likely to recall memories from the "self-exclusive" first-person perspective. In addition, they appear to be better able to put aside privileged knowledge available only to the self and assess how a situation would appear to a "naïve" person (Wu & Keysar, 2007), at least when they are not under cognitive load (Cohen & Hoshino-Brown, 2005). Thus, we humbly limit our claims in this chapter to individualist cultures. However, we encourage future researchers to consider exploring whether collectivist and individualist cultures have different starting points for perspective taking. Does perspective taking have the same effect in individualist and collectivist cultures, creating the same pattern of results, only with different mean levels? Or are members of collectivist cultures already performing at a perspective taking "ceiling" or some other qualitatively different starting point than members of individualist cultures?

Development and Mechanics of Perspective Taking

We have presented perspective taking so far as a remarkably simple strategy to increase prosocial behavior, and certainly it is less complicated than implementing, say, universal education or democracy. However, while perspective taking may seem to be a simple task for the adults reading this book, for the younger set, perspective taking constitutes a major developmental milestone. The famous cognitive developmental psychologist, Jean Piaget, included a visual perspective-taking task as one of his cognitive milestones (Piaget & Inhelder, 1956). Children looking at a 3D model of a landscape from one side were asked what someone viewing the landscape from the opposite side would see. Specifically, the task tested whether children would realize that mountains in the landscape obscured parts of the view from one vantage point, but not the other. The ability to perform such visual perspective-taking tasks has been linked, developmentally and conceptually, to social perspective-taking tasks and prosocial behavior (Flavell, 1963; Underwood & Moore, 1982). Although social perspective taking is the main focus of this chapter, perspective taking in general may represent a willingness to consider alternatives, which may potentially underlie the power of perspective taking and may be key in producing positive social change.

A rather dramatic social perspective-taking development takes place in children between the ages of about 3 and 5 years old, as they develop what is known as a "theory of mind." Children come to understand that people have minds, that the workings of these minds guide and influence people's behaviors, and that the contents of another person's mind (her thoughts, beliefs, desires) can differ from the contents of one's own mind. Although the changes associated with acquiring a theory of mind may not be as dramatically visible to a young child's parents as familiar milestones such as learning to walk or talk, the transition does leave the child qualitatively different – and possessing what some would argue constitutes the very essence of what distinguishes humans from other species (see, Povinelli & Vonk, 2003). Like many key early childhood developments, a theory of mind will emerge when the child is developmentally ready. Focused coaching or even the ear-lier development of other skills (Sabbagh, Xu, Carlson, Moses, & Lee, 2006) does not change the developmental trajectory substantially, although some developmental disabilities, like autism spectrum disorders, feature theory of mind deficits.

Ironically, a theory of mind can also improve some skills not considered to be prosocial. For example, a child may become a better liar by being able to take into account what information another person might consider in assessing the truthful-ness of a claim, such as being able to construct plausible answers to questions about exactly *why* there are cookie crumbs on the child's lap if he did not just eat a cookie. Although parents may not see their children's increased ability to lie convincingly as a positive development, it does represent an advancement in children's socialization when one considers that a large proportion of lies are told with an eye to avoiding other people's feelings from being hurt (DePaulo, 2002).

Once a young child has acquired a theory of mind, the work surrounding perspec-tive taking is not over. Other developmental progress allows for more complicated theory of mind tricks, such as the multi-level perspective taking involved in imagin-ing what Karyn thinks Ezra feels about Sean. However, the subsequent development of perspective taking appears to reflect more incremental progress, rather than the dramatic qualitative shift that occurs early on in life. And even though perspec-tive taking may become more sophisticated over developmental time, it can still be hard for grown ups. Intentionally trying to take another person's perspective acti-vates areas of the brain associated with effortful processing (Sabbagh & Taylor, 2000), focuses attention on certain pieces of information to the exclusion of others (Pichert & Anderson, 1977), and deteriorates under cognitive load (Keysar, Barr, & Horton, 1998; Rossnagel, 2000) and time pressure (Epley, Keysar, Van Boven, & Gilovich, 2004). As further evidence that perspective taking can be difficult, peo-ple's attempts to take other perspectives are less successful when they are offered fewer incentives to do it accurately (Klein & Hodges, 2001). Indeed, when people are praised for being good perspective takers, the admiration may be because of the perception that they have taken the effort to *try*, as much as any actual *success* they have at taking the other person's perspective (Hodges, Kiel, Kramer, Veach, & Villanueva, 2010)

If perspective taking ever does seem easy, it is probably when it does not need to be prompted by explicit intentions or instructions to take the other person's per-spective. Under these circumstances, it may not *feel* like perspective taking to the perspective taker, and thus it may not even be labeled as such by the person doing it. Repeatedly taking another person's perspective – such as a person whose opinion we care about (Baldwin & Holmes, 1987), someone with whom we must frequently coordinate, or even a fictional character (Taylor, Hodges, & Kohanyi, 2003) – may result in perspective taking becoming automatic (see Hodges & Wegner, 1997), in the same way that other often-repeated actions such as driving become automatic (e.g., Dreyfus & Dreyfus, 1986).

Some of the more effortless aspects of perspective taking may be handled out-side conscious awareness in neural structures specifically designed to link the self and others. Groundbreaking neuroscience research began to identify the presence of "mirror neurons" in non-human primates about 20 years ago (see Iacoboni, 2009, for a review) with analogous brain regions and functions also identified in humans. The hallmark of the mirror neurons in monkeys was that they fired both when the owner of the brain performed certain motor actions (the monkey reaching for raisins), and when the owner of the brain observed another primate performing the same motor action (the experimenter reaching for raisins).

In humans, the "mirror system" may play a fundamental role in emotional contagion: Seeing *your* emotional expression (e.g., fear) causes *me* to feel the same emotion (see, Carr, Iacoboni, Dubeau, Mazziotta, & Lenzi, 2003), although the concept of emotional contagion was around long before psychologists began to identify which neural areas might be involved in it (Hatfield, Cacioppo, & Rapson, 1993). As the name implies, emotional contagion is not considered an intentional strategy to increase perspective taking, although it may facilitate perspective taking: If both the perspective taker and the target of perspective taking are feeling the same emotion, the distance between their two perspectives may be shorter.

Something along the lines of "reduced effort" perspective taking may occur when the distinction between the perspective taker and the person whose perspective is taken is fuzzy, as is the case when representations of the self and representations of the other overlap or merge. When this occurs, some might argue that perspective taking is not occurring at all. If the self and other are the same, they have the same perspective and there is not really any new perspective to take (see, Batson, Sager, et al., 1997; Cialdini et al., 1997). However, there are striking parallels in terms of how people represent themselves and others, and how they allocate resources such as helping to others, that result both from an intentional attempt to take another person's perspective *and* from close associations with others (Batson, Sager, et al., 1997; Cialdini et al., 1997; Davis, Conklin, Smith, & Luce, 1996; Maner et al., 2002; Myers & Hodges, unpublished manuscript).

Taking the perspective of another person involves a complex interplay of multiple processes: projection ("What is my current perspective?"); adjustment ("How does her perspective differ from mine?"); stored knowledge and cognitive stereotypes and scripts ("What do single mothers feel?" "What generally happens when someone loses a parent?"); attention to individual cues provided by the target of perspective taking ("He looks nervous;" "She said she's not hungry because they ate on the road"); and imagination ("I wonder what he thinks about when he is alone?"). Although researchers are starting to identify how the various perspective-taking strategies interact (e.g., Ames, 2004a, 2004b; Davis et al.,2004; Epley et al., 2004; Gesn & Ickes,1999; Karniol & Shomroni,1999), identifying *which* strategies predominate *when* is an ongoing investigation.

Many studies – both those in the literature at large and those discussed in this chapter – have successfully manipulated perspective taking by explicitly instructing research participants to take another person's perspective (e.g., Batson et al., 1991; Toi & Batson, 1982). However, there are few easily identifiable "real life" analogues to an experimenter telling us to take another person's perspective, although explicit requests for perspective taking may come from people asking for understanding and sympathy ("Try to see it from my point of view;" "Just imagine how I felt when I read your letter"). Encouraging perspective taking as a habit may come from people trying to socialize children, such as parents who encourage their children to consider others' feelings (Krevans & Gibbs, 1996) or even institutionalized educational programs such as "Second Step" (Committee for Children, 1992) or the PATHS curriculum (Greenberg, Kusche, Cook, & Quamma, 1995). Perspective taking is entrenched in aphorisms ("walk a mile in another person's shoes") and moral and religions teachings (e.g., the "Golden Rule"). Perspective taking may also be "the result of prior similar experience or of attachment" (Batson, 1987, p. 91). Furthermore, manipulating similarity by telling people they have shared preferences and traits produces a similar pattern of effects on empathic concern and helping as do perspective taking instructions (e.g., Batson, Duncan, Ackerman, Buckley, & Birch, 1981; see also Goldstein & Cialdini, 2007).

In addition to being considered a variable that can be manipulated, perspective taking has also been treated as a tendency that varies in degree across individuals (e.g., Davis & Oathout, 1987; Galinsky, Maddux, Gilin, & White, 2008; Richardson, Green, & Lago, 1998; Richardson, Hammock, Smith, Gardner, & Signo, 1994, Studies 1 and 3): Greater perspective taking is assumed to occur among those scoring higher on scales such as the perspective-taking subscale of the Interpersonal Reactivity Index (IRI; Davis, 1983). Yet other lines of research do not explicitly manipulate or measure perspective taking, but rather focus on the processes related to perspective taking, like guessing what other people are thinking (Ickes, 2003), or the dynamics of close relationships, especially romantic ones, in which perspective taking is presumed to occur (Kilpatrick, Bissonnette, & Rusbult, 2002).

Exactly what triggers spontaneous perspective taking, how often the triggers occur, and whether people are consciously aware of them all represent frontiers yet to be charted in the perspective-taking landscape. Furthermore, we do not know whether the results of naturalistic perspective-taking prompts parallel the effects of explicit instructions from an experimenter. However, given the focus of this volume on mechanisms for social change, we want to make the encouraging statement that perspective-taking propensity is something that can be at least partially controlled, is affected by effort, and thus can potentially be increased. The following points support our position.

First, the beneficial outcomes associated with being dispositionally high in perspective taking do not look that different from those associated with manipulations that explicitly instruct people to perspective take. Researchers who have used both manipulated and measured perspective taking in conceptually similar studies find similar outcomes (e.g., Galinsky, Wang, & Ku, 2008; Galinsky, Maddux, et al., 2008). The difference just seems to be that people who score high in dispositional perspective taking do it without being told.

Second, dispositional *measures* of perspective taking look a lot like manipulated perspective taking *instructions*. A very commonly used measure of dispositional perspective taking (perhaps the most commonly used measure) is Davis's perspective-taking subscale of the IRI (Davis, 1983). As a self-report measure, it is largely a measure of people's self-perceived propensity and frequency to take others' perspectives (e.g., it includes items such as "I try to look at everybody's side of a disagreement before I make a decision" and "I sometimes try to understand my friends better by imagining how things look from their perspective") and *not* the range of their abilities (i.e., the items are not things like "I can read minds" or "I am particularly sensitive to what others are feeling"). In other words, the items on Davis's individual difference perspective-taking subscale could all be rewritten in the imperative and used as perspective-taking instructions!

Third, although dispositional perspective taking has been shown to be *somewhat* heritable, its heritability is lower than other components of empathy (Davis, Luce, & Kraus, 1994; Soenens, Duriez, Vansteenkiste, & Goossens, 2007), suggesting more potential room for environment and teaching to play a role. Finally, what people think about "naturally" when they encounter another person appears to resemble more what they think about when given explicit instructions to imagine how another person feels and looks a lot *less* like what people do when they are trying to inhibit perspective taking (Davis et al., 2004; see also Aderman, Brehm, & Katz, 1974). In fact, Davis et al. (2004) provocatively (and persuasively) argue that when differences are found in instructional sets for perceiving other people, it is less the "imagine self/other" sort of instructions (often portrayed as an experimental condition) that are facilitating perspective taking, and more the "observe carefully/objectively" sort of instructions (often portrayed as a control condition) that may actually inhibit perspective taking. Specifically, imagining what the other person is feeling may be a kind of default strategy in person perception and preventing oneself from trying to do this may be unnatural.

In sum, there is hope for all of us, individually and collectively, when it comes to harnessing perspective taking as a vehicle of positive social change. It is controllable, and when controlled, its effects are similar to the effects of being dispositionally high in perspective-taking propensity. Big questions about perspective taking do remain, but psychologists have already accumulated a substantial body of work demonstrating the link between perspective taking and behavior associated with positive social change. Rather than providing an exhaustive review of all these studies, our coverage is designed to give a sense of the breadth and variety of effects that perspective taking has on societally relevant behaviors and attitudes. We now turn to those findings.

Perspective Taking, Compassion, and Helpful Behavior

In surveying the positive results of perspective taking, we start with one of the most replicated and robust findings in social psychology: Taking the perspective of another person increases compassionate emotions (often called "empathic concern") toward that person (as just a sampling of references: Batson, 1987; Batson et al., 1991; Batson, Polycarpou, et al., 1997; Batson, Sager, et al., 1997; Klein & Hodges, 2001; Stotland, 1969).

The link between perspective taking and concern for others emerges early. When asked to imagine how victims in various scenarios felt, children in elementary school reported more concern for the victim (Thompson & Hoffman, 1980). And in support of Batson's (1987) claim that perspective taking is likely to occur between people who have had similar experiences, several studies have shown that people – at least children and adult women – have greater empathic concern for those who have had similar experience (Barnett, 1984; Batson et al., 1996; Hodges et al., 2010).

Many perspective-taking studies then go on to show the next step in Batson's "empathy-altruism" hypothesis (e.g., Coke, Batson, & McDavis, 1978), whereby empathic feelings lead to a valuing of the target's welfare, which motivates helping on their behalf (Batson et al., 1991; Batson, Polycarpou, et al., 1997; Batson, Sager, et al., 1997). As already alluded to, researchers have hotly debated whether the helping that results from perspective taking is motivated by truly altruistic concerns (i.e., no benefit to the self, and perhaps even some cost; Batson, Sager, et al., 1997) or whether it benefits a self that has been extended to include representations of others (Cialdini et al., 1997). However, designating a winner in that debate can be sidestepped for the purposes of this chapter, where we are more focused on outcomes than mechanisms, and the outcomes (empathic concern and helping as a result of perspective taking) are undisputed.

One important aspect of Batson's model that has been nicely resolved is the distinction between two kinds of empathic emotion – empathic concern and personal distress – that are evoked by perspective taking. The former is concern or compassion *for* the target of perspective taking; whereas the latter is distress felt *by* the perspective taker that is aroused by the target's plight. Slight, but meaningful, changes in perspective-taking instructions affect the balance of the two emotions. Asking research participants to imagine what *they* would feel in another person's situation ("imagine self" instructions) evokes both personal distress and empathic concern, whereas instructions to imagine what they think the *other person* is feeling ("imagine other" instructions) evokes only empathic concern (Batson, Early, & Salvarani, 1997). Related distinctions between the two sets of instructions have also been demonstrated by brain imaging studies (Lamm, Batson, & Decety, 2007), but it should be noted that for other behavioral outcomes, sometimes the results of the two sets of instructions are similar (Davis et al., 1996; Finlay & Stephan, 2000). Empathic concern is thought to be a more sophisticated empathic response than personal distress (Eisenberg & Fabes, 1990; Eisenberg, Wentzel, & Harris, 1998), emerging later developmentally (Hoffman, 1984; Zahn-Waxler & Radke-Yarrow, 1990; Zahn-Waxler, Radke-Yarrow, Wagner, & Chapman, 1992) and reflecting healthy emotion regulation (Eisenberg et al., 1996). Empathic concern is thought to do more of the heavy lifting, mediating the link between perspective taking and helping, whereas personal distress may interfere with addressing the target of perspective taking's needs, because the perspective taker becomes focused on resolving his own distress (Batson, 1987). This suggests that people might be more helpful after "imagine other" instructions than after "imagine self" instructions (Batson et al., 2003).

In another variation on perspective taking instructions, Oswald (1996) found that instructions to attend to a target person's *feelings* resulted in more willingness to help others similar to the target than did instructions to attend to the target's *thoughts*. The pattern of means for empathic concern in this study echoed those for helping. However, both forms of perspective taking instructions resulted in greater helping than instructions to attend to technical details of the film of the target person.

Perspective taking may also lead to more helping because the perspective taker is better able to provide help. In a psycholinguistics study by Traxler and Gernsbacher (1993), the researchers did not directly manipulate or measure perspective taking, but gave half of their participants access to another perspective by having them first play one role in a paired interaction, then play the other role, and then return to the first role. The interaction required one participant to describe complex geometric figures to the other, so that the other could then pick out which figure had been described from a set of distractors. The figures were complex and abstract enough that describing the target figure in such a way that would help another person distinguish it from the distractors was quite challenging (more challenging than most describers seemed to realize initially). Participants who first described the figures and were then given the other role of trying to pick which figure had been described showed marked improvements when they were asked to describe the figures to other people a second time, as compared to participants who were not given the experience of trying to pick out the figures. Thus, being temporarily put in someone else's shoes made people more effective helpers.

Perspective Taking, Similarity, and Self-other Merging

A variety of evidence supports the idea that perspective takers view the target of perspective taking in ways that resemble how they view the self. It is perhaps somewhat ironic that perspective taking is often associated with getting "outside" of one's self, and yet the self is highly involved (Davis et al., 2004; Galinsky & Moskowitz, 2000). However, the involvement of the self makes more sense when one considers what a valuable and useful proxy the self is when trying to comprehend something as complex and inaccessible as another person's mind (see, Ames, 2004a, 2004b; Dawes, 1990; Hoch, 1987) and also how perspective taking involves sharing with others the central spot in cognition and consciousness that is generally occupied by the self.

At the most basic level, perspective takers perceive greater similarity between traits they ascribe to themselves and traits they ascribe to the target of perspective taking. Perspective takers ascribe traits to the target of perspective taking that they previously used to describe themselves, such that perspective takers, relative to non-perspective takers, see a larger proportion of self-traits as also being traits belonging to the perspective-taking target (Davis et al., 1996; Myers & Hodges, unpublished manuscript). Perspective takers may also see smaller absolute differences between how they rate themselves on traits and how they rate the target of perspective taking on those same traits (Galinsky & Moskowitz, 2000; but see Batson, Sager, et al., 1997 for contradictory results). Perspective takers perceive trait similarity both when targets are generally similar to the perspective taker (e.g., college students taking the perspective of an average college student; Davis et al., 1996), and when targets are dissimilar (Myers, 2009) or are members of stereotyped outgroups (Galinsky &

Moskowitz, 2000). For example, Galinsky and Moskowitz (2000, Study 2) found that student participants taking the perspective of an elderly man showed less absolute difference between participants' self ratings on 85 traits and participants' ratings of the elderly as a group on those same traits.

In addition to perspective takers viewing the target of the perspective taking as more like the self, there is growing evidence that perspective takers also change their views of the *self* to be more similar to the target of perspective taking (Galinsky, Wang, et al., 2008; Goldstein & Cialdini, 2007). In a series of studies, Galinsky, Wang, et al. (2008) showed that people instructed to take the perspective of a stereotyped group (relative to people given instructions to remain objective) rated themselves, and even behaved, in ways that resemble the group's stereotype. For example, people asked to take the perspective of a cheerleader while writing about a day in her life subsequently rated *themselves* as more attractive and sexy (Study 1A). People asked to take the perspective of a professor rated themselves as more intelligent (Study 1B) and afterward performed better on standardized test questions designed to measured analytic ability (Study 2A). Even negative traits of the stereotyped group were attributed to the self more after taking the perspective of a representative of that group (Study 1C), with people rating themselves as weaker and less independent after taking the perspective of an elderly man. Galinsky, Wang, et al. (2008) assert that changing self-conceptions in a direction toward the group stereotype facilitates coordination with the target of perspective taking. Furthermore, they believe that perspective-taking instructions have a more powerful effect than merely priming traits associated with stereotyped group, although it must be noted that the mechanisms and effects involved appear to share common ground with those found in studies that prime stereotypes (e.g., Dijksterhuis & van Knippenberg, 1998) or create the anticipation of interactions with others who hold stereotyped views (e.g., Sinclair, Huntsinger, Skorinko, & Hardin, 2005).

Perspective-taking induced similarity in trait ascription is sometimes accompanied by greater global perceptions of similarity with the perspective-taking target (e.g., answers to the question, "How similar are you and the target?" Davis et al., 1996; Vorauer, Martens, & Sasaki, 2009, Study 4), but sometimes it is not (e.g., Galinsky & Moskowitz, 2000). Perspective taking also influences "inclusion of the other in self" (IOS), a construct introduced by Art Aron (e.g., Aron et al., 1992; Aron, Aron, Tudor, & Nelson, 1991) in the close relationships literature to describe how people perceive themselves as "merging" with close others or being interconnected with them in terms of their representations. The construct is often measured using the IOS scale developed by Aron et al. (1992) that presents seven pairs of side-by-side circles that increasingly overlap. It is striking that taking the perspective of a stranger – one who is often presented only via audiotape or videotape (Batson, Sager, et al., 1997, Study 2; Maner et al., 2002; Myers & Hodges, unpublished manuscript) – can result in people viewing themselves as joined to this stranger in a manner resembling the way long-term romantic couples see themselves as joined.

Thus, taking the perspective of another person seems to "align" the self with that person (see, Gentner & Markman, 1994), increasing the extent to which the perspective takers see the target of perspective taking as sharing their own traits; triggering perspective takers to take on traits of the target; and creating a shared representation of perspective taker and target. The social psychology literature is full of findings showing that similar others are liked better (Berscheid & Reis, 1998; Byrne, 1961, 1997; Griffitt & Veitch, 1974; Montoya, Horton, & Kirschner, 2008) and members of ingroups receive more favorable treatment and are viewed more charitably than outgroup members (Brewer, 1979; Tajfel, 1982; Tajfel & Billig, 1974). However, perspective taking seems to provide something beyond merely liking the target better (Davis et al., 1996; Galinsky & Moskowitz, 2000; Galinsky, Wang, et al., 2008; Gould & Sigall, 1977; Myers & Hodges, unpublished manuscript). It is as if the target of perspective taking is not just *liked* by the self, but somehow *joined* to the self. Not only does perspective taking extend the self, but also courtesies afforded to oneself are extended to the target of perspective taking as well, as we see in our next section when we turn to other perspective-taking outcomes that often accompany the two large classes of outcomes we have already discussed (empathic concern/helping, and similarity/merging). In many cases, researchers have not tested whether our "big two" mediate these other outcomes, but when those meditational results are available, we have tried to report them.

Perspective Taking and More Charitable Attributions

Although long held beliefs about attributional differences between actors and observers have recently been convincingly challenged (Malle, 2006), the classic claim that actors tend to explain their own behaviors in terms of factors external to themselves (e.g., aspects of the situation) and observers tend to explain the behaviors of others in terms of internal factors (e.g., personality) still holds for *negative* behaviors.[1] Thus, as an actor, when asked to explain why she failed her driver's test, Lulu is more likely to mention the uptight examiner or the ridiculously hard parallel parking spot she had to get into, whereas someone observing Lulu is likely to note that she simply did not practice enough. However, after perspective taking, observers make attributions more like actors, attributing negative outcomes to factors outside the agent's control.

In a classic example of perspective-taking observers making more charitable attributions for an agent's failures, Gould and Sigall (1977) asked observers to watch a target person try to make a positive first impression on another person. They

---

[1] Notably, although Malle's exhaustive meta-analysis shows no "traditional" actor–observer effect for positive behaviors, there are several oft-cited studies that report that perspective taking increases observers' external attributions even for positive or neutral behaviors, such as (Storms, 1973). However, Malle (2006) reports five published failures to replicate Storms' original attributional pattern among non-perspective-taking observers. Galper's (1976) study is also regularly cited. She labeled her manipulation as an "empathy" versus a control condition, but the instructions in the empathy condition are quite similar to "imagine self" perspective-taking instructions used in other studies. Additionally, it should be noted that Malle's meta-analysis only included studies that had actors and observers making attributions; studies that manipulated perspective taking but only for observer subjects were excluded.

gave the observers instructions to either imagine how the target person felt or care-fully observe the target. Observers were then told that the target either succeeded or failed at making a positive impression, and were asked to make attributions about the outcome. For observers instructed to "imagine the other," failures (i.e., nega-tive outcomes) were seen as more due to situational causes than were successes. Importantly, the perspective taking instructions did not affect how much observers liked the target, relative to observers in the control "observe" condition. Thus, the effects of perspective taking went beyond mere evaluation of the target.

Vescio, Sechrist, and Paolucci (2003) found that perspective-taking instructions ("imagine other") increased the extent to which White students made situational attributions for adjustment difficulties faced by an African-American student, rela-tive to students who received instructions to remain objective while hearing about the African-American student. Furthermore, Vescio et al. also found that the extent to which participants made situational attributions significantly mediated the effect of perspective taking on pro-African-American attitudes: Participants who took the target's perspective made more situational attributions, which in turn led to more pro-African-American attitudes.

In terms of perspective taking's effects on assigning blame and punishment, a study by Macrae and Milne (1992) asked participants to imagine a food-poisoning incident either from the perspective of the victim of food poisoning or from the perspective of the restaurant where the incident occurred. Participants' estimates of what the compensation and fines for the incident should be corresponded to their perspective: greater compensation when taking the victim's perspective and less compensation when taking the restaurant's perspective, relative to a control condi-tion with no assigned perspective. Participants' responses were amplified in these respective directions when the circumstances preceding the incident were out of the ordinary as opposed to routine (i.e., the diner went to a new restaurant instead of her regular haunt). The researchers also measured amount of sympathy felt for the victim, which appears to have mediated the financial award results.

In related work, Archer, Foushee, Davis and Aderman (1979) put perspective taking's attributional effects on trial. When instructed by a defense lawyer to take the defendant's perspective (using "imagine self" perspective-taking instructions), mock jurors saw the defendant's personality as having a less causal role in an aggres-sive bar room brawl (as long as they did not also hear a reminder from the judge to weigh only the facts in their deliberation). Taking the perspective of wrong-doers appears to have resulted in holding the defendant less responsible for the wrongdoing. However, a potentially even more effective way to get people to see a wrongdoer as less responsible is to have them recall a time when they engaged in similar wrongdoing (Takaku, Weiner, & Ohbuchi, 2001).

Of course, more sympathy or less blame for a particular party in a dispute does not *necessarily* lead to positive social change. More sympathy for a sham victim or truly guilty defendant may not be a good thing. However, in many con-texts, those who are disadvantaged (economically, socially, etc.) are not only more likely to be victimized, and victims are also often blamed for their misfortune (e.g., Branscombe, Owen, Garstka, & Coleman, 1996; Kaiser & Miller, 2003). Taking the perspective of the victim may remind us of the former and reduce the latter. Similarly, certain social and ethnic groups are more likely to be fingered as perpetrators and dealt with more harshly when found guilty (see Greene, Heilbrun, Fortune, & Nietzel, 2007). Taking their perspective may help counteract these biases. In both cases, perspective taking's effects on attributions may help level the playing field. Furthermore, perspective taking may simply result in attributions being made more carefully: In an attribution study by Malle and Pearce (2001), observers taking the perspective of others noticed and reported more actions being performed by those others.

Perspective Taking and Prejudice

Vescio et al.'s (2003) results that are discussed above foreshadow the idea that perspective taking not only makes us more charitable in our attributions about others whose perspective we have taken, but that perspective taking may also counteract culturally shared prejudices. In one set of very clear and illustrative results, Dovidio et al. (2004, Study 1) had college student participants watch a video clip from a documentary about discrimination against an African-American man. Beforehand, they received either perspective-taking instructions ("imagine other"), instructions to watch objectively, or no special instructions. Only those in the perspective-taking condition later showed a drop in prejudice toward African-Americans, relative to pretest scores collected earlier in the term using the same prejudice scale. Those in the perspective-taking condition also felt more of a sense of merging between themselves and the character in the video (using Aron et al.'s 1992 IOS scale), and reported a greater sense of injustice in response to the video, but only the latter appeared to mediate perspective taking's reduction of prejudice.

Using a different target of prejudice (gays), Karaçanta and Fitness (2006) found that perspective-taking instructions ("imagine other" instructions, relative to "remain objective" instructions) increased compassion for a gay target who discussed on video the harassment he had received for his sexual orientation. In another study, Johnson, Brems, and Alford-Keating (1997) measured dispositional differences in perspective taking with the perspective-taking subscale of Davis's IRI, rather than manipulating perspective taking, and found that higher perspective-taking scores predicted less homophobic attitudes.

Perspective taking for a particular stigmatized target may generalize to more positive attitudes toward the group as a whole, with the effect mediated by the empathic concern for the specific target (Batson, Polycarpou, et al., 1997). Batson, Polycarpou, et al. (1997) found this chain of events held generally, even when the specific target could be seen as somewhat responsible for the stigmatized fate (i.e., a homeless man who quit his job rather than being fired from it). In Batson, Polycarpou, et al.'s (1997) final study, where the stigmatized group was the decidedly unpopular category of "murderers," an ameliorative effect on attitudes toward the group was limited at first, but became more robust when attitudes toward prison reform and murderers were assessed a week or two later in an ostensibly unconnected survey. Finally in a closely related study, Batson, Chang, Orr, and

Rowland (2002) found that perspective takers not only reported more empathic concern for a convicted criminal and heroin addict, but they also recommended allocating more "Student Action Committee" funds to an addiction counseling program.

Perspective taking has been shown to reduce ingroup favoritism, even when the ingroup/outgroup distinction was novel to participants (Galinsky & Moskowitz, 2000, Study 3) – a result that appears to stem from a reduction in ingroup ratings *and* an increase in outgroup ratings. In at least one study, taking the perspective of ingroup member who experienced discrimination resulted in more positive attitudes toward members of *another* outgroup: Finlay and Stephan (2000) asked European-American participants to read a scenario about an American student (race not specified) who was discriminated against in Hong Kong. The participants were asked to either take the perspective of the student (using "imagine self" or "imagine other" instructions) or to follow control ("observe") instructions. Relative to participants in the control condition, participants who were asked to imagine the perspective of the student later reported more positive attitudes toward an outgroup (African-Americans), and less positive attitudes toward European-Americans (their own ingroup). However, these results may be limited to situations where the target of perspective taking is like the self and toward outgroups for whom prejudice is well-documented and easily brought to mind.

Perspective taking not only reduces prejudice, but also appears to reduce use of stereotypes. Galinsky and Moskowitz (2000) showed college participants a picture of an elderly man and asked them to write about a day in his life. Participants who were asked to imagine themselves as if they were the man in the photo wrote essays with content that was less stereotypic of the elderly and more positive in tone, relative to control participants. In a less serious context, Piper and Langer (1984) reported that people instructed to watch soap operas from the perspective of people in different professions ended up seeing the characters as more complex and less stereotypic.

Galinsky and Moskowitz (2000) explain their stereotype reduction results as being due to the fact that "perspective-taking nonconsciously increases the accessibility of the self-concept, which then diminishes the accessibility and application of the stereotype because only one construct tends to be dominant at any one time" (p. 720). This leads to an interesting paradox: On the one hand, perspective taking leads to a reduction in prejudice toward a group, which would seem consistent with abandoning the group's stereotype. On the other hand, it leads to viewing the self as having more in common with the stereotype of the group, which sounds consistent with embracing the group's stereotype. Despite an apparent surface contradiction, simultaneously obtaining both results is not impossible. After perspective taking, stereotypes are applied relatively less to members of the group (Galinsky & Moskowitz, 2000), but relatively more to the self (Galinsky, Wang, et al., 2008). The final piece of the puzzle that has to be reconciled is that past results have also shown that perspective takers ascribe more of their own traits to targets of perspective taking (Davis et al., 1996). In order to balance the equation, these self-traits would have to be traits that are inconsistent with the stereotype.

Of course, prejudice is a complex, thorny, and deeply embedded problem, and we should not expect any simple solutions, even with perspective taking. Further complicating matters are important boundary conditions to keep in mind, such as the perspective taker's view of the self. If, as we have asserted earlier, perspective taking results in sharing traits of the self with the target of perspective taking, then the positive effects of perspective taking on perceptions of another person might be expected to disappear if the self is not viewed favorably. Support for this idea comes from work by Galinsky and Ku (2004), who showed that perspective taking produces a reduction in prejudice toward a stereotyped group only when self-esteem is high. Furthermore, perspective taking may backfire in terms of reducing prejudice when the instruction to perspective take comes *from* a member of the stereotyped group and is directed toward people who are highly prejudiced against members of that group (Focella, Whitehead, Stone, & Schmader, 2010). In addition, Skorinko and Sinclair (2010) suggest an important moderator in perspective taking's ability to reduce the use of a group's stereotype in describing group members: When the group member strongly confirms to the group stereotype (such as an elderly man who is also clearly ill), perspective taking may actually increase stereotype use.

Finally, although perspective taking appears to improve beliefs and attitudes about other groups, work by Vorauer et al. (2009) demonstrates that perspective taking may backfire for certain people in actual social interactions. In four studies, university participants were asked to communicate with a person who was an ethnic minority (by writing, making an audiotape, or interacting face-to-face). Among those who took the perspective of their ethnic minority partner prior to the interaction, *lower* prejudice scores predicted *fewer* intimacy-building behaviors in their communication with their partner (Studies 1, 2, and 3) as well as interactions that were rated *less* positively by their ethnic minority partners (Study 4). Vorauer et al. explain these counterintuitive results by using a "divergent effort account": Low prejudice people assume that ethnic minorities will recognize their low prejudice beliefs, and thus they do not feel like they need to "work" to avoid being perceived as prejudiced. However, their non-prejudicial beliefs are *not* readily apparent to ethnic minorities, whereas their lack of work to convey positive attitudes apparently is. Ironically, higher prejudiced people may fair better after perspective taking – they do not assume that they will be perceived by the ethnic minorities in a positive manner and thus work harder to counteract negative perceptions. Clearly, although perspective taking is powerful weapon against prejudice, it is not perfect.

Perspective Taking and Aggressive Behavior

Perspective taking (either manipulated or measured as an individual difference) generally predicts less aggressive responses in a competitive laboratory task (although there appear to be boundary conditions, such as how threatening the task is; Richardson et al., 1998, 1994). In particular, people who score higher in dispositional perspective taking (using Davis's perspective-taking subscale of the IRI) respond less aggressively than do people who score lower, in response to interaction partners retaliating in a highly provocative way (Richardson et al., 1994, Study 3) or escalating in aggressiveness (Richardson et al., 1998). People who score high on perspective taking also report being more likely to seek out constructive strategies such as problem solving and discussion in potentially aggressive situations, and less likely to seek out aggressive tactics (Richardson et al., 1994, Study 1). However, perspective taking does not always lead to less aggression. When the perspective taken is that of a member of a group that is stereotyped as aggressive, such as African-Americans, perspective taking may lead to more aggressive behavior relative to taking the perspective of a member of a group that is not stereotyped as aggressive, such as the elderly (Galinsky, Wang, et al., 2008).

Perspective Taking and Social Interactions

People who score higher in dispositional perspective taking (using Davis's perspective-taking subscale of the IRI) appear to be more socially adept. They have higher self-esteem and show less social anxiety on a variety of measures (Davis, 1983). Greater perspective taking may increase the chances of reaching a deal in negotiations and lead to more creative solutions that result in gains for both parties (Galinsky, Maddux, et al., 2008; see also Neale & Bazerman, 1983), probably because they think more about what would satisfy the other party. In addition, Bernstein and Davis (1982) reported that people dispositionally high in perspective taking were better at a social perception task involving strangers. Participants were given three-word self-descriptions written by participants in a group discussion. After watching a videotape of the group discussion, people who were high in perspective taking were better able to match which self-description went with which group participant.

Perspective taking might be a particularly important component of successful close, long-term relationships (Davis & Oathout, 1987; Franzoi, Davis, & Young, 1985; Long & Andrews, 1990). Davis and Oathout (1987) found that when in close relationships, people who scored high in perspective taking reported more positive social traits (e.g., having a positive outlook) and fewer negative social traits (e.g., being untrustworthy) when describing themselves. Many of these self-reported traits were echoed in their romantic partners' perceptions, and some of those perceptions in turn led to reports of greater relationship satisfaction by the partners.

Perspctive Taking and the Environment

Can taking the perspective of something other than another person result in positive social change? A small collection of environmental science studies suggests that being asked to take the perspective of plants or animals that are pictured or described in text increases proenvironmental attitudes and commitment to helping the environment. Berenguer (2007) showed university students either a photo of trees that had been cut down, or a dead bird on an oil-covered beach. They were given instructions to either take the perspective of the trees or the bird, or to remain objective while viewing the photo. Perspective takers not only reported greater empathic concern after viewing the photos, but they also reported feeling more of a moral obligation to help the bird or trees and a greater desire to help nature as a whole (see also Shelton & Rogers, 1981, for conceptually similar results using whales as the perspective-taking targets). Furthermore, perspective takers advocated greater funding for environmental programs when asked to allocate money to student programs, a result that was mediated by how much empathic concern they reported feeling.

In a similar study, Berenguer (2010) asked some participants to perspective take while reading about a vulture being hit by a car and asked other participants to read the passage objectively. He found the same perspective taking induced empathic concern results as he did in the 2007 study. Furthermore, he found that when perspective takers were later asked to read environmental dilemmas and justify which course of action they would take, their answers contained more "ecocentric" reasons (i.e., reasons that referred to protecting nature for its own sake, rather than protecting it because of instrumental benefits to humans).

However, greater "ecocentrism" may be evoked by perspective taking only when the target of perspective taking in nature is being harmed. Schultz (2000) showed undergraduates photos of people in natural environments, animals in natural environments, or animals being harmed by human caused factors (e.g., a seal caught in a fishing net). Before viewing the photos, participants were given instructions either to take the perspective of the subject (human or animal in the photo) or to try to remain objective while viewing the photo. The two factors – type of photo and instructions – interacted, such that perspective takers who viewed animals being harmed reported more "biospheric concerns" – that is, concerns "based on a value for all living things" (p. 392), a construct similar to Berenguer's "ecocentrism."

Perspective Taking as Thinking Again, Thinking Differently

We detour now from concrete positive social outcomes associated with perspective taking to a more speculative path about how perspective taking may be generally related to flexible cognition. If nothing else, perspective taking makes us (a) think again and (b) think differently (see, Koehler, 1991), which can cause us to attend to new or different information. For example, participants reading a passage about a tropical island learned and recalled different information when they took the perspective of a florist looking for place to gather flowers than when they took the perspective of a shipwrecked person (Pichert & Anderson, 1977). Ginossar and Trope (1987) also found that asking people to take a different perspective caused them to attend to information to which they would not normally attend. In their study, they provided subjects with a hit-and-run scenario involving a taxicab. Subjects were asked to assess the likelihood that the taxicab was from one of two cab companies, the answer to which relied in part on the base rates of the number of cabs from the two companies. Subjects given this scenario usually ignore or under-utilize the base rate information (cf. Tversky & Kahneman, 1982), but when

Ginossar and Trope asked their subjects to judge the likelihood from the perspective of a lawyer involved in the case, their perspective-taking manipulation increased subjects' use of base rate information. In addition, thinking of alternative scenarios (which perspective taking seems to involve) results in making those alternatives more cognitively available (Koehler, 1991). Even though our initial construal (in this case, the self perspective) will probably still dominate, we may be less biased to doggedly defend it (Anderson, 1982; Bassok & Trope, 1984; Griffin, Dunning, & Ross, 1990; Lord, Lepper, & Preston, 1984).

Perspective taking may reduce people's unrealistic optimism about the likelihood of certain life outcomes happening. Weinstein and Lachendro (1982) found that asking students to list possible factors that would either increase or decrease their chances of a negative life event (e.g., cancer or heart disease) did not reduce their unrealistic optimism. However, asking subjects to either read another student's factor list or fill out the factor list from the perspective of a "typical" student did reduce optimism.

Ending Ideas

Even though we think we have gathered together a convincing collection of findings suggesting that perspective taking could play an important role in promoting positive social change, we don't want to leave the impression that we are "Pollyannas for perspective taking." Although we have already acknowledged a number of limitations on the positive potential of perspective taking within our section on prejudice and hinted at it in our section on attributions, there are other potential perspective taking pitfalls. For example, when Batson, Klein, Highberger, and Shaw (1995) asked participants to take the perspective of a target who had experienced a major life set back (a romantic breakup or a serious disease), they gave the targets preferential treatment when it came to allocating subsequent outcomes, even when that preferential treatment directly contradicted allocation guidelines and even when participants agreed it wasn't the fairest way to make the allocation (see also Batson et al., 1995).

Perspective taking can also backfire in zero-sum, competitive contexts where perspective takers have little information with which to generate another party's perspective, other than general theories of human behavior or their own tendencies. Epley, Caruso, and Bazerman (2006) reasoned that if participants who were asked to claim a part of a shared resource were also asked to take the perspective of other parties who were sharing that resource, they would assume the other parties would overclaim. They would then increase their own claim in order to counteract the predicted overclaiming by the other parties. In other words, if perspective taking leads people to draw negative conclusions about the target of perspective taking, then the perspective takers' subsequent behaviors may reflect retaliatory or self-protective behaviors that may impede positive social change. Perspective taking in zero-sum situations, particularly "winner takes all" scenarios (see Batson et al., 2003), may also highlight the costs to the self of behaving sympathetically toward the other.

Perhaps more sobering is that even when perspective taking is working at its best, it may fall short in counteracting some of the most noxious human behaviors. Perspective taking operates on a personal scale. Even though we have described studies where taking the perspective of an individual results in more positive outcomes for groups, there may be a bottleneck, given the limitations that we can take just one perspective at a time and that taking another perspective is effortful. When faced, for example, with a whole nation of victims, as in the case of genocide, perspective taking appears to be woefully insufficient (Slovic, 2007).

However, while we humbly acknowledge the limitations of perspective taking, we want to end this chapter on a positive note. Perspective taking has demonstrated a remarkable flexibility in its applications: It is like the duct tape of social interactions. And like duct tape, there may be ways we are – or could be – using perspective taking that have not yet been tried (or studied). If we can take the perspective of trees (Berenguer, 2007), could we take the perspective of other things – like a park, the department in which we work, or democracy – with similarly positive outcomes to the ones we have already covered? Here is a strategy that requires no special equipment or infrastructure and it is already endorsed by many of the world's religious, educational, and moral institutions. It is within the skill range of most people over the age of 5, and is perhaps close to the human default course of action in some contexts already (e.g., Davis et al., 2004). Most of us just need a bit of prodding to engage in it more often.

Acknowledgments The authors wish to acknowledge help on various sections of this chapter from Georgia Layton, Ezra Markowitz, Kathryn Oleson, Jennifer Pfeifer, Scott Sprague, and Joann Wu Shortt.

References

Aderman, D., Brehm, S. S., & Katz, L. B. (1974). Empathic observation of an innocent victim: The just world revisited. *Journal of Personality and Social Psychology, 29,* 342–347.

Ames, D. R. (2004a). Inside the mind reader's tool kit: Projection and stereotyping in mental state inference. *Journal of Personality and Social Psychology, 87,* 340–353.

Ames, D. R. (2004b). Strategies for social inference: A similarity contingency model of projection and stereotyping in attribute prevalence estimates. *Journal of Personality and Social Psychology, 87,* 573–585.

Anderson, C. A. (1982). Inoculation and counter-explanation: Debiasing techniques in the perseverance of social theories. *Social Cognition, 1,* 126–139.

Archer, R. L., Foushee, H. C., Davis, M. H., & Aderman, D. (1979). Emotional empathy in a courtroom simulation: A person-situation interaction. *Journal of Applied Social Psychology, 9,* 275–291.

Aron, A., Aron, E. N., & Smollan, D. (1992). Inclusion of other in the self scale and the structure of interpersonal closeness. *Journal of Personality and Social Psychology, 63,* 596–612.

Aron, A., Aron, E. N., Tudor, M., & Nelson, G. (1991). Close relationships as including other in the self. *Journal of Personality and Social Psychology, 60,* 241–253.

Baldwin, M. W., & Holmes, J. G. (1987). Salient private audiences and awareness of the self. *Journal of Personality and Social Psychology, 52,* 1087–1098.

Barnett, M. A. (1984). Similarity of experience and empathy in preschoolers. *Journal of Genetic Psychology, 145,* 241–250.

Baron-Cohen, S. (1997). *Mindblindness: An essay on autism and theory of mind.* Cambridge, MA: MIT Press.

Bassok, M., & Trope, Y. (1984). People's strategies for testing hypotheses about another's personality: Confirmatory or diagnostic? *Social Cognition, 2,* 199–216.

Batson, C. D. (1987). Prosocial motivation: Is it ever truly altruistic? In L. Berkowitz (Ed.), *Advances in experimental social psychology* (Vol. 20, pp. 65–122). San Diego: Academic Press.

Batson, C. D., Batson, J. G., Slingsby, J. K., Harrell, K. L., Peekna, H. M., & Todd, R. M. (1991). Empathic joy and the empathy-altruism hypothesis. *Journal of Personality and Social Psychology, 61,* 413–426.

Batson, C. D., Batson, J. G., Todd, R. M., Brummett, B. H., Shaw, L. L., & Aldeguer, C. M. R. (1995). Empathy and the collective good: Caring for one of the others in a social dilemma. *Journal of Personality and Social Psychology, 68,* 619–631.

Batson, C. D., Chang, J., Orr, R., & Rowland, J. (2002). Empathy, attitudes, and action: Can feeling for a member of a stigmatized group motivate one to help the group? *Personality and Social Psychology Bulletin, 28,* 1656–1666.

Batson, C. D., Duncan, B. D., Ackerman, P., Buckley, T., & Birch, K. (1981). Is empathic emotion a source of altruistic motivation? *Journal of Personality and Social Psychology, 40,* 290–302.

Batson, C. D., Early, S., & Salvarani, G. (1997). Perspective taking: Imagining how another feels versus imagining how you would feel. *Personality and Social Psychology Bulletin, 23,* 751–758.

Batson, C. D., Klein, T. R., Highberger, L., & Shaw, L. L. (1995). Immorality from empathy-induced altruism: When compassion and justice conflict. *Journal of Personality and Social Psychology, 68,* 1042–1054.

Batson, C. D., Lishner, D. A., Carpenter, A., Dulin, L., Harjusola-Webb, S., Stocks, E. L., et al. (2003). "... As you would have them do unto you": Does imagining yourself in the other's place stimulate moral action? *Personality and Social Psychology Bulletin, 29,* 1190–1201.

Batson, C. D., Polycarpou, M. P., Harmon-Jones, E., Imhoff, H. J., Mitchener, E. M., Bednar, L. L., et al. (1997). Empathy and attitudes: Can feeling for a member of a stigmatized group improve feeling toward the group. *Journal of Personality and Social Psychology, 72,* 105–118.

Batson, C. D., Sager, K., Garst, E., Kang, M., Rubchinsky, K., & Dawson, K. (1997). Is empathy induced helping due to self-other merging? *Journal of Personality and Social Psychology, 73,* 495–509.

Batson, C. D., Sympson, S. C., Hindman, J. L., Decruz, P., Todd, R. M., Weeks, J. L., et al. (1996). "I've been there, too": Effect on empathy of prior experience with a need. *Personality and Social Psychology Bulletin, 22,* 474–482.

Berenguer, J. (2007). The effect of empathy in proenvironmental attitudes and behaviors. *Environment and Behavior, 39,* 269–283.

Berenguer, J. (2010). The effect of empathy in environmental moral reasoning. *Environment and Behavior, 42,* 110–134.

Bernstein, W. M., & Davis, M. H. (1982). Perspective-taking, self-consciousness, and accuracy in person perception. *Basic and Applied Social Psychology, 3,* 1–19.

Berscheid, E., & Reis, H. T. (1998). Attraction and close relationships. In D. T. Gilbert, S. T. Fiske, & G. Lindzey(Eds.), *The handbook of social psychology* (4th ed., pp. 193–281). New York: McGraw-Hill.

Branscombe, N. R., Owen, S., Garstka, T. A., & Coleman, J. (1996). Rape and accident counterfactuals: Who might have done otherwise and would it have changed the outcome? *Journal of Applied Social Psychology, 26,* 1042–1067.

Brewer, M. B. (1979). In-group bias in the minimal intergroup situation: A cognitive-motivational analysis. *Psychological Bulletin, 86,* 307–324.

Brewer, M. B., & Gardner, W. (1996). Who is this "we"? Levels of collective identity and self representations. *Journal of Personality and Social Psychology, 71,* 83–93.

Byrne, D. (1961). Interpersonal attraction and attitude similarity. *The Journal of Abnormal and Social Psychology, 62,* 713–715.

Byrne, D. (1997). An overview (and underview) of research and theory within the attraction paradigm. *Journal of Social and Personal Relationships, 14,* 417–431.

Carr, L., Iacoboni, M., Dubeau, M. C., Mazziotta, J. C., & Lenzi, G. L. (2003). Neural mechanisms of empathy in humans: A relay from neural systems for imitation to limbic areas. *Proceedings of the National Academy of Sciences, 100,* 5497–5502.

Cialdini, R. B., Brown, S. L., Lewis, B. P., Luce, L., & Neuberg, S. L. (1997). Reinterpreting the empathy-altruism relationship: When one into one equals oneness. *Journal of Personality and Social Psychology, 73,* 481–494.

Cohen, D., & Gunz, A. (2002). As seen by the other... Perspectives on the self in the memories and emotional perceptions of easterners and westerners. *Psychological Science, 13,* 55–59.

Cohen, D., & Hoshino-Browne, E. (2005). Insider and outsider perspectives on the self and social world. In R. M. Sorrentino, D. Cohen, J. M. Olson, & M. P. Zanna (Eds.), *Cultural and social behavior: The Ontario symposium* (Vol. 10, pp. 49–76). Mahwah, NJ: Lawrence Erlbaum Associates Publishers.

Coke, J. S., Batson, C. D., & McDavis, K. (1978). Empathic mediation of helping: A two-stage model. *Journal of Personality and Social Psychology, 36,* 757–766.

Committee for Children. (1992). *Second step: A violence prevention curriculum* (2nd ed.). Seattle, WA: Committee for Children.

Davis, M. H. (1983). Measuring individual differences in empathy: Evidence for a multidimensional approach. *Journal of Personality and Social Psychology, 44,* 113–126.

Davis, M. H., Conklin, L., Smith, A., & Luce, C. (1996). Effect of perspective taking on the cognitive representations of persons: A merging of self and other. *Journal of Personality and Social Psychology, 70,* 713–726.

Davis, M. H., Luce, C., & Kraus, S. J. (1994). The heritability of characteristics associated with dispositional empathy. *Journal of Personality, 62,* 369–391.

Davis, M. H., & Oathout, H. A. (1987). Maintenance of satisfaction in romantic relationships: Empathy and relational competence. *Journal of Personality and Social Psychology, 53,* 397–410.

Davis, M. H., Soderlund, T., Cole, J., Gadol, E., Kute, M., Myers, M., et al. (2004). Cognitions associated with attempts to empathize: How do we imagine the perspective of another. *Personality and Social Psychology Bulletin, 30,* 1625–1635.

Dawes, R. M. (1990). The potential nonfalsity of the false consensus effect. In R. M. Hogarth (Ed.), *Insights in decision making: A tribute to Hillel J. Einhorn* (pp. 179–199). Chicago: University of Chicago Press.

DePaulo, B. M. (2002). The many faces of lies. In A. G. Miller (Ed.), *The social psychology of good and evil* (pp. 303–326). New York: Guilford Press.

Dijksterhuis, A., & van Knippenberg, A. (1998). The relationship between perception and behavior, or how to win a game of trivial pursuit. *Journal of Personality and Social Psychology, 74,* 865–877.

Dovidio, J. F., Vergert, M. T., Stewart, T. L., Gaertner, S. L., Johnson, J., Esses, V. M., et al. (2004). Perspective and prejudice: Antecedent and mediating mechanisms. *Personality and Social Psychology Bulletin, 30,* 1537–1549.

Dreyfus, H. L., & Dreyfus, S. E. (1986). *Mind over machine.* New York: The Free Press.

Eisenberg, N., & Fabes, R. A. (1990). Empathy: Conceptualization, measurement, and relation to prosocial behavior. *Motivation and Emotion, 14,* 131–149.

Eisenberg, N., Fabes, R. A., Murphy, B., Karbon, M., Smith, M., & Maszk, P. (1996). The relations of children's dispositional empathy-related responding to their emotionality, regulation, and social functioning. *Developmental Psychology, 32,* 195–209.

Eisenberg, N., Wentzel, M., & Harris, J. D. (1998). The role of emotionality and regulation in empathy-related responding. *School Psychology Review, 27,* 505–521.

Epley, N., Caruso, E., & Bazerman, M. H. (2006). When perspective taking increases taking: Reactive egoism in social interaction. *Journal of Personality and Social Psychology, 91,* 872–889.

Epley, N., Keysar, B., Van Boven, L., & Gilovich, T. (2004). Perspective taking as egocentric anchoring and adjustment. *Journal of Personality and Social Psychology, 87,* 327–339.

Finlay, K. A., & Stephan, W. G. (2000). Improving intergroup relations: The effect of empathy on racial attitudes. *Journal of Applied Social Psychology, 30,* 1720–1737.

Flavell, J. H. (1963). *The developmental psychology of Jean Piaget.* Princeton, NJ: Van Nostrand.

Focella, E., Whitehead, J., Stone, J., & Schmader, T. (2010). *Target empowerment: Can targets use perspective taking to reduce bias?* Poster presented at the 2010 meeting of the Society of Personality and Social Psychology.

Franzoi, S. L., Davis, M. H., & Young, R. D. (1985). The effects of private self-consciousness and perspective taking on satisfaction in close relationships. *Journal of Personality and Social Psychology, 48,* 1584–1594.

Galinsky, A. D., & Ku, G. (2004). The effects of perspective-taking on prejudice: The moderating role of self-evaluation. *Personality and Social Psychology Bulletin, 30,* 594–604.

Galinsky, A. D., Maddux, W. W., Gilin, D., & White, J. B. (2008). Why it pays to get inside the head of your opponent. *Psychological Science, 19,* 378–384.

Galinsky, A. D., & Moskowitz, G. B. (2000). Perspective-taking: Decreasing stereotype expression, stereotype accessibility, and in-group favoritism. *Journal of Personality and Social Psychology, 78,* 708–724.

Galinsky, A. D., Wang, C. S., & Ku, G. (2008). Perspective-takers behave more stereotypically. *Journal of Personality and Social Psychology, 95,* 404–419.

Galper, R. E. (1976). Turning observers into actors: Differential casual attributions as a function of empathy. *Journal of Research in Personality, 10,* 328–335.

Gentner, D., & Markman, A. B. (1994). Structural alignment in comparison: No difference without similarity. *Psychological Science, 5,* 152–158.

Gesn, P. R., & Ickes, W. (1999). The development of meaning contexts for empathic accuracy: Channel and sequence effects. *Journal of Personality and Social Psychology, 77,* 746–761.

Ginossar, Z., & Trope, Y. (1987). Problem solving judgments under uncertainty. *Journal of Personality and Social Psychology, 52,* 464–474.

Goldstein, N. J., & Cialdini, R. B. (2007). The spyglass self: A model of vicarious self-perception. *Journal of Personality and Social Psychology, 92,* 402–417.

Gould, R., & Sigall, H. (1977). The effects of empathy and outcome on attribution: An examination of the divergent-perspectives hypothesis. *Journal of Experimental Social Psychology, 13,* 480–492.

Greenberg, M. T., Kusche, C. A., Cook, E. T., & Quamma, J. P. (1995). Promoting emotional competence in school-aged children: The effects of the PATHS curriculum. *Development and Psychopathology, 7,* 117–136.

Greene, E., Heilbrun, M., Fortune, W. H., & Nietzel, M. T. (2007). *Wrightsman's psychology and the legal system.* Belmont, CA: Thompson Wadsworth.

Griffin, D. W., Dunning, D., & Ross, L. (1990). The role of construal processes in overconfident predictions about the self and others. *Journal of Personality and Social Psychology, 59,* 1128–1139.

Griffitt, W., & Veitch, R. (1974). Preacquaintance attitude similarity and attraction revisited: Ten days in a fall-out shelter. *Sociometry, 37,* 163–173.

Haidt, J. (2003). The moral emotions. In R. J. Davidson, K. R. Scherer, & H. H. Goldsmith (Eds.), *Handbook of affective sciences* (pp. 852–870). Oxford: Oxford University Press.

Hall, J. A., & Bernieri, F. J. (2001). *Interpersonal sensitivity: Theory and measurement.* Mahwah, NJ: Lawrence Erlbaum Associates.

Hatfield, E., Cacioppo, J. T., & Rapson, R. L. (1993). Emotional contagion. *Current Directions in Psychological Science, 2,* 96–99.

Hoch, S. J. (1987). Perceived consensus and predictive accuracy: The pros and cons of projection. *Journal of Personality and Social Psychology, 53,* 221–234.

Hodges, S. D., & Biswas-Diener, R. (2007). Balancing the empathy expense account: Strategies for regulating empathic response. In T. F. D. Farrow & P. W. R. Woodruff (Eds.), *Empathy in mental illness and health* (pp. 389–407). Cambridge: Cambridge University Press.

Hodges, S. D., Kiel, K. J., Kramer, A. D. I., Veach, D., & Villanueva, B. R. (2010). Giving birth to empathy: The effects of similar experience on empathic accuracy, empathic concern, and perceived empathy. *Personality and Social Psychology Bulletin, 36,* 398–409.

Hodges, S. D., & Wegner, D. M. (1997). Automatic and controlled empathy. In W. Ickes (Ed.), *Empathic accuracy* (pp. 311–339). New York: Guilford.

Hoffman, M. L. (1984). Interaction of affect and cognition in empathy. In C. E. Izard, J. Kagan, & R. B. Zajonc (Eds.), *Emotions, cognition, and behavior* (pp. 103–131). Cambridge: Cambridge University Press.

Iacoboni, M. (2009). Imitation, empathy, and mirror neurons. *Annual Review of Psychology, 60,* 653–670.

Ickes, W. (2003). *Everyday mind reading.* Amherst, NY: Prometheus Books.

Johnson, M. E., Brems, C., & Alford-Keating, P. (1997). Personality correlates of homophobia. *Journal of Homosexuality, 34,* 57–69.

Kaiser, C. R., & Miller, C. T. (2003). Derogating the victim: The interpersonal consequences of blaming events on discrimination. *Group Processes and Intergroup Relations, 6,* 227–237.

Karaçanta, A., & Fitness, J. (2006). Majority support for minority out-groups: The roles of compassion and guilt. *Journal of Applied Social Psychology, 36,* 2730–2749.

Karniol, R., & Shomroni, D. (1999). What being empathic means: Applying the transformation rule approach to individual differences in predicting the thoughts and feelings of prototypic and nonprototypic others. *European Journal of Social Psychology, 29,* 147–160.

Keysar, B., Barr, D. J., & Horton, W. S. (1998). The egocentric basis of language use: Insight from a processing approach. *Current Directions in Psychological Science, 7,* 46–50.

Kilpatrick, S. D., Bissonnette, V. L., & Rusbult, C. E. (2002). Empathic accuracy and accommodative behavior among newly married couples. *Personal Relationships, 9,* 369–393.

Klein, K. J. K., & Hodges, S. D. (2001). Gender differences, motivation and empathic accuracy: When it pays to understand. *Personality and Social Psychology Bulletin, 27,* 720–730.

Koehler, D. J. (1991). Explanation, imagination and confidence in judgment. *Psychological Bulletin, 110,* 499–519.

Krevans, J., & Gibbs, J. C. (1996). Parents' use of inductive discipline: Relations to children's empathy and prosocial behavior. *Child Development, 67,* 3262–3277.

Lamm, C., Batson, C. D., & Decety, J. (2007). The neural substrate of human empathy: Effects of perspective-taking and cognitive appraisal. *Journal of Cognitive Neuroscience, 19,* 42–58.

Long, E. C. J., & Andrews, D. W. (1990). Perspective taking as a predictor of marital adjustment. *Journal of Personality and Social Psychology, 59,* 126–131.

Lord, C. G., Lepper, M. R., & Preston, E. (1984). Considering the opposite: A corrective strategy for social judgment. *Journal of Personality and Social Psychology, 47,* 1231–1243.

Macrae, C. N., & Milne, A. B. (1992). A curry for your thoughts: Empathic effects on counterfactual thinking. *Personality and Social Psychology Bulletin, 18,* 625–630.

Malle, B. F. (2006). The actor-observer asymmetry in attribution: A (surprising) meta-analysis. *Psychological Bulletin, 132,* 895–919.

Malle, B. F., & Pearce, G. E. (2001). Attention to behavior events during interaction: Two actor-observer gaps and three attempts to close them. *Journal of Personality and Social Psychology, 81,* 278–294.

Maner, J. K., Luce, C. L., Neuberg, S. L., Cialdini, R. B., Brown, S., & Sagarin, B. J. (2002). The effects of perspective taking on motivations for helping: Still no evidence for altruism. *Personality and Social Psychology Bulletin, 28,* 1601–1610.

Markus, H. R., & Kitayama, S. (1991). Culture and the self: Implications for cognition, emotion, and motivation. *Psychological Review, 98,* 224–253.

Montoya, R. M., Horton, R. S., & Kirchner, J. (2008). Is actual similarity necessary for attraction? A meta-analysis of actual and perceived similarity. *Journal of Social and Personal Relationships, 25,* 889–922.

Myers, M. W. (2009). *Self-other overlap and its relationship to perspective taking: Underlying mechanisms and implications.* Unpublished doctoral dissertation, University of Oregon, Eugene.

Myers, M. W., & Hodges, S. D. (unpublished manuscript). *Looking for overlap: Are measures of self-other merging tapping the same construct?* University of Tokyo.

Neale, M. A., & Bazerman, M. H. (1983). The role of perspective taking ability in negotiating under different forms of arbitration. *Industrial and Labor Relations Review, 36,* 378–388.

Oswald, P. A. (1996). The effects of cognitive and affective perspective taking on empathic concern and altruistic helping. *Journal of Social Psychology, 136,* 613–623.

Piaget, J., & Inhleder, B. (1956). *The child's conception of space.* London: Routledge and Kegan Paul.

Pichert, J. W., & Anderson, R. C. (1977). Taking different perspectives on a story. *Journal of Educational Psychology, 69,* 309–315.

Piper, A., & Langer, E. (1984). Aging and mindful control. In M. Baltes & P. Baltes (Eds.), *Aging and control.* Hillsdale, NJ: Erlbaum.

Pizarro, D. (2000). Nothing more than feelings? The role of emotions in moral judgment. *Journal for the Theory of Social Behavior, 30,* 355–375.

Povinelli, D. J., & Vonk, J. (2003). Chimpanzee minds: Suspiciously human? *Trends in Cognitive Sciences, 7,* 157–160.

Richardson, D. R., Green, L. R., & Lago, T. (1998). The relationship between perspective-taking and nonaggressive responding in the face of an attack. *Journal of Personality, 66,* 233–256.

Richardson, D. R., Hammock, G. S., Smith, S. M., Gardner, W., & Signo, M. (1994). Empathy as a cognitive inhibitor of interpersonal aggression. *Aggressive Behavior, 20,* 275–289.

Rossnagel, C. (2000). Cognitive load and perspective-taking: Applying the automatic-controlled distinction to verbal communication. *European Journal of Social Psychology, 30,* 429–445.

Sabbagh, M., & Taylor, M. (2000). Neural correlates of "theory of mind" reasoning: An event-related potential study. *Psychological Science, 11,* 46–50.

Sabbagh, M. A., Xu, F., Carlson, S. M., Moses, L. J., & Lee, K. (2006). The development of executive functioning and theory of mind: A comparison of Chinese and U.S. preschoolers. *Psychological Science, 17,* 74–81.

Schultz, P. W. (2000). Empathizing with nature: The effects of perspective taking on concern for environmental issues. *Journal of Social Issues, 56,* 391–406.

Shelton, M. L., & Rogers, R. W. (1981). Fear-arousing and empathy-arousing appeals to help: The pathos of persuasion. *Journal of Applied Psychology, 11,* 366–378.

Sinclair, S., Huntsinger, J., Skorinko, J., & Hardin, C. D. (2005). Social tuning of the self: Consequences for the self-evaluations of stereotype targets. *Journal of Personality and Social Psychology, 89,* 160–175.

Skorinko, J., & Sinclair, S. (2010). *Perspective taking and stereotyping: The role of stereotype content.* Poster presented at the 2010 meeting of the Society of Personality and Social Psychology, Las Vegas, NV.

Slovic, P. (2007). "If I look at the mass I will never act": Psychic numbing and genocide. *Judgment and Decision Making, 2,* 79–95.

Smith, J. L., Ickes, W., Hall, J., & Hodges, S. D. (in press). *Managing interpersonal sensitivity: Knowing when – And when not – To understand others.* New York: Nova Science Publishers.

Soenens, B., Duriez, B., Vansteenkiste, M., & Goossens, L. (2007). The intergenerational transmission of empathy-related responding in adolescence: The role of maternal support. *Personality and Social Psychology Bulletin, 33,* 299–311.

Storms, M. D. (1973). Videotape and the attribution process: Reversing actors' and observers' point of view. *Journal of Personality and Social Psychology, 27,* 165–175.

Stotland, E. (1969). Exploratory investigations in empathy. In L. Berkowitz (Ed.), *Advances in experimental social psychology* (Vol. 4, pp. 271–314). New York: Academic Press.

Tajfel, H. (1982). Social psychology of intergroup relations. *Annual Review of Psychology, 33,* 1–39.

Tajfel, H., & Billig, M. (1974). Familiarity and categorization in intergroup behavior. *Journal of Experimental Social Psychology, 10,* 159–170.

Takaku, S., Weiner, B., & Ohbuchi, K. (2001). A cross-cultural examination of the effects of apology and perspective taking on forgiveness. *Journal of Language and Social Psychology, 20,* 144–166.

Tangney, J. P., Stuewig, J., & Mashek, D. J. (2007). What's moral about the self-conscious emotions? In J. L. Tracy, R. W. Robins, & J. P. Tangney (Eds.), *The self-conscious emotions: Theory and research* (pp. 21–37). New York: The Guilford Press.

Taylor, M., Hodges, S. D., & Kohanyi, A. (2003). The illusion of independent agency: Do adult fiction writers experience their characters as having minds of their own? *Imagination, Cognition and Personality, 22,* 361–380.

Thompson, R. A., & Hoffman, M. L. (1980). Empathy and the development of guilt in children. *Developmental Psychology, 16,* 155–156.

Toi, M., & Batson, C. D. (1982). More evidence that empathy is a source of altruistic motivation. *Journal of Personality and Social Psychology, 43,* 281–292.

Traxler, M. J., & Gernsbacher, M. A. (1993). Improving written communication through perspective-taking. *Language and Cognitive Processes, 8,* 311–334.

Tversky, A., & Kahneman, D. (1982). Evidential impact of base rates. In D. Kahneman, P. Slovic, & A. Tversky (Eds.), *Judgment under uncertainty: Heuristics and biases* (pp. 153–178). Cambridge: Cambridge University Press.

Underwood, B., & Moore, B. (1982). Perspective-taking and altruism. *Psychological Bulletin, 91,* 143–173.

Vescio, T. K., Sechrist, G. B., & Paolucci, M. P. (2003). Perspective taking and prejudice reduction: The meditational role of empathy arousal and situational attributions. *European Journal of Social Psychology, 33,* 455–472.

Vorauer, J. D., Martens, V., & Sasaki, S. J. (2009). When trying to understand detracts from trying to behave: Effects of perspective taking in intergroup interaction. *Journal of Personality and Social Psychology, 96,* 811–827.

Weinstein, N. D., & Lachendro, E. (1982). Egocentrism as a source of unrealistic optimism. *Personality and Social Psychology Bulletin, 8,* 195–200.

Wu, S., & Keysar, B. (2007). The effect of culture on perspective taking. *Psychological Science, 18,* 600–606.

Zahn-Waxler, C., & Radke-Yarrow, M. (1990). The origins of empathic concern. *Motivation and Emotion, 14,* 107–130.

Zahn-Waxler, C., Radke-Yarrow, M., Wagner, E., & Chapman, M. (1992). Development of concern for others. *Developmental Psychology, 28,* 126–136.

Chapter 13
Investing in Others: Prosocial Spending for (Pro)Social Change

Lara B. Aknin, Gillian M. Sandstrom, Elizabeth W. Dunn, and Michael I. Norton

Imagine the following: It is a Saturday morning in December and you have decided to have breakfast at your local diner. You take a seat in a booth by the window and order the usual – a mushroom and cheese omelet with a side of hash browns and a coffee. As you enjoy your omelet, you consider your plans for the day. You have a long list of errands to attend to before heading to a friend's place tonight, so as soon as you finish your meal, you summon your waitress for the check. She makes her way to your table and tells you that your check has been paid by another customer who just left the diner and then adds, "Happy Holidays." Your bill was not large, but you are emotionally moved by the kindness of this generous act. You reach for your wallet anyway and tell the waitress you would like to pay the check for the next table. You leave $20 and head out the door with a smile. And just like that, a favor has been paid forward.

This may sound more like a scene from a movie than real life, but this is just what happened in a Philadelphia diner in the winter of 2009 (Johnson, 2009). The positive chain reaction was initiated by an unknown couple who paid for their bill and the bill of another customer. The couple did not leave their names or phone number, but simply asked that the waitress wait until they had left the restaurant before informing the other customer that their tab had been paid. This act inspired others to do the same. For the next 5 h, dozens of customers continued to pay the favor forward. The staff at the diner were amazed by the string of generous spending, so much so that one waitress reported that the "magical" event brought tears to her eyes.

This occurrence provides a poignant example of how *prosocial spending*, that is, spending money on others, can lead to positive outcomes for the people spending the money, those receiving it, and even other individuals nearby. In this chapter, we unpack and explore the possibility of prosocial spending as a mechanism for positive social change. After providing some background, we review our research on the happiness benefits of prosocial spending. We discuss the impact of prosocial spending at four levels, starting first with the happiness benefits of prosocial spending for individuals, and then extending this discussion outward to dyads, to

E.W. Dunn (✉)
University of British Columbia, Vancouver, BC, Canada
e-mail: edunn@psych.ubc.ca

R. Biswas-Diener (ed.), *Positive Psychology as Social Change*,
DOI 10.1007/978-90-481-9938-9_13, © Springer Science+Business Media B.V. 2011

teams, and to organizations. Finally, we offer several practical strategies for utilizing this prosocial spending research, applying the findings of some of our newest
research to propose ways in which prosocial spending can produce the largest
benefits.

The Relationship Between Money and Happiness

Scholars ranging from economists and psychologists to sociologists and philosophers have explored the relationship between money and happiness (e.g., Diener &
Seligman, 2004; Kahneman, Krueger, Schkade, Schwarz, & Stone, 2006; Layard,
2005; Oswald, 1997; Veenhoven, 1991). Understanding this relationship is important because many people spend a large part of their lives working to accumulate
wealth, driven in part by the belief that income is closely related to happiness
(Ahuvia, 2008; Kahneman et al., 2006). The majority of studies conducted over the
past several decades examining the link between money and happiness have used
correlational designs, and suggest that money has a small but significant effect on
happiness within developed nations (e.g., Diener & Biswas-Diener, 2002; Frey &
Stutzer, 2000). Interestingly, however, it seems that people overestimate how much
happiness money can bring: When we asked a nationally representative sample of
Americans to predict how happy they would be at various levels of income, participants envisioned a much steeper relationship between money and happiness than
the actual data revealed (Aknin, Norton, & Dunn, 2009). Yet, while absolute levels
of income may not matter as much for happiness as most people may believe, we
suggest that *how* people spend their money may be as important for their happiness
as how much they earn. Indeed, while there are several reasons why income may
have a weak effect on well-being, one possibility is that people choose to invest
their increased wealth into spending choices that provide little in the way of lasting
happiness gains. As economist Robert Frank (2004) has suggested, money *might* be
able to increase well-being if people were to spend it wisely. Thus, instead of using
increased wealth to buy material purchases, like bigger homes and faster cars, we
suggest – and our research demonstrates – that people should spend their money in
service of goals that have been shown to increase happiness, such as investing in
other people through kind or generous acts.

   Whereas wealth has been shown to have a relatively small impact on happiness, an emerging body of research suggests that engaging in prosocial behavior
can increase well-being. This relationship has been well-documented through correlational methods (Aderman, 1972; Cunningham, Steinberg, & Grev, 1980; Lucas,
2001; Rosenhan, Underwood, & Moore, 1974; Williams & Shiaw, 1999) and, more
recently, with experimental design (Lyubomirsky, Sheldon, & Schkade, 2005). For
example, Lyubomirsky and colleagues showed that students assigned to perform five
random acts of kindness a week for 6 weeks were happier than those in a no-action
control group. Given that prosocial behavior has been shown to increase happiness,
our work has sought to test whether using money to this end could increase happiness as well. Specifically, we hypothesized that prosocial spending, through gift

giving and charitable donations, would lead to higher happiness levels than spending money on oneself.

Prosocial Spending at the Individual Level

Initial Evidence. In an initial study, we asked a nationally representative sample of Americans to rate their general happiness and to estimate their monthly personal and prosocial spending (Dunn, Aknin, & Norton, 2008). Specifically, participants reported the funds they devoted in a typical month to personal spending (bills, expenses, and gifts for themselves) and to prosocial spending (gifts for others and donations to charity). Individuals who spent more money in a typical month on prosocial spending reported greater happiness, whereas personal spending was unrelated to happiness. Importantly, this relationship remained even when controlling for annual household income. While these results provide a promising first step in linking prosocial spending and happiness in the population, the correlational nature of this study does not allow us to ascertain the direction of the relationship; it is possible that, instead of indicating that prosocial spending leads to happiness, the relationship simply shows that happier people are more likely to engage in prosocial spending.

Therefore, we next used an experimental design to examine whether spending money on others leads to higher happiness levels than spending money on oneself (Dunn et al., 2008). Participants were approached in person during the morning hours in public places and reported their baseline happiness level. After doing so, participants were randomly assigned to one of four spending conditions, receiving either $5 or $20 to spend on either themselves or others. Participants in the personal spending condition were asked to spend their windfall on a bill, expense, or gift for themselves, while participants in the prosocial spending condition were asked to spend their windfall on a gift for someone else or a donation to charity. Participants were asked to spend the money before the end of the day, when a research assistant would call them with a series of follow-up questions. As predicted, participants who spent their windfall prosocially were happier at the end of the day than participants who spent the windfall on themselves. Interestingly, the amount of money that participants received ($5 or $20) did not influence happiness levels, suggesting that *how* people spent their money was more important than *how much* money they spent. Therefore, this experimental study provides support for the causal claim that spending money on others leads to higher happiness than spending money on oneself.

While it is not surprising that people devote a large portion of their income to personal spending – after all, people need to pay the bills – we explored whether the relative infrequency with which people engaged in prosocial spending might be linked to a misunderstanding of its emotional benefits. We examined whether people recognize that spending money on others will make them happier than spending money on themselves by asking another group of participants to read brief descriptions of the four conditions in the experimental study and predict which spending condition would make them happiest (Dunn et al., 2008). A significant majority of participants reported believing that spending money on themselves would make them happier than spending the money on someone else, suggesting that people overlook the happiness returns associated with prosocial spending.

International Replication. While the studies discussed above demonstrate that spending money on others leads to higher happiness than spending money on oneself, it is important to note that these studies were conducted in North America. Because previous research has shown that the relationship between money and happiness can vary depending on a country's wealth (Deaton, 2008; Diener & Biswas-Diener, 2002), a critical question is whether prosocial spending will lead to similar happiness increases when disposable income is limited. To examine this question, we examined the responses of over 230,000 participants drawn from 136 countries in the Gallup World Poll (Aknin et al., 2010). Respondents reported their overall well-being and whether or not they had donated money to charity in the past month. The relationship between prosocial spending and well-being was positive in 122 out of 136 countries around the world, even after controlling for individuals' household income. Importantly, the relationship was unrelated to the average income of each country, suggesting that donating money to charity has emotional benefits in rich and poor countries alike. Given the large number of countries showing a positive relationship between prosocial spending and well-being, this research highlights the possibility that the emotional benefits associated with spending money on others are universal.

Beyond Immediate Mood Benefits. The data described above suggest that the emotional benefits of prosocial spending can be detected around the globe, but another important question concerns the endurance of the mood boosts associated with prosocial spending. Our initial experimental investigations focused on the short-term benefits of spending money on others by comparing participants' self-reports from the morning and evening of a single day. Given the possibility that the mood benefits resulting from prosocial spending could quickly fade, some of our more recent work has examined whether the mood benefits can accrue over time; when people think back to a time when they engaged in prosocial spending, do they experience increased happiness from that remembered utility? We asked a sample of more 600 participants from Canada and Uganda to recall and describe in detail the last time they spent a small sum of money on themselves or someone else (Aknin et al., 2010). After describing this spending experience, participants reported their current level of happiness. Participants who recalled a time they spent money on others reported higher levels of happiness than participants who recalled a time they spent money on themselves. Thus, the emotional benefits of prosocial spending persist beyond the hours immediately following spending, and are accessible when thinking back at a later time. Importantly, the lasting emotional benefits of prosocial spending have been shown in both Canada and Uganda, again suggesting that these findings are not limited to participants in North America.

Sustainable Happiness: A Positive Feedback Loop between Happiness and Prosocial Spending. The research described above demonstrates that engaging in and recalling an act of prosocial spending both lead to higher levels of happiness, but do higher levels of happiness, in turn, promote acts of prosocial spending? Classic work by Isen and colleagues (e.g., Isen, 1970; Isen & Levin, 1972) showed that experimentally induced positive moods – produced by receiving cookies or finding a dime – led to higher levels of helping in a subsequent task. More recent work has shown this is also the case with naturally occurring moods: Happier people are more likely to give a donation in an anonymous economic exchange (Konow & Early, 2008). Indeed, research on volunteering and prosocial behavior suggests that the relationship between prosocial behavior and happiness may be bidirectional. That is, happier people are more likely to engage in helping behavior and to experience higher levels of happiness from doing so (e.g., Piliavin, 2003; Thoits & Hewitt, 2001). Given that prosocial spending represents one form of prosocial behavior, we wondered whether happiness and prosocial spending may also reinforce one another in a positive feedback loop. Specifically, we examined whether recalling a previous act of prosocial spending made people happier and whether higher levels of happiness lead people to select a prosocial spending act in the future.

To investigate this question, we asked participants to think back and describe, in as much detail as possible (Strack, Schwarz, & Gschneidinger, 1985), the last time they spent either $20 or $100, either on themselves or on someone else (Aknin, Dunn, & Norton, 2010, unpublished data). After describing this experience, each participant reported their current level of happiness. Next, each participant was asked to select the future spending behavior they thought would make them happiest: spending either $5 or $20, either on themselves or on someone else. As observed before, participants who were asked to recall a time they spent money on someone else were happier than parrticipants who were asked to recall a time they spent money on themeselves, regardless of the amount of money spent. To test for the existence of a postive feedback loop between happiness and prosocial spending, we also examined whether these elevated levels of happiness were associated with future spending choice. Analyses confirmed that higher levels of happiness significantly predicted a preference for future prosocial spending. Thus, these data suggest that prosocial spending and happiness mutually reinforce each other in a postive feedback loop.

Health Outcomes. Given that prosocial spending is consistently linked with emotional well-being, we sought to investigate whether prosocial spending might also hold downstream consequences for physical well-being. Previous research has demonstrated that emotional responses to stress represent a pathway through which psychosocial variables can influence physical health (e.g., Cohen & Pressman, 2006; Polk, Cohen, Doyle, Skoner, & Kirschbaum, 2005). In addition, emotional responses to psychosocial events have been shown to activate the hypothalamic–pituitary–adrenal (HPA) axis (Polk et al., 2005), which regulates the release of the stress hormone cortisol. While elevated levels of cortisol secretion in response to stress may be adaptive in the short-term, frequent or prolonged elevation of cortisol in response to stress can inhibit immune functioning and increase the likelihood of disease (McEwen, 1998). Because the emotional responses provoked by stress shape the secretion of cortisol (Dickerson & Kemeny, 2004; Polk et al., 2005), we wondered whether generous and stingy economic decisions could influence emotional responses and thereby shape cortisol levels.

To examine whether physiological responses are sensitive to the economic decisions people make, we measured participants' feelings and cortisol levels before and after participation in a well-studied economic game called the "dictator game" (Dunn, Ashton-James, Hanson, & Aknin, 2010). Students in a large undergraduate class reported their general happiness and provided a baseline sample of cortisol by chewing on a cotton roll. Afterward, half the participants were informed that they had been randomly assigned to the decision-maker role in the upcoming economic game and were given ten $1 coins that they could keep for themselves or share with a yoked recipient in the classroom. Decision makers delivered the funds to the recipient and informed the recipient of the donation amount. After delivering their donations, decision makers immediately reported their current affect levels and then provided cortisol samples 15 and 45 minutes after the exchange. As expected, larger donations were associated with higher positive affect and lower negative affect and shame. Importantly, these findings held even when accounting for pre-exchange happiness ratings, which means that the size of the donation predicted post-exchange affect over and above initial happiness levels. Analyses confirmed our prediction that stingy economic decisions resulted in higher post-exchange cortisol levels by increasing shame. That is, to the extent that low donation amounts led decision makers to feel shame, they were likely to show elevated levels of cortisol. Thus, taken together, these results suggest that personal and prosocial spending, as measured by selfish and generous dictator game decisions, may have downstream consequences for health.

Putting the "Social" in Prosocial Spending: The Importance of Social Connection in Prosocial Spending. In several studies, spending money on others has been shown to lead to higher levels of happiness than spending money on oneself; but what is it about prosocial spending that leads to these happiness gains? Only a handful of studies have investigated this question, but the results suggest that the increased social connection encouraged by prosocial spending may be critical. That is, when spending money on others fosters positive interpersonal contact, prosocial spending is particularly likely to enhance well-being.

A recent study we conducted examined happiness levels after giving to charity (Aknin, Dunn, Sandstrom, & Norton, 2010, in preparation). Participants reported their happiness and then viewed a printed ad for a charity that helps bring fresh water to the people of Africa and were asked if they would like to donate to the cause. Some participants were told that the charity was of special importance to the research assistant. In another condition, no link was provided between the research assistant and the charity, and donations were made anonymously by putting the desired donation amount in a sealed envelope. Finally, participants again reported their well-being, on a different measure. When the research assistant was personally connected to the cause, participants who gave larger donations reported higher levels of happiness after giving, over and above their initial happiness levels. However, larger donations given to the research assistant with no connection to the charity did not lead to an increase in happiness.

The importance of social contact for the mood benefits of prosocial spending has also been replicated with person-to-person spending (Aknin et al., 2010, in preparation). We contacted participants in the morning hours and gave them a Starbucks gift card to spend by the end of the day. We asked participants to spend the gift card on someone else in a way that either maximized or minimized social contact. When participants were contacted on the same evening, they reported the highest happiness when the gift card was used to maximize social contact. That is, participants who spent the gift card on both themselves and someone else by visiting Starbucks together were happiest at the end of the day. Taken together these results suggest that the happiness benefits of prosocial spending are greatest when giving occurs in a social fashion.

In summary, spending money on others has been linked to a variety of positive outcomes for the spender. At the emotional level, prosocial spending has been shown to cultivate happiness gains immediately after giving, at the end of the day, and when an act of prosocial spending is reflected upon later. Moreover, these findings are not limited to North America; the well-being benefits of prosocial spending appear consistently in most countries around the world. Further, it seems that happiness and prosocial spending may mutually reinforce one another in a positive feedback loop, such that prosocial spending increases happiness and happiness increases prosocial spending. At the physiological level, generous and stingy monetary decisions have been shown to impact the body's stress response. Finally, it seems that the emotional benefits of prosocial spending are greatest when the giving is linked to an interpersonal context.

Prosocial Spending at the Dyadic Level

Having discussed the benefits of prosocial spending for the spender, we now consider the effects of prosocial spending for the recipient. Indeed, considering that the mood benefits of prosocial spending for the giver seem to hinge upon interpersonal interaction with the receiver, examining the impact on that receiver is a logical next step.

There are theoretical reasons to suspect that acts of prosocial spending may have positive benefits for the recipient. At the most basic level, receiving gifts may increase the recipient's well-being through the experience of gratitude. Gratitude is a positive emotion produced when someone feels they have benefited from the intentional, costly, and voluntary actions of someone else (Emmons & McCullough, 2003; McCullough, Kimeldorf, & Cohen, 2008). Expressions of gratitude have been shown to produce emotional benefits (Emmons & McCullough, 2003) and to encourage future acts of prosocial behavior in both the giver and the recipient (McCullough, Emmons, & Tsang, 2002; McCullough, Kilpatrick, Emmons, & Larson, 2001). Importantly, gratitude may increase positive affect by creating and strengthening social bonds (Algoe, Haidt, & Gable, 2008; Emmons & McCullough,

2003). In addition, a recipient's happiness may fluctuate with the happiness of others around them (Fowler & Christakis, 2008). Indeed, people have been shown to catch and match the emotional states of others in even brief interactions through processes such as emotional contagion and mimicry (Hatfield, Cacioppo, & Rapson, 1993). Therefore, if spenders perform acts of prosocial spending that allow for contact with the recipient, happiness may spread from the spender to the recipient.

To investigate whether prosocial spending has positive outcomes for the recipient, we measured the happiness of both givers and receivers in an experiment using the dictator game (Aknin et al., 2010, in preparation). Participants were given a short questionnaire to report their baseline happiness and were randomly assigned to either the dictator or receiver role in the upcoming monetary exchange. Dictators were given ten $1 coins and were asked to decide how much of this $10 sum, if any, they would like to keep for themselves and how much they would like to share with their yoked receiver. Importantly, half of the dictators makers were told that they would have to deliver the donation in person and notify the receiver of the amount. Dictators in the other condition were told that a research assistant would deliver their donation. Once recipients received their donations, all participants reported their current affect levels.

To examine whether prosocial spending led to happiness gains for receivers, we tested whether receiving larger donations predicted greater happiness. However, we suspected that the happiness benefits of prosocial spending might hinge upon whether the donation was received directly from the dictator (direct social contact) or by way of a research assistant acting as an intermediary. That is, just as prosocial spenders reported increased happiness after giving in a truly social context, so too might receivers reap the largest emotional benefits of receiving money when the funds are given through direct social contact. Supporting the importance of social connection for happiness, analyses revealed that larger donations were only associated with higher happiness for the recipient when the giving took place in an interpersonal fashion. These findings suggest that it is not simply the experience of receiving a gift or money that increases happiness: Prosocial spending appears to have emotional benefits for the receiver if monetary gifts are transferred in a way that allows direct social contact.

Prosocial Spending at the Team Level

We now move beyond the dyad level of analysis and examine whether prosocial spending has benefits for teams and small groups. Having established that emotional gains of prosocial spending are experienced by both spenders and recipients when spending occurs in a dyadic context, we go one step further and examine whether spending money on others can produce measurable benefits for entire teams of individuals. Previous research has demonstrated that happiness can spread through large social networks (Fowler & Christakis, 2008); indeed, the happiness of one individual can spread up to three degrees of separation, influencing the happiness of one's friends' friends' friends. Within a single team, the moods and happiness of members are often linked, and are associated with subjective ratings of member performance (Totterdell, 2000). Therefore, we explored whether assigning team members to spend money on a teammate could lead to greater team success.

To investigate this question we recruited intramural dodge ball teams and pharmaceutical sales teams to complete a study on teams and emotions (Norton, Aknin, Anik, Dunn, & Quoidbach, in preparation). Each team was randomly assigned to either the personal or prosocial spending condition. On teams assigned to the personal spending condition, one to four team members (approximately 20–35% of the team) were randomly selected to receive $20 (or €15) to spend on themselves in the next week. On teams assigned to the prosocial spending condition, one to four team members (approximately 20–35% of the team) were randomly selected to receive $20 (or €15) to spend on a randomly assigned teammate.

We measured performance for both dodge ball and sales teams before and after the spending intervention. In both contexts, prosocial spending teams were more successful than personal spending teams after the spending intervention; dodge ball teams won a higher percentage of their games and sales teams sold more product. Importantly, personal spending teams did not perform more poorly over time; rather it was the prosocial spending teams whose performance improved. Thus, these findings suggest that while personal spending may not influence team outcomes, prosocial spending may improve team success. Indeed, a closer look at the prosocial spending pharmaceutical sales teams shows that the money invested for teammates to spend on each other was returned twofold in team sales.

Prosocial Spending at the Organizational Level

The previous section discusses the benefits prosocial spending can have for sports and sales teams, but do the positive outcomes extend even further? Small work teams are situated within larger organizations, raising the possibility that if large establishments were to facilitate prosocial spending, similar rewards may materialize for the employee and organization.

To investigate the benefits of engaging in prosocial spending at the organizational level, we conducted a study with employees at an Australian bank (Norton et al., in preparation). Participants completed an online survey, reporting their baseline happiness and job satisfaction. Two weeks later, participants randomly assigned to the prosocial spending conditions were informed that their company had given them either a $50 or a $100 voucher that they could donate to the charity of their choice, via a website where they could select from over 100 charitable causes. Participants in both conditions then completed a final survey in which they reported their current job satisfaction and happiness.

Participants who allocated $100 to charity reported a significant gain in happiness over the 2-week period. However, participants in the control condition and those that allocated $50 did not show the same increase in happiness. Similarly, participants who allocated $100 to charity reported a significant increase in job satisfaction, whereas participants in the control condition and those that allocated $50 did not show the same job satisfaction increase. While it is unclear why the happiness and job satisfaction gains would only materialize for participants who allocated $100 to charity, it is interesting to note that neither of these effects were influenced by tenure with the company. Thus, it appears that the benefits associated with engaging in larger acts of prosocial spending are equally accessible to all employees, regardless of length of employment.

These data show that prosocial spending can have benefits in the workplace. Employees assigned to donate a relatively large monetary sum to charity on behalf of their employer reported increased happiness and job satisfaction. These findings may be particularly pertinent given the current economic climate, with the percentage of Americans reporting dissatisfaction with their job at an all time high; in a 2009 survey, only 45% of American workers said they are satisfied in their current position (Aversa, 2010). Given that prosocial spending provides such a simple way to increase employee happiness and satisfaction, this strategy may be a worthwhile and cost effective intervention for companies. Further, this study demonstrates that prosocial spending interventions need not be an economic burden for companies. Simply allowing employees to distribute a firm's allotted charitable funds through personalized donations can lead to positive results.

Onward and Outward

Could acts of prosocial spending spiral outward? After benefiting from an act of prosocial spending in an everyday transaction, are people more likely to engage in prosocial behavior themselves? To find out, we went to the drive-thru at a local coffee shop and paid for the order of randomly selected customers behind us in the drive-thru line up (Aknin et al., 2010, in preparation). Because the coffee shop was collecting donations for a children's charity that day, all customers were asked if they would like to donate to this particular cause. Customers who found out that their bill had been paid were significantly more likely to donate to charity. Of course, customers who received an act of prosocial spending may have been more likely to donate money because they had just received their order for free; these customers may have simply donated the money they had already mentally allocated for their order. While this is a possibility, almost half of the participants who received an act of prosocial spending donated more than the price of their bill. These findings offer some preliminary evidence to suggest that being the beneficiary of prosocial spending may inspire individuals to pay the favor forward, leading to positive outward spirals of prosocial behavior.

Given the positive outcomes associated with giving and receiving prosocial spending described above, it should come as no surprise that companies have tried incorporating these principles in creative ways (Anik, Aknin, Norton, & Dunn, 2010). For example, in fall 2009, Banana Republic stores in New York City invited representatives from various charities to mingle with their customers and offer information on ways to get involved (Wilson, 2009). This campaign, coordinated by ServiceNation, was designed to pair potential donors and volunteers with a cause suited to their interest. Banana Republic sees value in this campaign, according to their president, Jack Calhoun, because they believe their customers care about things other than fashion (Wilson, 2009). Indeed, helping individuals find a cause to which they can contribute is only one way companies have aligned themselves with prosocial behavior. Other companies have taken to offering consumers the chance to donate to causes through the purchase of specific products. For example, MAC Cosmetics, Apple, and Motorola have all sold specialty products with partial proceeds dedicated to philanthropic causes, such as AIDS research (Barbaro, 2009). Thus, these examples present a glimpse at some of the many ways companies have assimilated prosocial programs into their business practices.

Why Does Prosocial Spending Increase Happiness? New Theoretical Questions and Applications

Having reviewed our program of research on prosocial spending, we now consider *why* prosocial spending may increase happiness. While no study has isolated a single feature of prosocial spending responsible for the observed effects, clues may be gleaned by returning to earlier findings reported in this chapter. Specifically, several studies demonstrated that acts of prosocial spending such as giving a donation or gift card lead to the greatest happiness gains when the giving allowed for positive interpersonal contact. Thus, these findings suggest that one reason prosocial spending produces hedonic gains is because spending money on others, when done in a social manner, can contribute to and facilitate the development of social relationships. This interpretation dovetails with previous research demonstrating that strong social relationships are a key predictor of happiness (Myers, 2000). Indeed, very happy people report having more satisfying relationships than their peers (Diener & Seligman, 2002), and having a number of positive and supportive social relationships may also serve to satisfy our fundamental need to belong (Baumeister & Leary, 1995; Deci & Ryan, 1985; Ryan & Deci, 2000). Of course, engaging in acts of prosocial spending cannot guarantee that an individual will have strong social relationships. However, to the extent that spending money on others encourages positive social interactions, prosocial spending may foster social networks.

The relationship between prosocial spending and happiness may be further elucidated by the Broaden and Build theory of positive emotions (Fredrickson, 1998, 2001, 2004). According to this theory, positive emotions produce favorable outcomes in the present and future. Parallel to theories examining the action tendencies triggered by negative emotions, the Broaden and Build theory suggests that positive emotions serve to broaden an individual's thoughts and build enduring resources. Happiness, a positive emotion, may broaden one's mindset and promote the building of future resources through the formation and augmentation of social relationships. Support for this argument can be seen in the mutually reinforcing nature of happiness and prosocial spending. For instance, the finding that higher levels of happiness encourage a future willingness to spend on others suggests that happiness may expand an individual's mindset beyond the typical preference for personal spending (Dunn et al., 2008) to incorporate thoughts of others. Further, happiness, in turn, leads people to build their present and future resources by strengthening their social bonds through acts of prosocial spending. Thus, prosocial spending leads to higher levels of happiness when conducted in social ways that facilitate social bonding, which fuels a mutually reinforcing positive feedback cycle.

This theoretical explanation fits with real-world examples of how people choose to engage in prosocial spending and suggests applications for how best to invest in others (Aknin et al., 2010, in preparation). A desire for positive interpersonal contact helps explain why the majority of prosocial spending occurs between two acquainted individuals. For example, less than 1% of the money raised by charitable organizations in 2008 was collected from online donations, suggesting that donors may prefer to make donations in more socially significant ways, such as donating to friends, family, or co-workers raising money for the cause (Barton & Wasley, 2009). Further, fewer than 2% of donations by college alumni to their alma mater are made in an anonymous fashion (Glazer & Konrad, 1996). Finally, these findings coincide with reports suggesting that one of the most common reasons donors offer for their charitable behavior is personal experience with the recipient (Schervish & Szanto, 2006) or because they were asked by someone (Independent Sector, 1999).

Thus, these studies suggest that applications of prosocial spending should encourage increased social connection. One easy way for this to occur is to promote face-to-face prosocial spending whenever possible. If someone decides to make a donation or give a gift, they should try to give directly to the recipient or someone with a vested interest. For example, taking a friend out for a birthday dinner would lead to higher levels of happiness than mailing your friend a restaurant gift card for an equivalent amount. This direct act of prosocial spending will not only produce happiness gains for the spender, but will lead to higher happiness for the receiver as well. When this type of direct giving is not possible, it may be beneficial to increase connection in other ways. For example, the online charity organization DonorsChoose.org connects contributors to their selected classroom charity project with student and teacher thank you notes as well as pictures of the classroom. Through these forms of interaction, donors feel connected to the cause, can see the results of their donation, are more likely to feel the hedonic boosts of giving, and may be more likely to give again in the future.

Of course, the extent to which prosocial spending increases happiness hinges upon other factors as well. For instance, the mood benefits associated with prosocial spending may depend upon the degree to which the act affirms one's values. This notion, from (Lyubomirsky et al., 2005) theory of person-activity fit, suggests that an individual's preferences, strengths, and interests predispose some people to benefit most from certain happiness-increasing interventions. Therefore, the degree of consistency between an individual's values and those of the prosocial spending beneficiary may influence whether and how much happiness is gained from prosocial spending. Thus, giving to an individual or cause that one believes important or deserving may lead to larger emotional boosts. Similarly, the *method* in which prosocial spending is enacted may also enhance or inhibit happiness gains. That is, while acts of prosocial spending made in a social context may increase happiness for most people (as observed in several of the studies presented here), other individuals may prefer to give in a more private setting. Finally, alternating the ways in which prosocial spending is conducted may also be important. Research conducted by Sheldon, Boehm, and Lyubomirsky (in press) has shown that participants who committed kind acts for others over the course 10 week intervention showed the greatest well-being gains when these behaviors were enacted in a variety of ways. Thus, when implementing extended prosocial spending interventions, it may be wise to utilize multiple means of giving. For example, companies who want to increase the happiness and job satisfaction of their employees should try incorporating several strategies, such as offering employees a small amount of money to spend on their colleagues as well as the opportunity to allocate the company's charitable funds.

Conclusion

This chapter explored prosocial spending as a mechanism for positive social change. To do so, we began reviewing our research that demonstrates the positive mood and health outcomes associated with prosocial spending for the individual spender. We then extended our discussion to include an examination of the effects of prosocial spending for other individuals, such as the recipient and others nearby: Recipients are happiest after receiving an act of prosocial spending that facilitates positive interpersonal contact. Further, we demonstrated the positive impact of prosocial spending on job satisfaction, team success, and company sales. Finally, we also presented data showing that prosocial spending may provide a route to sustainable happiness for the spender and encourage similar outward spirals of prosocial behavior in others. Indeed, just as the happiness one experiences after engaging in or recalling an act of prosocial spending encourages a future willingness to spend on others again, benefiting from an act of prosocial spending may spur individuals to pay the favor forward. In sum, our research on prosocial spending offers further support for the notion that the findings of *positive psychology* can reach beyond the individual and inspire positive outcomes on a greater scale.

References

Aderman, D. (1972). Elation, depression, and helping behavior. *Journal of Personality and Social Psychology, 24*, 91–101.

Ahuvia, A. (2008). If money doesn't make us happy, why do we act as if it does? *Journal of Economic Psychology, 29*, 491–507.

Aknin, L. B., Barrington-Leigh, C. P., Dunn, E. W., Helliwell, J. F., Biswas-Diener, R., Kemeza, I., et al. (2010). Prosocial spending and well-being: Cross-cultural evidence for a psychological universal. Unpublished data.

Aknin, L. B., Dunn, E. W., & Norton, M. I. (2010). Positive feedback loop between prosocial spending and happiness. Unpublished data.

Aknin, L. B., Dunn, E. W., Sandstrom, G., & Norton, M. I. (2010). Putting the social in prosocial spending. Manuscript in preparation.

Aknin, L. B., Norton, M. I., & Dunn, E. W. (2009). From wealth to well-being? Money matters, but less than people think. *Journal of Positive Psychology, 4*, 523–527.

Algoe, S. B., Haidt, J., & Gable, S. L. (2008). Beyond reciprocity: Gratitude and relationships in everyday life. *Emotion, 8*, 425–429.

Anik, L., Aknin, L. B., Norton, M. I., & Dunn, E. W. (2010). Feeling good about giving: The benefits (and costs) of self-interested charitable behavior. In D. M. Oppenheimer & C. Y. Olivola (Eds.). *Experimental approaches to the study of charitable giving* (pp. 3–13). London, England: Psychology Press.

Aversa, J. (2010). *Americans' job satisfaction falls to an all time low*. Retrieved January 5, 2010, from http://finance.yahoo.com/news/Americans-job-satisfaction-apf-1483464009.html?x=0&sec=topStories&pos=3&asset=&ccode=

Barbaro, M. (2009). *Candles, jeans, lipsticks: Products with ulterior motives*. Retrieved December 12, 2009, from http://www.nytimes.com/2006/11/13/us/13retail.html

Barton, N., & Wasley, P. (2009). Online giving slows. *Chronicle of Philanthropy*. http://philanthropy.com/free/articles/v21/i14/14001701.htm

Baumeister, R. F., & Leary, M. R. (1995). The need to belong: Desire for interpersonal attachments as a fundamental human motivation. *Psychological Bulletin, 117*, 497–529.

Cohen, S., & Pressman, S. D. (2006). Positive affect and health. *Psychological Science, 15*, 122–125.

Cunningham, M. R., Steinberg, J., & Grev, R. (1980). Wanting to and having to help: Separate motivations for positive mood and guilt-induced helping. *Journal of Personality and Social Psychology, 38*, 181–192.

Deaton, A. (2008). Income, health, wellbeing around the world: Evidence from the Gallup World Poll. *Journal of Economic Perspectives, 22*, 53–72.

Deci, E. L., & Ryan, R. M. (1985). *Intrinsic motivation and self-determination in human behavior*. New York: Plenum.

Dickerson, S. S., & Kemeny, M. E. (2004). Acute stressors and cortisol responses: A theoretical integration and synthesis of laboratory research. *Psychological Bulletin, 130*, 355–391.

Diener, E., & Biswas-Diener, R. (2002). Will money increase subjective well-being? A literature review and guide to needed research. *Social Indicators Research, 57*, 119–169.

Diener, E., & Seligman, M. E. P. (2002). Very happy people. *Psychological Science, 13*, 81–84.

Diener, E., & Seligman, M. E. P. (2004). Beyond money: Towards an economy of well-being. *Psychological Science, 5*, 1–31.

Dunn, E. W., Aknin, L. B., & Norton, M. I. (2008). Spending money on others promotes happiness. *Science, 319*, 1687–1688.

Dunn, E. W., Ashton-James, C. E., Hanson, M. D., & Aknin, L. B. (2010). On the costs of self-interested economic behavior: How does stinginess get under the skin? *Journal of Health Psychology, 15*, 627–633.

Emmons, R. A., & McCullough, M. E. (2003). Counting blessings versus burdens: An experimental investigation of gratitude and subjective well-being in daily life. *Journal of Personality and Social Psychology, 84*, 377–389.

Fowler, J. H., & Christakis, N. A. (2008). Dynamic spread of happiness in a large social network: Longitudinal analysis over 20 years in Framingham heart study. *British Medical Journal, 337*, a2338.

Frank, R. H. (2004). How not to buy happiness. *Daedalus, 133*, 69–79.

Fredrickson, B. L. (1998). What good are positive emotions? *Review of General Psychology, 2*, 300–319.

Fredrickson, B. L. (2001). The role of positive emotions in positive psychology: The broaden-and-build theory of positive emotions. *American Psychologist, 56*, 218–226.

Fredrickson, B. L. (2004). The broaden-and-build theory of positive emotions. *Philosophical Transactions of the Royal Society, 359*, 1367–1377.

Frey, B. S., & Stutzer, A. (2000). Happiness, economy and institutions. *The Economic Journal, 110*, 918–938.

Glazer, A., & Konrad, K. A. (1996). A signaling explanation for charity. *American Economic Review, 86*, 1019–1028.

Hatfield, E., Cacioppo, J. T., & Rapson, R. L. (1993). Emotional contagion. *Psychological Science, 2*, 96–99.

Independent Sector. (1999). *Giving and volunteering in the United States.* http://www.independentsector.org/GandV/default.htm

Isen, A. M. (1970). Success, failure, attention and reaction to others: The warm glow of success. *Journal of Personality and Social Psychology, 15*, 294–301.

Isen, A. M., & Levin, P. F. (1972). Effect of feeling good on helping: Cookies and kindness. *Journal of Personality and Social Psychology, 21*, 384–388.

Johnson, D. (2009). *Mystery couple starts "magical" chain reaction.* Retrieved December 14, 2009, from http://www.nbcphiladelphia.com/news/local-beat/Mystery-Couple-Pay-It-Forward-79179347.html?yhp=1

Kahneman, D., Krueger, A. B., Schkade, D., Schwarz, N., & Stone, A. A. (2006). Would you be happier if you were richer? A focusing illusion. *Science, 32*, 1908–1910.

Konow, J., & Earley, J. (2008). The hedonistic paradox: Is homo economicus happier? *Journal of Public Economics, 92*, 1–33.

Layard, R. (2005). *Happiness: Lessons from a new science.* London: Penguin Books.

Lucas, R. E. (2001). Pleasant affect and sociability: Towards a comprehensive model of extraverted feelings and behaviors. *Dissertation Abstracts International, 61*(10-B), 5610, UMI No. AAI9990068.

Lyubomirsky, S., Sheldon, K. M., & Schkade, D. (2005). Pursuing happiness: The architecture of sustainable change. *Review of General Psychology, 9*, 111–131.

McCullough, M. E., Emmons, R. A., & Tsang, J. (2002). The grateful disposition: A conceptual and empirical topography. *Journal of Personality and Social Psychology, 82*, 112–127.

McCullough, M. E., Kilpatrick, S. D., Emmons, R. A., & Larson, D. B. (2001). Is gratitude a moral affect? *Psychological Bulletin, 127*, 249–266.

McCullough, M. E., Kimeldorf, M. B., & Cohen, A. (2008). An adaptation for altruism? The social causes, social effects, and social evolution of gratitude. *Psychological Science, 17*, 281–285.

McEwen, B. S. (1998). Protective and damaging effects of stress mediators. *New England Journal of Medicine, 338*, 171–179.

Myers, D. G. (2000). The funds, friends, and faith of happy people. *American Psychologist, 55*, 56–67.

Norton, M. I., Aknin, L. B., Anik, L., Dunn, E. W., & Quoidbach, J. (2010). Prosocial spending increases employee satisfaction and job performance. Manuscript in preparation.

Oswald, A. J. (1997). Happiness and economic performance. *The Economic Journal, 107*, 1815–1831.

Piliavin, J. A. (2003). Doing well by doing good: Benefits for the benefactor. In C. L. M. Keyes & J. Haidt (Eds.), *The life well-lived* (pp. 227–247). Washington, DC: APA.

Polk, D. E., Cohen, S., Doyle, W. J., Skoner, D. P., & Kirschbaum, C. (2005). State and trait affect as predictors of salivary cortisol in healthy adults. *Psychoneuroendocrinology, 30*, 261–272.

Rosenhan, D. L., Underwood, B., & Moore, B. (1974). Affect moderates self-gratification and altruism. *Journal of Personality and Social Psychology, 30*, 546–552.

Ryan, R. M., & Deci, E. L. (2000). Self-determination theory and the facilitation of intrinsic motivation, social development, and well-being. *American Psychologist, 55*, 68–78.

Schervish, P., & Szanto, A. (2006). Wealth and giving by the numbers. Excerpts from Wealth & Giving Forum Gatherings, Issue 2. Published Fall 2006.

Sheldon, K. M., Boehm, J. K., & Lyubomirsky, S. (in press). Variety is the spice of happiness: The hedonic adaptation prevention (HAP) model. In I. Boniwell & S. David (Eds.), *Oxford handbook of happiness.* Oxford: Oxford University Press.

Strack, F., Schwarz, N., & Gschneidinger, E. (1985). Happiness and reminiscing: The role of time perspective, affect, and mode of thinking. *Journal of Personality and Social Psychology, 49,* 1460–1469.

Thoits, P. A., & Hewitt, L. N. (2001). Volunteer work and well-being. *Journal of Health and Social Behavior, 42,* 115–131.

Totterdell, P. (2000). Catching moods and hitting runs: Mood linkage and subjective performance in professional sports teams. *Journal of Applied Psychology, 85,* 848–859.

Veenhoven, R. (1991). Is happiness relative? *Social Indicators Research, 24,* 1–34.

Waldfogel, J. (1993). The deadweight loss of Christmas. *The American Economic Review, 83,* 1328–1336.

Williams, S., & Shiaw, W. T. (1999). Mood and organizational citizenship behavior: The effects of positive affect on employee organizational citizenship behavior intentions. *Journal of Psychology, 133,* 656–668.

Wilson, E. (2009). *Shopping for clothing, donating time.* Retrieved December 11, 2009, from http://www.nytimes.com/2009/11/12/giving/12BANANA.html?_r=1&ref=givin

Part VI
Positive Psychology and Social Change Interventions

Chapter 14
How Does Coaching Positively Impact Organizational and Societal Change?

Sunny Stout Rostron

Introduction

This research study incorporates stories and self-reflexive inquiry from a small sample of leading coach practitioners, consultants and executive leaders working with coaching in their organizations. I have gathered the following stories with a focus on the challenges in organizational and institutional environments, to help us understand if and how coaching has influenced organizational and societal change. Executive coaching practice far outstrips its evidence base of knowledge as coaching continues to grow as an international phenomenon. Organizations today are challenged by the complexity and swiftness of change within business, social and political environments, and leaders are expected to quickly adapt their skills and competence in volatile and often crisis-driven markets and societies (Stout Rostron, 2009:19–22).

I have interviewed a range of top leaders and managers who use coaching within their organizations, as well as the coaching consultants, practitioners and researchers, coaching psychologists, and human resources (HR) and organizational development (OD) specialists whose work I knew had made a difference. Their stories and the knowledge that they have gained from coaching highlight a way forward using individual and team coaching to empower individuals, organizations and communities. For me, this research activity has proved to be a useful snapshot of how coaching is working globally, as well as what work still needs to be done. Every one of the participants in this research study insisted that coaching is the way forward out of the difficulties and conflicts that we face as fellow human beings in the twenty-first century. Whether you agree with them or not, I hope you will find their thinking and their work inspiring.

The questions I asked the participants in this study were

- Can you describe your work, and what drew you to your current work?
- How has being coached helped you with this work?

S. Stout Rostron (✉)
Manthano Institute of Learning (Pty) Ltd, Cape Town, South Africa
e-mail: express@iafrica.com

R. Biswas-Diener (ed.), *Positive Psychology as Social Change*,
DOI 10.1007/978-90-481-9938-9_14, © Springer Science+Business Media B.V. 2011

- How have you used coaching in your work?
- As a result of your work, what differences would you like to see (and/or have you seen) in terms of social and organizational change? Can you tell me a story that relates to this?
- What are the main challenges that you have overcome in your work as it relates to societal/organizational change, both in relation to yourself and those with whom you are working? Can you tell me a story that relates to this?
- Is there anything else you would like to share with me as far as how coaching has helped you in your work for social/organizational/institutional change?

How Is Coaching Making a Difference in Organizations and Society?

I asked each coaching leader to describe what drew them to their current work, and how they personally experience and use coaching in their work. Second, they shared the differences they have seen as a result of their work, and what they would still like to see in terms of social and organizational change. There are some dramatic stories, even some radical views on the potential of coaching as a force for change. Personally I feel enthralled and energized by the freshness, enthusiasm and originality expressed by these practitioners, all leading experts in their fields.

What comes through clearly, from the following stories, is a passionate belief in the potential and power that coaching can unleash. Here then are some of the most dynamic and innovative voices within the "coaching process" today. I will let them speak directly for themselves. We should listen very carefully to them.

Nancy Kline: Independent Thinking to Create Societal Change

Nancy Kline is President of Time to Think Inc., a leadership development company specializing in the Thinking Environment®. Time to Think is currently developing consultants, facilitators and coaches in the United Kingdom, USA, South Africa, Ireland, Sweden and Australia. Author of Time to Think *(1999) and* More Time Think *(2009). Kline's Thinking Partnership® is based on the "chosen philosophical view that human beings are by nature good: intelligent, loving, powerful, multi-talented, emotional, assertive, able to think through anything, imaginative and logical". Kline says that "behaviour to the contrary is seen as the result of assumptions generated over a lifetime by events, conditions and attitudes in a person's environment" (Kline, 2005, p. 4). One of the key theories which determines how we work with clients in the "coaching conversation" is that of "positive philosophical choice".*

I teach, coach, write about and research the Thinking Environment® – having been drawn to my work through one observation and one question. The observation, dry but chilling, is that the quality of everything we do depends on the quality of the *thinking* we do first. The question that arises from this observation is, "How can we

help each other to think *for ourselves* with rigour, imagination, courage and grace"?
I think I became interested in this question when I was 7 years old. My mother, a
quiet, understated woman who never shouted at anyone, 1 day charged through the
living room with her fist in the air shouting, "There is no greater crime than the
waste of a single human mind", then disappeared down the hall. I was mystified;
but as children do, I stored that memory, filing it under "I" for incomprehensible but
immensely important.

Ten years later when I was 17, I was sitting with my father going through his
old papers. I picked one up, began to read it and then to cry; it was a speech he
had delivered when *he* was 17, in which he called for complete equality for African-
Americans. That was in 1920 in Tennessee when black people were segregated from
white people by law. I marvelled at his courage and asked, "Dad, how did you ever
get permission to deliver this speech? Weren't you scared?" He looked it over and
said, "Well, honey, I didn't ask for permission. I just asked myself the question,
'What is the most important issue facing my generation?' I immediately knew the
answer, so I asked myself another question: 'If I weren't afraid, what would I say
about that issue in my speech?' As I was delivering it at the graduation ceremony,
about halfway through, I looked out at the audience of faculty, student body, parents,
board of trustees – and noticed that they had all stood up and were walking out.
As I stood there, looking out at the empty auditorium, I decided I needed to do
only two things with my life. One: to keep thinking for myself, and two: not get
killed."

Those are two of the earliest experiences of my being drawn to the importance
of independent thinking. Over the years I decided somewhere inside of me that I
would pursue the question, "How we can help each other to think for ourselves"?
I was also drawn to this work because of an increasing awareness that most of
what wasn't working in human life and in organizations could probably be traced
to the conformity, inaccuracies and inhumanity of people's thinking. I wanted to
contribute to a core level of change by seeing if independent thinking could make
a difference. I soon found myself growing interested in organizational and societal
transformation.

My coaching sessions each week are vital to the development of my work.
Coaching allows me to refine the capacity to be clear in my own thinking, to be
focused on what matters most to me. It helps me in my work to be able to listen
in a particular way to people. And I think that perhaps most of all, coaching keeps
me curious about one of the core questions in my work, "How far can people go
in their *own* thinking before they need mine?" My coaching keeps me courageous,
and it keeps me from getting lost in my fears or unwarranted reluctance to go to
the cutting edge. It helps me to be less concerned about myself, and more focused
on generating others' independent thought. And I also think it keeps me physically
healthy. I wouldn't want a life without coaching; it lets the streams run clear.

And on the issue of transformation, it seems to me that at the heart of societal change is the resurgence of pride in our own group identities. As a female, a
New Mexican, and a woman over 60, I think my coaching indirectly and sometimes directly helps me to be more of *myself*. This matters because we can think

for ourselves only if we can think *as* ourselves. Finally, coaching is the key to my work because I think that it is only out of our own breakthroughs that we can offer a breakthrough process to others with confidence.

When we teach the Thinking Partnership® programme and the Thinking Environment® coaching and supervision programmes, we are expressly using coaching. But I think that any time two or more people are thinking together, with all ten components of a Thinking Environment® present, there is a coaching element in the conversation. This is because we are both interested in what the other person truly thinks and feels. So, in that sense you could say that everything that I do is a form of coaching. This work, however, didn't start as a coaching process. It was embraced by the coaching world because it generates independent thinking in people. The important question I think coaches need to be asking is: *what more can we do in this moment to help people to think for themselves*? The emerging answers to that question do contribute to an efficacious coaching framework, and I feel personally very excited by what is now developing in the search for better and better answers to that question. Also, I've seen the Thinking Environment® process create coaching results widely: in one-to-one relationships, in groups, in corporate cultures as well as in organizations that are focused on societal change, and in neighbourhoods, hospitals, families and communities.

From the beginning, my work has been motivated by a passion for a world that works beautifully for everyone. I would like to see a world in which every human being knows that they matter, that their thinking and their contributions are central to our success as a society, and a world in which every human being lives well. I would like to see a world of work in which people come home with a spring in their step because they have spent all day knowing that their thinking was valued. I would also like to see a world in which war is a thing we learn about only through our history books, a thing that seems an outrageous aberration of human activity. Many years ago I began to wonder what might be one change that could change everything else. I reasoned that because everything depends on the quality of the thinking we do first, creating structures in which people could think for themselves might have a chance of helping to bring about some significant, human changes in society.

One story comes from work this year when I was working with a professional multi-disciplinary patient team. The issue the team was considering was "best patient service". Even before the meeting started we turned the issue into a question. Because the mind works best in the presence of a question, this practice of turning agenda items into questions immediately brings elements of a coaching culture to the meeting. The question they crafted was, "How can the patient team coordinator keep the patient at the centre?" This group was made up of experts, all of whom live in their own silos of arrogance. They included the social worker, the key doctor, the physiotherapist, the radiologist and the psychologist. Their behaviour in meetings typically focused on having the loudest voice and the final say, and taking the least amount of time to be seen as the most important person. Not until that day did they consider putting the patient at the centre of their meetings and decision-making. We used the Thinking Environment® processes throughout, and everyone had an uninterrupted turn to address the question.

We went round the group systematically so that people knew when their turn was; the chair didn't determine who spoke first and people kept attention on the person whose turn it was. As a high level of respect for each person became palpable, arrogance began to dissipate and silos began to break down. Ease prevailed so that people could think afresh, without interruption or urgency. As a result the thinking accelerated.

Within an hour they came up with new ideas easily implementable by the lead professional. They agreed, for example, that the patient should be asked how they would like to interact with these experts so that they would not feel infantilized or frightened. The patient would be invited to ask questions of these professionals; they would be key in shaping the building of the relationship with the professional. The professionals also agreed to ask themselves when in patient meetings, "Is this patient at the centre of this meeting, and if they aren't, how can we restore them to that central position?" For this team it was a radical idea to listen to each other without interruption and to learn from each other, regarding each other *and the patient*, as thinking equals throughout. This was a step right outside of their too often me-centred culture. A particularly societal-change focus of this outcome, also, was that the patient group was adolescents. In the meeting, the professionals had effectively discarded their own prejudices against young people as thinkers. They began to operate instead on the assumption that young people can think brilliantly, for themselves, if they are offered a thinking environment. Through that meeting the patient had moved firmly into the centre.

Certainly one of my greatest challenges has been sustaining a thinking environment in conflict. A key question is: how can we keep each other thinking well for ourselves when the message we are delivering is hard, and when it is born of anger or fear? How do we express difficult things so that the person can *keep thinking* while we are expressing it?

I saw this challenge handled beautifully recently. One of the members of a team was feeling discriminated against by his colleagues. It had to do with his not being selected to deliver some of the work others were delivering. He wanted to understand the selection criteria and he was angry. He called together a teleconference of the team. He consciously created a thinking environment. He said, "I would like to speak and say everything I want to say as if I am handing you the moon. And then I would like everyone to have a chance to speak as if you were handing me the moon." And he did exactly that. He talked about the things that were upsetting him; his tone was loving, he was not urgent; no one interrupted and at the end of the turn he felt different and more open to hearing what the others were saying. The others weren't feeling threatened by him, and they spoke calmly and intelligently. As we went round the circle, there was an accumulation of accurate information about how the people had been selected, information that hadn't been communicated during the selection process. He was satisfied with the criteria, and they decided that in the future they would communicate all criteria in particular ways, creating transparency to prevent the perception and the experience of marginalization. At the end, this man spoke again, generating his freshest thinking, which was useful to everyone; then everyone appreciated him, and he appreciated them. In my view, what took place in that 45 min probably prevented a year of misunderstanding.

Mark Rittenberg: Theatre Practices to Develop Holistic, Authentic Leaders

Dr. Mark Rittenberg has worked as an executive coach all over the world for the last 20 years. In addition to coaching leaders from Fortune 500 companies, he acts as master coach for consultants from the major US consulting firms, and has been instrumental in instituting organizational coaching programmes to grow emerging and aspiring leaders. He was invited to participate as both master coach and mediator in Level 3 of the Middle East Peace Process. An award-winning actor and director, he teaches at a number of business school faculties including the Kellogg School, Olin School of Business and Haas School of Business of the University of California at Berkeley, where he is the designer and senior consultant for the Executive Coaching Institute. He divides his time between Berkeley and Johannesburg, South Africa, where he is an executive coach and designer of internal coaching programmes working with the new black leadership in several South African institutions.

His programmes coach leaders in the practices of Active Communicating[®] based on four principles which distinguish effective and high-performing teams from ineffective and dysfunctional ones: show up and choose to be present; pay attention to what has heart and meaning; tell the truth without blame or judgement and be open to outcome, not attached to outcome.

I was drawn to my current work after having been an actor and theatre director for many years. In 1984, I won an award at the Jerusalem Festival for a play called "Life or Theatre", and I was subsequently invited to direct it at Harvard University. I recast the play with a group of Harvard MBA students who shared with me that this was "the most profound leadership development" they had ever experienced, despite their current MBA classes. Their request was that I facilitate similar theatre-based work with their peers and colleagues at the Harvard Business School – for them this work was about authentic leadership.

When I asked what they liked about the work, they said that I was coaching them holistically, as an actor, in voice, body and individual leadership. They said, "You're not afraid to go deep, yet somehow you create a safe space for each individual to find their own authentic, true voice. We have all changed as a result of this rehearsal process, and we believe that this work will greatly impact on leaders who want to motivate their work groups and become authentic, inspirational leaders." From that moment in the mid-1980s, the theatre-based Active Communicating[®] work began. We coached several teams at Harvard Business School, and those already successful, final-year MBA students invited us into their companies to facilitate theatre-based workshops on the Art of Leadership Presence.

These teams were particularly interested in one-on-one coaching. So began a massive amount of work at Pacific Bell, AT&T and Levi Strauss in the USA, putting groups of managers alongside their rank-and-file employees to work, not just on interpersonal communication skills, but to become true communicators and ambassadors for their brand. The one-on-one coaching impacted their work groups and peers, emphasizing how they themselves could be forces for change within the workplace.

At the moment I have three coaches, because when working with others in a generous, compassionate and empathetic way, I need a baseline of where I as a coach can take someone. I need to understand where I am willing or not willing to go on a certain journey, and I must overcome my own barriers. Being in a coaching relationship gives me a baseline of what I will do myself, helping me to develop competence and the right to work with others in a similar way. My coaches have always asked my permission before opening up a conversation around a leadership behaviour that I need to change. I have adopted this in my coaching approach to ensure that the work we do together is meaningful, helping them to fulfil their aspirations and their dreams.

My coaching practice encompasses three areas. First, my private coaching practice of 12 individuals who are each taking part in an executive team-coaching programme. Second, I have personally trained a group of executive coaches who work in my Active Communicating® team. Third, at the Center for Executive Education at the University of California at Berkeley, we facilitate open enrolment and customized programmes for the "Leader as Coach". In this programme, managers and emergent inspiring leaders who want to grow themselves and others, experience the Active Communicating® theatre-based skills of "coaching behaviour". This theatre-based methodology enables them to coach their own direct reports more easily. The coaching tools we look at include what it means to be an excellent listener, how to listen and facilitate in a group dialogue, and to truly engage their group in problem-solving and consensus-building.

Finally, at the Center for Executive Education at Haas Business School, we launched the Executive Coaching Institute (ECI) for three specific markets. The first wish to become better coaches; perhaps they are changing profession, changing their role within the organization or even setting up their own executive coaching practice. Some are already successful coaches; however, due to our methodology using actors' skills to train coaches, these students add techniques and evolve their own repertoire. A second group refers to the current trend in the field of coaching where organizations are developing in-house coaches; they send these internal coaches to us to learn theatre-based coaching techniques. The third group are senior executives who don't want to train as an executive or internal coach, but want to adopt a coaching leadership style. This executive is someone who facilitates learning, problem-solving and employee growth.

As a result of the work that I'm doing, I want to see leaders who operate from the head and the heart, becoming more in touch with themselves and others. If more in touch with others, they are more tolerant, understanding that people have different work and learning styles – i.e. one size doesn't fit all. But what does it mean to embrace a variety of learning and leadership styles? One of the stories that spring to mind is an executive I coached for a number of years; he was a command-and-control leader in a large American multinational corporation.

As a result of the coaching process he became an extraordinary visionary – an exceptional individual who could see and act on the future of his company. Although many people in his workforce were intelligent, diligent and hard-working individuals, they could not meet his high expectations. During the second year of the coaching relationship, he shared his concerns about succession planning, worrying that there was no one to take his place or that of the other vice-presidents.

As one of his coaching goals was to pay attention to succession planning, we created a leadership institute within the company; he put his most aspiring leaders through an intensive, high-level leadership development programme to give them the skills and competence to become "leaders of tomorrow". I made an observation that what was missing was his "relationship" with those leaders, even though he had created the programme. To open the Institute's first morning, I asked him and the other seven vice-presidents serving as faculty to create their individual leadership story and share it with the audience. The stories were to illustrate how they became the leaders they are today. He exclaimed, "I don't have a leadership story; I don't even know what I want to say". I suggested, "Why don't you speak about the events in your early life that really touched and challenged you? I think that should be the context of your leadership story".

He resisted for a long, long time. On the opening day he told his story: "I am not a storyteller and so will have to share my story with you in three sentences. My father died when I was six, and from that moment my mother had to go out each night, after her day job, to work in the wealthy homes of people who lived in the next neighbourhood. She cleaned their houses every evening to provide school uniforms for myself and my five brothers. My mother will be 89 next month and she remains my greatest hero." The entire room dissolved in tears. The barrier that had always been between him, his direct reports and the entire workforce disintegrated. >From the moment he told his story, the leadership team began to rise to the occasion as he had wanted them to. Somehow previously they had been too intimidated or too frightened to do so. Everything he wanted began to happen. And the reason was because he too had began to show his vulnerability.

The main challenge that I've overcome in my work has been to overcome my own fear of being able to really help a leader who desperately wants to commit to personal change. As an external consultant I am very conscious that there is a certain protocol to be observed inside each organization. The idea of taking a CEO and turning him or her into a storyteller when giving an annual report is generally taboo! Leaders move away from traditional corporate stereotypical roles when they get in touch with what people want to hear, and with what really motivates and inspires them. I have seen such miracles happen by not being afraid myself, helping a leader to open their own creative possibilities through storytelling. This means encouraging leaders to talk about their failures and challenges through their own stories. For years, I've had a curious relationship with those in very senior leadership positions; often they insist that the leaders and the teams are not ready to work on building relationships, becoming powerful communicators or engaging in building trust through partnership and collaboration. Often, building trust is not even on the radar screen of work to be done with leaders. Although I haven't committed these acts of "civil disobedience" deliberately, when I conduct a leadership study I ask the sponsor, "If you were his coach what would you be working on?" Or, "What are the three things as a workplace community that you would like to become in the next year?" I hear things like, "We need to be better communicators and partners in the building process, able to understand what makes each other tick. We've never had time to build relationships with each other. In addition, we'd like our leaders to communicate with us, to let us know what is happening, and what challenges lie ahead that keep the leadership awake at night". Internal communication between leader and staff continues to rank as the loudest "positive change" employees want to see in their workplace.

When I hear the voices of the people echo these themes, it removes my fear and gives me the courage to do things in coaching conversations and in facilitating workshops, which might normally be the least-chosen alternative. The results are often the release of untapped potential in people, where trust is built between leadership and staff in a way that allows individual passion, talent and true selves to come forward.

Lee Salmon: The Entrepreneurial Go-To Place for Executive Coaching

Lee Salmon is an executive coach and management consultant with the Federal Consulting Group of the US Department of the Interior in Washington, DC. He provides professional services in organizational development, change management, executive and personal performance coaching. He is a practice leader for executive coaching, leadership development and mentoring programmes to agencies in the Federal government on strategic planning, change management, leadership and organization development, executive coaching, meeting facilitation, teambuilding, and human capital development. He also specializes in coaching executives in scientific and technical organizations for career transitions, change management, leadership development and performance management. He represents the International Consortium for Coaching in Organizations (ICCO), a group of senior-level coaches who are committed to working in public and private organizations to have a positive impact.

I started to make a shift into organizational change, human development and the softer side of change in 1995. I was working at the Environmental Protection Agency (EPA) as a senior scientist and health physicist. At that time, I was given an opportunity to reinvent my career due to downsizing which took me out of management. I was asked to figure out what I wanted to do with my career, and I decided to work with organizational transformation, working with the skills I had used in teams, presenting and teaching. I started to make that shift in 1995, which led me to explore coaching in government, which was new at that time. More and more, as we shifted to teamwork environments with small group practitioners, I could see that people were having difficulties working effectively in teams. I could see how to make those teams function and be effective from the beginning, and it was then that I started full facilitation work: in meetings with senior officials, and with colleagues in the EPA.

I worked as team leader for the science teams until I reached a turning point in 2000. It was then that I joined Federal Consulting Group, a small internal government-consulting group that serves only government agencies. We are a unique hybrid, working in government with an entrepreneurial model yet with government constraints. We bring in outside consultants and coaches to assist us in our work, but we are the ones who take care of customers, contracts and get the results that government wants. Our focus is to transform government so that it can provide services the public trusts and has confidence in. We've been in existence 22 years with only ten of us in the group, doing $12 million worth of business each year. When I arrived at Federal Consulting Group, coaching was contracted at senior executive level only, and quietly executed through human resources (HR) departments. In the last 10 years, I have created and built a coaching and consulting practice that serves all government agencies. We provide extraordinary coaches and consultants to help in personal and organizational transformation, having built a reputation as the "go-to place" for executive coaching.

Coaching has helped me to accomplish my particular personal goals – to affect the quality of leadership in the organization, and be able to create a government that serves the needs of society. From a stewardship or "servant leadership" perspective, which I believe in, one of the ways I can be a more effective servant leader is to develop my skills in coaching, process and facilitation. This means engaging in one-to-one work, and working with teams to influence the ways they collaborate, communicate and make government work. In meeting a large range of people who have a similar or like-minded focus, I have slowly begun to build a community of coaches and consultants where we can share our learning and experiences. This means we are not so isolated, and have more impact in the areas in which we work and serve.

In using coaching in my work, I've contracted individual coaching assignments for myself and other coaches who form part of our network of coaches. I have also started working with other government agencies to help them develop coaching programmes for future leaders in their organizations. It's only now that we have the capability to provide coaching services from individual assignments, to full organizational and systemic coaching programmes that play an ongoing part of leadership and succession planning. I can best illustrate this with a case study from the Centers for Disease Control and Prevention (CDC University) in Atlanta, Georgia. CDC deals nationally and globally with health care systems, global pandemics and other huge issues that affect public health. The Director of CDC University had long wanted to do some work with coaching. Together we developed a coaching programme that served groups of 30–35 small executives annually. We started with the top senior executives, working across the organization, hitting management systemically across all the different offices in CDC. It has been very successful, and we've coached over 100 executives and senior managers within CDC, including all of their functional areas.

We have had phenomenal results in terms of the impact and the way leaders show up, engage others and have impact in their organizations. For example, in clearer communication, effectiveness in activity, partnering and reaching out to other organizations, and in the leaders' ability and capacity to be adaptable and flexible in times of crisis and change. That's the impact of the work we've done in CDC, which has been nominated a couple of times for the International Coach Federation's (ICF) annual PRISM award.

There's something else. We realized the work we needed to do in changing these leaders and making them more effective was to build their emotional and social skills – with a strong focus on emotional intelligence, working in areas that relate to emotional effectiveness. We used the work of Reuven Bar-On, which is one of the most heavily researched 360 instruments (Bar-On is an internationally known expert and pioneer in the field of emotional intelligence, and has been involved in defining, measuring and applying various aspects of this construct since 1980. He coined the term "Emotional Quotient" or "EQ" in 1985 to describe his approach to assessing emotional and social functioning). We administer the EQ360 Instrument at the very beginning of each coaching programme, using that to help guide the developmental work of our clients.

Lately, we have been using the Kouzes and Posner leadership profile to help complement the EQ work for the last 6–9 months (the Kouzes and Posner approach is that, leadership is a measurable, learnable and teachable set of behaviours. The leadership practices inventory (LPI) is a 360° assessment instrument based on 25 years of research. It allows participants to test Kouzes and Posner's five practices model for leadership behaviour, and provides a tool that helps leaders assess the extent to which they actually use those practices). What we've seen is a dramatic improvement in the leaders' emotional and social intelligence scores, along with critical factors relating to "change resilience" leadership.

The evaluation results vary from the individuals themselves, depending on how transformational this has been in their lives, how they have changed their way of being and how they are engaging in their relationships with others. As people in the organization are reporting remarkable changes in their leaders due to this work, it seems that positive organizational change is occurring and we are continuing to focus on creating positivity. Our coaches are positive psychology-focused, and use the work of Martin Seligman and Barbara Frederickson on the power of positive psychology.

What I would like to see, however, is more work with leaders around transition. It seems that not only are leaders willing to get used to change, but they live in a sea of constant change. All of them need to develop flexibility in their leadership style and competence, with the ability to adapt to a rapidly changing world. The big challenge is to get people to actually take part in the coaching intervention, and to integrate their learning into their existing leadership style. That sustainable long-term perspective on leadership is yet to be recognized by most organizations. Also, we see constant change in administrations, with political leaders stepping into their roles without much strength in terms of emotional competence. They tend to try to whip people into shape, thinking they can push a button, telling them that what's been done before has been terrible, instead of building upon what has been successful. They push the great "undo" button, which means that they try to undo everything that's gone before, often without understanding how to work with people through a process of change. This means they basically dismantle people's lives: "Well, we're going to be doing something different, so get on with it", without realizing that if you don't engage the heart and souls of people nothing will be sustainable.

I'm in the process of writing a new paper that is coming out in the ICCO journal looking at how coaching can support leadership during times of crisis. It's looking at government institutions in the financial arena through my and other coaches' experiences as to how we have supported leaders during times of crisis, and how we have started to build leaders' capability to tackle change in the moment. This entails stepping back to understand how to build change resilience in these leaders. We know change is constant, and that government leaders will continue to move from one crisis to another. This area of crisis leadership is coming to the fore. For social and emotional effectiveness, how can we build practices and capability to help leaders step up to these crises, to survive, thrive and lead organizations and people in times of extraordinary change? I believe that a new consciousness is emerging.

We have obtained funding from four different programme offices in the EPA, and have been able to stay below political levels of scrutiny so that no one sits on us. We've been given full range to address environmental leadership, stewardship, sustainability, global climate change and how to create "change-resilient" leadership from the ground up. Seeing that there is something larger emerging that I am now a part of, I can let it emerge without trying to force it. That is part of my stewardship role to connect people and create resources. We're looking to offer this service using IP TV so that other government departments can also participate using social networking technology to bring more people into the conversation.

Lew Stern: Positively Influencing Leadership for Global Sustainability

Dr. Lew Stern is president of Stern Consulting and Founder and executive director of the Foundation for International Leadership Coaching. Lew is a licensed psychologist in Massachusetts, and since 1977 has served as a leader, executive and leadership coach, and consulting psychologist. Lew has coached and consulted to senior leaders of private- and public-sector organizations around the world. He serves as senior advisor to the Institute of Coaching at McLean Hospital, Harvard Medical School and has a faculty appointment as clinical instructor at Harvard Medical School. On the board of advisors of the International Consortium for Coaching in Organization (ICCO), he is an editorial board member of Coaching: An International Journal of Theory Research and Practice. *He chaired the Working Group on Education and Development at the Global Coaching Convention (GCC). He has authored or co-authored many articles and handbooks in coaching including* Executive Coaching: A Working Definition; The Executive Coaching Handbook; *and* Executive Coaching: Building and Managing Your Professional Practice. *Lew has a passion for bringing the power of leadership coaching to leaders around the world who are committed to global sustainability.*

I have three different areas in which I currently work, although I will focus on the Foundation for International Leadership Coaching. The first two areas are in organizations, coaching senior leaders and their teams, and as a senior advisor to build and achieve the mission for the Institute of Coaching at Harvard/McLean. This is to help develop coaching as a professional discipline. The Foundation's mission is most important right now, to have an impact so that leadership coaching can change the future of our world. I feel passionately that our world is headed in the wrong direction, and that government and NGO leaders are in control of funds, policies and resources that, if shifted, coaching could positively influence global sustainability, for the environment, international peace and worldwide quality of life. I believe coaching can positively influence our world leaders and their impact on our future.

However, most coaches aren't hitting that. Instead, they are helping large corporations make more money to improve the lives of the people working in those organizations, but they are not making a difference to our global society. What's drawing me to it? I'm a grown-up hippie; a pacifist; an environmentalist; I truly love children; I believe in the democratic process and in equality of human rights and freedom. So much of the work I've done in the past had little impact on any of that. What I hope to do now is help bring the world's leading coaches together to build the leadership capacity of international leaders and ultimately to shift the direction of our planet.

Other people coaching me has helped me with my work, and I'm fortunate to work with people like you. My colleagues coach me; my friends and colleagues are generous with their feedback, confronting me, acting as devil's advocate to ensure that I balance my health and my life. They question me if I am doing too much or too little, and bombard me daily with positive coaching. I've been truly stretched in this last year, seeing the world from a global perspective, seeing my own ethnicity from a larger perspective, seeing myself as a person with continuous needs for personal and professional development, helping me to be more humble, yet see the influence I can have. Coaching has changed my whole outlook on life, on my profession and on my place in the world.

More specifically, I use coaching in my daily routine as I coach global leaders in the corporate and the non-profit world. In the last 2 weeks I have shared coaching conversations with executives from Russia, Mexico, Asia, Europe and the USA. I have been working with potential CEOs of organizations and leading executives in government and educational institutions. I see coaching more as a process than a profession: it is the process of stepping back and helping people to look at themselves in a positive way, helping them to leverage their strengths, identifying what they want to accomplish while they work with others to remove personal barriers in order to unleash the power of what they want to do. I use coaching in everything I do, whether it is with other coaches, colleagues, leaders, building affiliations and collaborations.

As a result of my coaching work, the biggest story is yet to be told, because right now there's very little coaching taking place with the world's leaders. Most of them have stepped into their positions through technical capability, political affiliation or other reasons than being effective leaders. I'm looking at the Foundation project as a 5-year plan to make an impact on society rather than just on individuals. We need to gather many leaders together to collaboratively address societal and planetary change albeit in a different way, as opposed to winning elections, money and power. It is time to think about future generations, and the impact of what we are doing today in the world. This story is not yet told. I would like us to help these leaders to be leaders! Recently, I spoke in Scottsdale, Arizona to 100 consulting psychologists at the Society for Consulting Psychology (Division 13 of the American Psychological Association). The audience was made up of doctoral-level experts with many years' experience in their field. When I explained the vision and mission of the Foundation, many wanted to sign up immediately.

Almost everyone I speak to, including coaches, teachers, leaders and individuals from many different perspectives, see the need to build international leadership capability. All view the potential of positive psychology and coaching as having the capacity to build leaders who can build the future of our world. I am told leadership stories from day-to-day and am asked, "What can we do?" Many organizations have similar exciting missions in different parts of the world. Some focus on organization development, another takes coaching to third world villages; others work with leadership development for government leaders; others bring leaders together across international boundaries – e.g. the Center for Creative Leadership (CCL) and their Leadership Beyond Boundaries Programme. There are many different voices. For example: the Coach Initiative, the Coaches Alliance for Social Action, Coaching in Philanthropy Project, Coaching Beyond Boundaries, Coaching for a Cause, Coaching the Global Village, the Global Coaching Community; there is a separate Group for Societal Change; the Mirus Coaching for Social Change; International Coach Federation who offer *pro bono* grants for coaching and education; Root Cause, the Kennedy School of Leadership; the Clinton Foundation who send coaches to Ethiopia to work on AIDS; Mexican ICF: Social Initiative for Social Change.

There are many organizations trying to build world leaders in their own way. We are collaborating, reaching out to as many organizations as possible to leverage each other's resources. There's another group with whom we speak regularly, which is interested in facilitating the coach's impact on social change in the United Kingdom, the USA and many other countries. Worldwide, many different organizations are forming to make an impact and to leverage social change. This is a very exciting story, and it gives me hope that many people really want to make a difference in a positive way. I know I sound idealistic, but I don't mind idealism!

Italia Boninelli: Global Mining and Its Impact on Communities and Society

Italia Boninelli is senior vice-president, human resources of Gold Fields, and is the chairperson of the Gold Fields Leadership and Business Academy. Previously group human resources director of Netcare, the largest private healthcare organization in South Africa, and HR director and marketing director at Standard Bank, Italia has more than 20 years' experience in human resources, marketing, communications, customer relationship management and business transformation in a variety of industries. A registered industrial psychologist, she is a founder member of the National Human Resources Research Initiative of the South African Board for

Personnel Practice, which is setting the agenda for research into strategic human resources practices.

Italia has lectured at business schools and for national bodies such as the Institute for Personnel Management; she is passionate in her support for women's leadership development programmes and the development of strategic business skills in HR practitioners. She received the "HR Director of 2008" award from the Institute for People Management of South Africa and the "SA Most Influential Women in Business and Government" award for the Mining Sector for 2009 from CEO Magazine *together with Wits Business School. She is the author of numerous publications including two books:* Building Human Capital, *and* Conversations in Leadership: South African Perspectives, *which are used as set works at various universities.*

I head up human resources (HR) and training and development for the Gold Fields Group. We have mining operations in South Africa, Ghana, Australia, Peru and exploration sites in 16 other countries. My work is setting the strategic direction for HR, and current focus areas include negotiating wage demands and other significant issues with multiple unions, stakeholder management, maintaining and developing the talent and skills pipeline, managing the leadership development portfolio and driving a significant investment in organizational design and culture change. What drew me to my work is the ability to make large-scale systemic changes and to turn an organization around, which is part of my track record. I was attracted to Gold Fields by a visionary CEO who had a very clear idea of what he wanted a new Gold Fields to become. In this job, what appeals to me is that I operate at a different level of work that involves huge organizational change with international exposure and the ability to influence across other countries as well.

Besides providing a sounding board (it is always "lonely at the top" in an executive role), coaching has helped me with my own personal transition to a new level of work. It has also helped with the adjustment to a new industry and culture. I moved from the Netcare environment in the healthcare industry where the staff was 84% female, to Gold Fields, which is in the mining industry with a 95% male workforce. Gold Fields is a very large organization, with about 50,000 permanent employees and 16,000 contract staff. The traditional hierarchical structure and paternalistic yet authoritarian management style has meant that organizational and culture change occur slowly and require great effort. There is often resistance in the ranks to new initiatives. I've used coaching of key executives and senior managers inside the organization to help transition people to higher levels of work and to develop a critical mass of people who are starting to think in a new way. That helps to leverage change.

Very specifically in the HR arena, I have used coaching to support particular programmes; for example specific women's programmes to bring women into mining and to progress women through the ranks. Second, we have Mining Charter obligations and need to find ways to accelerate black talent with leadership potential. Due to the skills shortage, we also need to accelerate young graduates and technical specialists into managerial roles much more quickly than might have been the case in the past. The scarcity of key mining skills has been an issue for more than 20 years, but in the past we had old experienced hands that were internal mentors.

As retirement, emigration and other factors have depleted their ranks, coaching has been used to fill part of that gap. The third area where coaching has played a key role is in support of our leadership development programme. Leadership in large organizations emerges when three sets of conditions are met: where people have the analytical and problem-solving skills together with the technical and business knowledge required to address that industry's challenges; where they have the personal passion, purpose, stress resilience and risk propensity to take up the challenge; and lastly where the context requires leadership, i.e. there is some pressing issue or "burning platform" that requires bold action. Executive coaches help people to confront their personal limitations, understand their risk preferences and leadership styles, and enable them to make the transition to being a real leader, and not just a manager. And this can occur at all levels of the organization!

One of the interesting developments I have seen is how the use of coaching to support leadership development has resulted in broader social and organizational change than just the person being coached. We have seen greater personal empowerment for those who are receiving coaching, and they have transferred their coaching skills into the workplace, coaching their colleagues and subordinates. This has impacted other parts of the organization, where those being coached have used their personal insights and coaching skills to coach young graduates across the other disciplines; this has broadly impacted and started to change organizational culture. Once we have created "critical mass" thinking and behaving in a new way from their coaching experience, our managers have started to positively influence hundreds of other managers who have not yet been through this experience. Some of the coaches have also applied their coaching skills to our community investment projects. Our employees are thus involved in an expansion of coaching outside of the organization.

What are our challenges? Like many companies in the mining industry, Gold Fields as an organization has focused on production costs and efficiencies. But the complexity of the challenges we face is rising exponentially. Many traditional managers do not necessarily have the skills or awareness of the more complex challenges which a mining organization faces today. We need to manage new stakeholder groupings that pose new challenges. For example, the green movement and community groups are challenging companies like ours on the environmental impact we have. The focus on safety and health factors is high on the agenda of workers, unions and government. Any of these issues can potentially impact the continuation of mining activities, and might even force the closure of a mine. The challenge is to get staff who have functioned very successfully at an operational level to understand the increasing complexity of the world in which we live, and to assist them in improving their own skills to deal with these challenges. In all the countries in which we operate, we support very broad corporate social investment initiatives.

Shani Naidoo: Coaching and Social Networking

Shani Naidoo is managing director of human resources for Foschini Group in South Africa. She has spent the last 20 years in human resources practice. She joined the Foschini Group in 1990 and developed competence in recruitment and selection; psychometrics; counselling, and training and development. She then joined BMW South Africa as general manager, human resources. During her career she has led small, medium and large teams, worked across multi-level international and national organizations, and led projects from performance management to remuneration and transformation. She rejoined the Foschini Group in 2005 as general manager of the human resources division, and was appointed to the board as managing director, human resources in 2006. She is known for her well-developed technical expertise in human resources, her vision in developing world-class solutions and pursuing a sound understanding of the business she works in to deliver these solutions. As a senior industrial psychologist, she mentors psychology internship candidates and continually pushes the boundaries of HR practice in business. Not willing to wait and see what business requires, her motto is to predict and develop solutions before it is needed in business. She has served 3 years as the chairperson of the Retailers' Association, where her work involved developing sound HR practice in retail, and engaging retail stakeholders on transforming business and HR policy.

My work is to develop the best people solutions in support of the business achieving its goals. These people solutions involve the entire human value chain in the organization, and my job is to optimize, research and diagnose the business issues as they relate to people, finding solutions that are business and people appropriate. What drew me to this work is its complexity. There is more than just one business unit, and there are quite distinct cultural attributes, even a different DNA within individual business units. When I arrived, these business units were quite disparate, and one of my roles has been to realign them. Retail is a fast moving, dynamic, people-focused business, and because human resources is a critical and strategic function in Foschini, I wanted to work in an organization where people are important.

Coaching has helped me as an individual leader to think and diagnose without emotion, to talk something through, to see the wood for the trees, to create space in my mind to see the picture clearly. Through working with a coach, I have been able to develop distance and perspective and improve my decision-making as a result.

In my work, coaching has helped me to improve individual and company acceleration towards a goal. For example, coaching has helped individual executives find solutions quickly, and coaching has helped individual executives when they have been stuck – helping them think something through, finding a solution. Sometimes coaching has resulted in clear change and achievement of an individual's objectives. Coaching has also been used for longer-term interventions to grow and develop an individual's certain weaker attributes, as well as to assist them in improving and building new relationships. I think coaching has even helped our leadership to appreciate the value of coaching; it has helped our very senior executives develop a greater awareness of the nexus between individuals and the achievement of business objectives.

The difference that I would like to see as a result of coaching is collaboration, particularly greater collaboration between silos. There has been social change between business units who previously worked very separately. But now we have chat rooms where individuals in Foschini get together across business functions and units to develop relationships and business solutions. This is due to the need for change processes to be bedded down quickly. We are currently experiencing an economic slowdown, and we need to identify what processes require improvement, which requires people to work across functions and to create new processes. Change in itself is requiring us to change our practices. The other area that is still new for me is social networking. Facebook and Twitter have affected how our business operates internally and externally, and is changing the social interaction of our employees and with our customers. If you want to interact with people on Facebook, it can be in real time; people respond and make comments on your wall, and this is definitely starting to filter into our business! We will post a business problem and it can be debated and blogged using social networking technology. We will soon be trialling that technology with my performance management tool. Having developed a paper-based tool in the last 3 years, we will use some of the aspects of social networking to optimize performance management in our business. Social networking is changing how we engage, communicate and tell stories inside the organization.

One of my main challenges is that this organization is so fragmented. When I arrived it was unusual to find a coordinated strategy where people worked together on common issues. The same problem was being solved in different places but with differing levels of quality, and the organization didn't benefit as a result. That has been a challenge that we have addressed using cross-company collaboration (CCC). CCC is there to help us to change the organization, but I think other societal changes such as an increased legislative environment has played a major role. We have had to adhere to a wide range of social changes: BBBEE (Broad-Based Black Economic Empowerment); amendments to corporate law; the King Commission's third set of recommendations on corporate governance; the National Credit Act and Consumer Protection Act; changes to labour equity law – all of these changes have forced us to work together as one unit, instead of disparate companies within one group.

Willem de Jager: Leadership and Innovation for Social Projects

Willem de Jager is leadership and organizational culture specialist for Resolve Encounter Consulting, a leading consulting firm in South Africa. He completed his Ph.D. in executive leadership development from a systems psychodynamic stance in 2002 with the University of Johannesburg/Tavistock Institute. He has extensive experience in the design, development, consultation and facilitation of leadership development programmes for global and national organizations. He developed and implemented ABSA Bank's organization development consultation model, and played an instrumental role in the Barclays/ABSA high-performance leadership culture turnaround strategy.

Willem regularly leads cross-cultural executive and team-based coaching interventions, and currently manages the Resolve Group Executive Coaching and Mentoring Service Line; he has developed the largest coaching services panel in Africa, in which he project-leads major coaching and mentor development initiatives in South Africa. Willem has presented and published nationally and internationally on the topics of leadership development and group dynamics, and is a member of the Centre for Creative Leadership's international coaching panel.

At the moment I am senior coach consultant for the Resolve Group, which means that I develop proposals for coaching tenders and work on leads for business development in the executive coaching market. I lead the executive coaching service line branding for Resolve, coordinating our major executive coaching projects, project managing and supervising our executive coaches to ensure quality delivery and the achievement of organizational leadership development strategic aims. I custom-design executive and group or team coaching initiatives to ensure that executive coaching assignments are aligned with organizational talent management architecture, and retention and development strategies. We package executive coaching initiatives for wellness coaching, appointment of executives into new roles, performance coaching, alignment of leadership behaviours with organizational values, succession pool initiatives, and cross-cultural coaching for expatriates.

All coaching assignments are custom-designed to meet client organizations' leadership development aims as part of their overall talent management retention and development planning. Individual executive coaching initiatives are often supplemented with group or team coaching which we custom-design. All members of the Resolve coaching panel are required to be registered with COMENSA and the ICF to ensure continuous professional development, supervision and development towards classification as "master coaches". I also run an internship programme for young black qualified executive coaches to ensure that Resolve always have a well-represented and diversified panel from which clients can select their potential coaches.

I have been coaching (executive face-to-face, group or team coaching) for the past 15 years, and worked on many large-scale coaching contracts with teams of executive coaches, including continuous supervision of coaches on coaching assignments. This has helped me with my own personal mastery, to be more effective as a leader, stepping into my personal power and authority when I lead large coaching projects with multiple organizations at a time. My role is complex, as I deal with many different sectors and clients; this requires a certain personal autonomy and self-authorization from the coaches and organizational clients with whom I work. Coaching has also helped me to understand the covert human response, and organizational collective covert resistance, to change in leadership culture and transformational change initiatives. I have developed insight and skills as a result of my own coaching to work effectively with transformational change and oversee coaching initiatives towards high-performance leadership culture.

I see coaching as a leadership style and leadership culture in organizations. Whether you are a situational leader, change leader or high-performance leader, coaching is the next-generation leadership style. Adopting a leadership coaching style has helped me to lead an executive coaching panel of 110 executive coaches who coach on multiple projects at a time. I try to adopt a coaching style with all of my clients, particularly in large project interventions, to help my clients feel empowered. Part of the process is to be as collaborative as possible, empowering the coaches and clients with whom I work. The back office supports me with finance and administration, and I also follow a coaching style with them so that they can feel empowered in their work.

One of our greatest success stories is a coaching contract that we are delivering for the Leadership and Innovation Network for Collaboration (LINC) in the children's sector. Resolve developed a custom-designed executive coaching methodology to work collaboratively with multiple service providers in leadership development and systemic problem-solving, to address the South African crisis with orphaned and vulnerable children. Resolve's Executive Coaching for Fellows – carefully selected from government, NGOs, business donors and the private sector – was implemented during 2008. Today the total number of Fellows on this national project has reached 150. All Fellows receive executive coaching and are part of a group coaching initiative across the country, contributing to the development of innovations to make a difference to South Africa's orphaned and vulnerable children.

All Fellows who are part of this incredible journey take on multiple roles in their journey with LINC and the Department of Social Services, and have achieved numerous successes at the level of societal change.

- *Building community* – funding proposal for the development, testing and instutionalization of a model for 16–18-year olds to access a foster care grant, support a household, stay in the community, and access support and develop skills.
- *Building local government* – funding proposal to involve municipalities in improving community participation and becoming more sensitive to hearing children's voices.
- *Coordinating the children's sector* – funding proposal and mandate letter received to develop the cooperative governance structures which are responsible for children.
- *Department of Social Services Children's database* – database developed by the Department of Social Services to track maternal orphans (the database did not exist before).
- *Donors* – establishment of a national donor forum to increase collaboration between donors which has resulted in the publication of research results on the AIDS Buzz Website; successful donor dialogue meetings and a national donor forum are being created.
- *Education* – research and assessing the approach to increase parental and community involvement in the education of children that has reached crisis proportions in South Africa; the result is a proposal for funding to support proposed work.
- *Media* – research for a funding proposal for mass mobilization campaigns to increase the focus on children in need.

The second success story relates to executive coaching for Volkswagen South Africa (VWSA). Resolve developed a 360° feedback survey for leadership culture behaviours which was aligned to VWSA's company values. In 2009, all executives and senior leaders were assessed using the 360° VWSA leadership-alignment survey. Individual and divisional survey results were used in an executive coaching assignment (twelve 90-min sessions a month) to turn around leadership behaviour in alignment with company values. A significant development in leadership behaviours was reported in post-assessment results, and in the leadership development initiative through executive coaching. This programme is nominated as a global leadership best practice in the VW Group worldwide. As a result of the effectiveness of the Resolve executive coaching approach, VWSA has decided to continue with the coaching process during 2010 with a focus on team coaching at divisional level, to further embed leadership behaviours in alignment with company values.

My challenges, and what I have gained in the LINC project, are that what seemed to be an impossible task proved to be very successful. I think the other challenges we are normally faced with as providers of executive coaching interventions, stem from organizations splitting coaching contracts to make use of multiple service providers. The company's executive committee is often split from the rest of the organization in terms of its leadership development, and is often working with a different coaching provider to other levels of management. Working across the gap becomes challenging, particularly in regard to sustaining the very leadership behaviours that are required to transform as a result of coaching assignments. It is challenging for coaches to deliver high-quality and effective coaching interventions when the corporate system is neither transparent nor working collaboratively; it often maintains the "dysfunctionality" in the system.

Roger Maitland and Brett Anderson: Coaching for Wellness and HIV/AIDS Awareness

Roger Maitland is a founding member and director of LifeLab. He specializes in leadership coaching and organizational change, consulting to blue-chip corporations in South Africa and internationally. Roger lectures on the M.Phil. programme in coaching at the University of Stellenbosch Business School. He has a special interest in the development of transformational leadership practices that effectively address complex sustainable development issues.

Brett Anderson is also a founding member and director of LifeLab. His work focuses on enabling leaders and organizations to innovate by reframing change. He coaches and consults to facilitate performance enhancement, sustainable leadership and workplace wellness. He is a well-regarded international HIV/AIDS activist, and a UN fieldworker who provides strategic business insight with a creative edge.

Brett Anderson

My interest in human development arose from my own personal journey in discovering that I had HIV. In that first year, it was through the deeper learning about myself and what was made possible through the horrendous situation of being HIV-positive, that I became fascinated by human potential through tragedy – it took various courses. In terms of behaviour change: some people die, and some resist behaviour change; I determined to change direction. For my own personal journey, I became curious about how other people's tragedies held them back, and I used coaching to help others to go to that deeper place to review what needed to change. I love to learn by jumping right in, and finding out what takes people to their next level. As a coach and a change consultant, I am the catalyst to help people identify their way ahead. But I don't believe you have to go through tragedy to create change.

Having HIV/AIDS is what got me curious; and working in the field of coaching, I have had a number of mentors and coaches who have helped me to identify things I hadn't yet seen. Observing the techniques that these mentors and coaches used with me, I noticed a pattern and could see how I could help others. When Roger began his masters in Executive Coaching, it was a catalyst for me, going through it with him. What always stands out in our work today is not to get stuck in one methodology – every client presents a different issue and problem. They either need a spanner or a star screwdriver, and so I need tools to help the client achieve their goals. Having qualified as a counsellor early in my career, coaching is the next step in problem-solving; how can I help my clients to make their next decisions? Coaching has helped me and my clients – it has helped my clients to overcome obstacles when they discover they are HIV-positive. We ask, "What can we do?", rather than being defeated by the problem.

This led us at LifeLab to present a coaching methodology to VirginActive in South Africa to support people with manageable diseases and relationship issues. How could coaching help people to find solutions, like a traffic light, helping them to think through their options? How could coaching allow the client or the group to see more options than they presently see? We worked with VirginActive in 86 fitness clubs scattered across the country, and we trained up 86 internal coaches to work primarily with "wellness" and support issues in the workplace.

I believe there is a huge developmental need in South Africa, and I can see how coaching helps to broaden the possibilities, options and solutions – to solve some of the many problems we are seeing. My interest rose from my own personal one, but I would like to see more coaches play a bigger role, helping South Africans to overcome the many challenges we have. It's not that the challenges don't have solutions, it's that we need a different way of looking at the solutions, with LifeLab's work in coaching, and through the mentoring where I work at the Medical School at the University of Cape Town. This deeper process of self-reflection, identifying my risks and through mentoring helping others to open the door to a new way of seeing solutions – knowing that through tragedy brings new possibilities. That's the analogy I use in helping people to see and overcome their own personal obstacles. Rather than running away, I enjoy coaching to help them face it. The opportunities are endless because there are so many needs.

Roger Maitland

My work is in coaching, but I see it more broadly than that. For me, the core competence for coaching is to help organizations and individuals make transitions. That takes various forms, and what I enjoy is interacting within a range, from working in a rural town to working in a corporation, or with an individual leader going through substantial leadership change. What drew me to my work? I was studying towards being a psychologist and was frustrated in my career. I heard about coaching, experienced it as a client, and saw how powerful the coaching paradigm was. I had always wanted to be involved in making a positive contribution, so coaching was a good fit for me. My work has diversified, but it is always to do with change – practical change, and the quality of thinking around change.

From the beginning, I developed an understanding of the tacit knowledge around the process of change. I began to get a sense of the process of change, particularly going through it in a coaching relationship where I was supported. It helped me to have more self-insight, which makes it easier for me to withhold judgment. I think for me it has been coupled with therapy – two support structures have supported my process. It's interesting that both of those experiences have been quite different, and both have made a powerful contribution to my life. We get drawn into the helping professions, even if we consider that work in the corporate sector is commercial. Coaching has also helped me to accept my sexual orientation, and my personal crisis after coming out of the closet, as the internal battle took time to work through that internalized repression. Understanding those motivational roots and making them part of my value system, allowed me to separate my issues from the client, learning to use myself as the instrument of practice, although I don't get that right all the time! Coaching was an early influence in my career; it influenced how my practice developed, and is now integrated across the board in the way I work. The coaching and learning principles that support coaching have shaped how I design interventions for the client. Aside from delivering coaching for example in VirginActive, the need was around HIV training. What I have seen through many years of experience in this field is that standard training models don't lead to behaviour change. Coaching, however, can help to create support structures inside organizations, empowering people to have conversations and explore their own attitudes, behaviour patterns and the situations in which they find themselves and that inhibit them from helping themselves. When designing training programmes, even the way we design the daily sessions involves peer coaching to help people to make changes in their lives and their work. We use coaching in individual and group coaching interventions, moving towards creating a coaching culture, helping teams to work across boundaries or silos.

I would like to see people harness their strengths more, identifying and utilizing internal resources they hadn't noticed before. We did some work with an insurance company, within the legal services department of that company, where I was coaching several managers. One story stood out for me – the coachee was a man in his mid- to late-40s, a lawyer by training. He was working in a compliance function in that company, and was despondent as he had been trying for a promotion for over 5 years without success. He struggled to make decisions, and I had noticed very little progression; robust conversations did not create much movement. We decided to take him through the neuro-science inventory that I work with; it is related to Jung's model, with the key difference being that it can pick up falsification (Benziger). Essentially it looks at competence, and at an individual's lead strength in the brain.

This is found to be 100 times more efficient than the other regions of the brain. My client had studied law, but had barely graduated. He did not see himself in the court-room, and ended up in the compliance function in the corporate sector, which was the safety net of administration.

We picked up falsification; he had a frontal-right dominance (spatial creative thinking), and had wanted to be an architect (working in the opposite region of the brain!). With that framework, and building that into our coaching, we started to see the root cause of his difficulties. We began to see where his strengths were; essentially our competences might not be our core talents (i.e. dominance in the cerebral cortex). Sometimes, after many years of falsification, the competences and dominance can be difficult to distinguish; it just gives a guide to where his talents actually lie. I supported him through a coaching intervention, harvesting his strengths in a natural way. Preliminary data shows us that falsification rates may be higher in South Africa than in the rest of the world, and may be due to the post-apartheid context.

There's one other example that might be interesting about a woman of mixed race working in the financial information technology sector. We were engaged in a broad coaching intervention in the company at her level. In our coaching conversations, I noticed a pattern that she constantly spoke of feeling that her peers and subordinates did not accept the value of her work and her contribution. This was her perception, sometimes noticed in conflict situations, sometimes in other ways. At some point our coaching conversations began to deepen. She started to talk about her experiences as a student during her days at university. She came to the end of her studies and to the graduation. She had studied with a very small class, and some of those 30–40 people with whom she had studied for 4 years didn't even know her name; she felt invisible, and that she hadn't been valued as a person. Other, similar stories emerged from our coaching conversations, which highlighted her constant questioning of her own value, asking "Am I really good enough?" She struggled academically, but socially she really struggled, coming out of the strained race relations in apartheid South Africa.

This is the "internalized mediocrity" Paolo Freire refers to when people are marginalized – their voice becomes internalized, and it becomes an internal mechanism (which Ngũgĩ wa Thiong'o referred to in terms of the need for "decolonizing the mind"). As we named it, the internal work became so important – through the conversation we started to name it, and as that dynamic came into place, she started to see other elements of the conversation that she had been missing. She started to see that it was the opposite of what she believed to be true; she began to see (e.g. she was in a peer conflict with a white male, vying for the same position), and she was worried she would get the job just because she was black and female; she also thought he would get it because she wasn't valued. She began to see that people really valued her. What she was picking up was quite distorted. This is a positive psychology domain – the road to draw on those positive psychology tools is quite a process. Importantly, I wasn't doing therapy; we were trying to make progress using a coaching agenda. This led to delving in a practical way into these fundamental beliefs. It radically changed the way my client could operate socially in her business network and ultimately deliver results. She experienced a fundamental shift and growth in self-esteem.

Another story that pops out is due to doing quite a bit of work in continental Africa, and encountering the perception that South Africa is the "America of Africa". South Africans who work in the African continent tend to go in with an arrogance and an attitude of "knowing better" and adopting a rather autocratic way. In delivering services and starting up businesses, we South Africans have got ourselves a bit of a tarnished reputation. We had to overcome this in our coaching and training work, using our own vulnerability as coaches and facilitators to connect and build bridges. Through this, even in the town of Rundu, on the border between Angola and Namibia, on the battlefield where South Africa was occupying Namibia and invaded Angola during the mid-1970s and early 1980s, it is possible to make an even deeper and more real impact as a result of our history.

In coaching local business leaders in Africa, a similar dynamic existed where South African expatriates have sometimes treated locals very autocratically, as if they were "less than". We learned to name this dynamic, offering a mutual learning environment in which we act as partners, taking a coaching position, working respectfully within their values system and context, rather than in a neo-colonial fashion. And I think often the other element is trying to understand and locate the need for change, within the paradigm of a nation, trying to link or frame the way that the intervention is used by using local dynamics and local knowledge. In Namibia, where we were working with HIV, we used a training model in alignment with coaching conversations. We used the theme of their political independence and their struggle. We used visualization (taking delegates back to their feeling and memories of Independence Day) and coaching processes to harness the strengths they had learnt from the struggle, and used those to figure out how to fight HIV. It was inspired through our coaching practice, and provided an opportunity for them to harness Namibian solutions rather than us as South Africans providing the models, and in an emotive way – they danced to their own music. The quality of input that was referred to later on when we worked with them in smaller groups was that they figured out their own solutions, which was profound.

Marilyn Johnson: Coaching for Leadership and Community Awareness

Marilyn Johnson, an African-American born in Tennessee, has nearly 30 years of corporate experience contributing to the profitability of organizations through various procurement, operations and sales/marketing leadership roles. Her strategic and tactical know-how lends itself to the development and implementation of wide-scale organizational change initiatives while successfully managing to business objectives. Currently, Marilyn combines her functional expertise in an expatriate assignment as general manager – Africa, in Johannesburg, South Africa, for the US-based Cummins Inc., a $14 billion, Fortune 206 manufacturing company.

Whether growing a business utilizing innovative methods, enhancing operational efficiencies through a disciplined approach, or improving the communities in which she works via creative interventions, Marilyn demonstrates high-energy, tireless passion and a results-oriented focus. Marilyn received her Master of Business Administration from the University of Tennessee – Knoxville, and Bachelor of Science in biochemistry from Tennessee State University. She serves on the Board of the Center for Women's Health Research at Meharry Medical College, and is a member of Alpha Kappa Alpha Sorority, Inc., a public service organization.

Coaching has helped to keep me grounded; it allows me to step back and think strategically and in a focused manner to accomplish my goals. Specifically coaching has helped me get to the end game by giving me different perspectives on how to manage the business. But for me coaching is not just about work: it's about my overall being and ensuring positive results when making tough decisions. It allows me to look at things from a different viewpoint and stretches me mentally. Coaching is also a good networking opportunity; it broadens my capacity to reach further when making career decisions.

As the general manager of Africa for the Filtration Division of Cummins Inc., the scope of my work includes business development, leading and executing business strategy, analysing, measuring and tracking market sales potential, community social responsibility, and financial responsibility for the entire profit and loss of the business. My role also encompasses human relations – i.e. skills and leadership development through coaching. In South Africa it's about the transfer of skills.

Before coming to South Africa, my line manager convinced me that she recognized what she thought were natural abilities to become a general manager. The position has given me an opportunity to experience all facets of the business, from sales to finance, manufacturing, operations and logistics, as well as involvement with the key parameters, particularly human relations, that make Cummins Filtration a successful business.

The opportunity to work in Africa meant stepping into the role of an expatriate; living and working in a new country, and experiencing and learning a wide range of African cultures. This experience has given me the opportunity to contribute and to make a difference. I want to leave a legacy, so that the generations to come will benefit from some of the work that I and my team have contributed to the continent in my role as general manager. Some of the key corporate social responsibility initiatives that I have led, and consider rewarding for the organization and the local communities are as follows:

- Building a Habitat for Humanity home in Pietermaritzburg.
- Building the Masakhane crèche, a crèche for young children born to parents with HIV/AIDS.
- Awarding a significant contribution to the SOS Children's Village in Pietermaritzburg.
- Leading a committee to secure a Cummins Foundation grant of R4.3 million ($325,000) for the Ithemba Institute of Technology in Soweto (for high school

grades 10–12; learnerships and skills training programmes for unemployed youths and young adults and trade courses for adults in mechanics, computer science and welding).

During the past 7 years, Cummins has joined with other corporate partners to support Ithemba in developing skills that can be used within Cummins and other major Fortune 500 companies; this is part of the skills transfer.

I use coaching and mentoring with my direct reports. When I recognize my managers may be going off track, I step in to coach them back on track. I use different approaches, from one-on-one mentoring-type conversations to offer guidance, or exposing them to different views through team coaching. My intention is always to use coaching to help my staff become better managers and leaders. I also use coaching for goal setting, and to manage my expectations of them, helping them to think through processes through questions and discussion.

I even coach my customers! I believe the success of my customers depends upon the relationship they have with us at Cummins. In Africa, the business practices are quite different from those used in the United States. I've spent a lot of time transferring processes and skills to my customers e.g. providing marketing support and participating in joint marketing campaigns, making observations to help their business, engaging them in leadership development opportunities so that they can better develop their staff. We have hosted business/sales conferences that are phenomenal in educating customers, not only on our product line but also on sales techniques. Sharing best practices has helped customers develop their team. The positive results are shown through customer loyalty.

A great example is when we had to temporarily shut down one of our manufacturing plants in France. Our customers were challenged with poor delivery service, and had an opportunity to go to our competitors. Instead, they didn't leave us because of our strong relationship; they were confident that we would help them work through the challenges. Yes, we certainly had challenges in getting product to them. But, instead of relying on that particular plant, we looked at other sourcing avenues (e.g. China, India, Brazil and Australia) to get product to them so that they could deliver to their customers. In using a coaching style with them, we kept open the lines of communication, keeping them informed of events that were taking place. Good communication was the key in helping to manage our customers' anxieties.

As a result of my work, the differences that I would like to see are success in managing conflict and diversity issues. For example, because of persisting racial division, difference and conflict within the management team, I brought in a facilitator to work with the managers, and also brought the shopfloor employees and the managers together. I used team coaching to help them to understand each other as individuals. The result was to help them to understand each other, because they were simply working in silos. They discovered that "We've got something in common; I can talk to you, and you aren't going to bite my head off". It raised self-awareness, and now they are working together more as a team; managers are getting input from shopfloor people when decisions are to be made, and shopfloor employees are more willing to participate. They built self-esteem and grew their interpersonal skills – so coaching helped both the organization in terms of performance, and the individual from an interpersonal development point of view.

My greatest challenge when I first arrived in South Africa was the fear factor. I had a driver who also acted as my bodyguard when I first arrived, and he wouldn't allow me to go out alone. There were also certain places and events he would not allow me to attend. For example, I couldn't go to a soccer game unless I had box seats – from a safety standpoint he was very cautious, as his job was to protect this expatriate American. Eventually, my need for independence outweighed the fear factor. I purchased a global positioning satellite (GPS) navigation system, had my car windows shatter-proofed and relieved my driver/bodyguard of his duties. I have not had any problems, and am in control of my own destiny.

Another instance was when I imagined that someone had put *muti* (bad magic) on me. In my flat there was under-carpet heating. The heating element was underneath my bed, and during the night it had burned through the carpet leaving a burnt, melted spot. The next morning I woke up with ash on my bed from the flames, and I thought, "What is this? Who has come in and sprinkled *muti* in my room"? I was pretty scared and called the owner of the apartment that Saturday morning not knowing what was going on. Finally he looked underneath the bed and there it was, the burnt-out heating element . . . My fear factor had caused my imagination to work overtime!

It was coaching that helped me to overcome the fear factor. On first arriving in South Africa, a colleague came with me, stepping into the role of director of operations and logistics. He left when my line management changed. The biggest challenge when he left was to maintain stability in the operations facility and to achieve targets without having his support. I had to step in and take over the role myself. To cope, I promoted two of the individuals on-site to substitute for the one that my colleague previously held, and I started to work more closely with the plant. This was actually a major organizational change; I had altered the infrastructure, putting people into roles they weren't ready for. But I had no choice, as I could not get approval to recruit or hire any more people. I realized that I had to work very closely with them to get them to perform at an acceptable level. So we worked together, one-on-one, relying for extra support from our functional directors in the United States and Europe. To transfer skills I used on-line training and worked in a coaching style with each of my managers in bi-weekly meetings by phone and in monthly face-to-face meetings, giving each individual time to talk through their challenges. It also allowed me an opportunity to help them with their challenges by sharing past experience and best practices. This process yielded positive results as each manager stepped into their own ability to think and lead, working more closely with other managers. The organizational restructure has given them confidence in their own personal abilities, and is strengthening the relationship between them and me. And we have met our performance objectives.

Nonkqubela Maliza: Driving the Transformation Agenda

My work as director for corporate and government affairs for Volkswagen South Africa (VWSA) is to advance corporate objectives and priorities while enhancing and promoting relationships at all levels of government and in the community. I drive the transformation agenda, the Black Economic Empowerment (BEE) codes, company strategy and the transformation budget. I also drive the transformation agenda, and champion stakeholder engagement for corporate affairs and social investment. I was drawn to the company because I wanted to work for a multi-national firm that is an icon in its industry. VWSA is known to be the best at what it does, and I wanted to work with the best in the big league. It's very meaningful work as it's about transformation, which is of crucial importance to the nation and the company. I'm drawn to the work of corporate social investment as a contribution to development, and the transformation agenda serves national priorities and national objectives. It is about development rather than charity, is a strong way of contributing to development in communities that are underdeveloped. There is the potential to do meaningful work that can leave a positive change legacy and a development legacy.

My own coaching has helped me to do my job better, more effectively because it has created a supportive environment for me. I feel less alienated, and in my coach I've had a thinking partner to test ideas on. Coaching has helped me to feel more self-confident, and has helped me to be more competent in going about my work. I have tried to use coaching with my stakeholders and my team, as well as in my other roles chairing various boards and steering committees. I am drawn to creating a thinking environment, creating an empowering environment where people's thoughts and problem-solving skills are honoured and encouraged. This makes the teams more effective, and makes the work more joyful and qualitatively better. That people's minds are ignited, that is my goal.

My story is a mentoring story, and to simply encourage people to think for themselves. We are starting a mentoring programme in Midrand, and are about to set one up in the Eastern Cape, in our own plant. This is inspiring, as people feel they are making a personal contribution. I love the flyer, which said, "You give nothing when you give your possessions; when you give of yourself that is when you truly give". With mentoring you can make a difference to someone's life. If you impact one person in a family, they will impact the rest of the family, and that starts to make a difference in communities. There are a couple of challenges in the social development space. I manage VWSA's Community Trust; but you have to walk with the community – they must own the process so that they can drive it. I don't live in their community, they do. We need to get the community to own the projects so that they can drive them and lobby and help them to grow and grow and grow, and to get other benefits we might not have thought of. We constantly have to work with them.

One of the projects in Uitenhage is to build an early childhood centre, a preschool for very young children in that community. It is very exciting. Employees have been giving the equivalent of 1 h of their monthly wages for the project for the past 3 years. We are using these people's money for the project, which we call "One Hour for the Future". This is money they have contributed every month; they have a vested interest in the project and are supportive and proud of it. For this project we have partnered with local government, who gave us the land for free. We are setting up a world-class infrastructure, including environmentally friendly aspects such as solar power for heating and insulation, because in South Africa access to electricity is an issue. My learning is to work alongside the community and have them take an active part in the project.

Conclusion

I hope you have found food for thought in the achievements, concerns and insights of your colleagues working in the field of coaching today. It is still a radical thought to encourage people to think for themselves in organizations and institutions, and coaching is pioneering this "civil disobedience". The impact of coaching is far wider reaching than any of us have yet to realize, and as the field of coaching and practitioner research grows, we will begin to see the results of these "inspiring conversations" which just may begin to change the way we perceive and manage our world.

References

Kline, N. (1999/2004). *Time to think: Listening with the human mind*. London: Ward Lock.
Kline, N. (2005). *The thinking partnership® programme: Consultant's guide*. Wallingford, CT: Time to Think.
Kline, N. (2009). *More time to think*. London: Ward Lock.
Stout Rostron, S. (2009). *Business coaching international: Transforming individuals and organizations*. London: Karnac.

Chapter 15
Positive Psychotherapy and Social Change

Antonella Delle Fave and Giovanni A. Fava

Defining the Unknown: Mental Health in Clinical Psychology

The debate around health and well-being is increasingly expanding in our societies, among professionals, researchers, policy-makers, non-profit organizations, and political movements. This phenomenon reflects the relevance of this issue, at the same time shedding light on the ambiguities it endorses and the contradictory attitudes of society towards the conceptualization of mental health. We can identify at least three aspects of this debate that highlight these ambiguities and contradictions.

The first contradiction concerns the dichotomy between definition of mental health and clinical intervention. WHO (2004) defined mental health as "a state of well-being in which the individual realizes his or her own abilities, can cope with the normal stresses of life, can work productively and fruitfully, and is able to make a contribution to his or her community". This definition includes terms such as well-being, abilities, coping, work performance, and social contribution that are widely used in positive psychology research. However, in the same year the last version of DSM was published, in which clinical intervention was strictly confined within the pathology-focused model of disorders, symptoms, and their diagnostic classification. No reference can be found in it to resource development, personal growth, self-actualization, meaning-making, strengths and assets of the individuals.

The second ambiguity concerns the term "well-being". The WHO definition is substantially focused on individuals' performance, within a narrow Western pragmatist perspective. Well-being means doing, working, making. What about being? In this definition there is no trace of the mental health dimensions that research in the last 20 years had already identified among the basic fuel that feeds human action. The need for relatedness, positive emotions such as love and gratitude, identity building through the search for meaning, strengths such as spirituality, wisdom and equanimity find no place in WHO's definition.

A. Delle Fave (✉)
Università degli Studi di Milano, Milan, Italy
e-mail: Antonella.dellefave@unimi.it

R. Biswas-Diener (ed.), *Positive Psychology as Social Change*,
DOI 10.1007/978-90-481-9938-9_15, © Springer Science+Business Media B.V. 2011

Moreover, many terms in the WHO definition are discriminatory towards some categories of citizens. Can we really consider a person who is unable to work because of quadriplegia or multiple sclerosis as lacking mental health? Can we assume that a 90-year-old woman, living in a residential community and spending her time talking with the other guests, waiting for the visits of her beloved ones and writing her memoirs is affected by some kind of mental disorder? Do we consider a hermit who spends most of his time practicing meditation, rituals, and prayer as a mentally disturbed person? And – on the contrary – what about people with Down Syndrome, labelled as mentally retarded, who are fond of gardening, work productively and fruitfully, go to the movies with their friends, and devote their free time to a non-profit organization?

Seligman (2002) proposed a definition and operationalization of *positive mental health*, by taking into account the variables and dimensions addressed by positive psychology. Similarly, the crucial conceptualization of flourishing versus languishing developed by Keyes (2003, 2007) brought the difference between presence of mental health and absence of mental illness into focus. Maddux (2008) claimed the necessity to overcome the illness ideology, deeply rooted in the biomedical model, which is still dominant in clinical psychology. This process requires a systematic overhaul of the basic assumptions underlying classification of disorders and treatment models. The findings accumulated in the last decade by researchers and professionals in positive psychology suggest that this process is not only necessary, but that the instruments to start it are already available to the clinical community.

On the basis of the empirical evidence gathered through studies in positive psychology, in the following sections we will focus on some key issues to be included in a positive mental health model, moving from the premise that health and well-being can only be evaluated by assessing the dynamic interplay between individual and environment.

Building Positive Mental Health: The Bricks

A growing number of theoretical and empirical studies in positive psychology are shedding light on the dimensions that should be considered and evaluated in clinical intervention in order to promote positive mental health. We will briefly outline the major ones.

Opportunities and Constraints

The amazing increase in facilities, material goods, pharmacological treatments, and behavioural possibilities offered by the explosion of technology has instilled in citizens of the Western world the feeling that everything can be achieved. However, this is not true, and we have to accept that various aspects of our life, environment, health, and society cannot be modified. Therefore, in line with what Epictetus said 2,000 years ago, the pathway towards happiness includes ceasing to worry about the things we cannot change. This is a crucial point to be discussed with patients in the psychotherapy process, particularly when using a positive approach. Situational constraints can be related to any aspect of daily life. We will briefly exemplify some of them: the work and leisure settings; the health conditions; the experience of traumatic events.

In post-industrial countries the evolution of technology, the growing flexibility in work organization, and the demand for highly specialized job skills pose new challenges to the individuals as concerns job choices and work-related stress (Maslach, 1982; Maslach, Schaufeli, & Leiter, 2001; Rifkin, 1995). During the last two decades, however, theoretical and empirical studies have also explored the role of work in promoting well-being and life satisfaction (Danna & Griffin, 1999; Donaldson, Berger & Pezdek, 2006; Karasek & Theorell, 1990; Linley & Joseph, 2004; Schaufeli & Bakker, 2004; Sivanathan, Arnold, Turner, & Barling, 2004; Warr, 1999). In addition, changes in the workplace in Western countries have brought about an increasing amount of free time, and the enormous proliferation of leisure opportunities. The relationship between work and leisure is not homogeneous within a given society, but it depends on people's occupation (Parker, 1997). In particular, people involved in creative and autonomy-supporting jobs, such as artists, scientists, and specialized professionals, tend to extend their skill cultivation and level of satisfaction from work to the other areas of life. People enrolled in risky and damaging jobs compensate with leisure the frustrations and constraints of work. Finally, the great majority of today's workers, employed in neither particularly creative nor dangerous jobs, perceive work and leisure as two independent life domains, with no mutual influences (Parker, 1997).

Several studies show that active engagement in daily tasks can be used as an index of complexity and predictor of future goals and activity cultivation (Greene & Miller, 1996; Higgins & Trope, 1990). In particular, when daily activities are perceived as sources of rewarding and complex experiences, their selective cultivation provides the individual with increasingly higher challenges and skill refinement, fostering personal growth and development (Delle Fave, 2007). However, not all workers can enjoy creativity, autonomy, and engagement in their daily tasks, and work organization posits various constraints which are not always modifiable. For this reason, a more practicable way to foster complexity, self-expression, and well-being is the promotion of engagement in "serious leisure" activities (Stebbins, 1997), providing opportunities for personal growth and social awareness, and preserving an ethical dimension that has been obscured by consumer culture (1995). This strategy is also consistent with the previously described importance of finding a balance between the perceived quality of life in different domains.

Situational constraints are also experienced by people with chronic diseases and physical or mental disabilities. The disadvantages they face in daily life are not related to their biological impairments only, but also to the social attitude towards such limitations, as well as to material and organizational constraints (Delle Fave & Massimini, 2005a; Ingstad, 1999). Many people with disabilities perceive themselves as ordinary persons coping with extraordinary circumstances (Saravanan, Manigandam, Macaden, Tharion, & Bhattacharji, 2001). Supporting them in the process of adjustment to disease and to its consequences is a demanding task, and it has to be designed according to the bio-psycho-social aspects of the specific situation: psychological features, family and social support, material and economic resources, educational background, cultural representations, and social policies (Üstün et al., 2001). It thus behooves psychotherapists and, indeed, all health workers to be aware of *all* of these factors and to take them into account in their intervention, helping the patient distinguish between aspects that can be modified (within the person, but also in the environment) and aspects that have to be accepted as they are.

A similar approach has to be adopted in the case of traumatic events. It is impossible to deny or to modify their negative nature, as well as their dramatic consequences on the person's life. As suggested by Tedeschi and Calhoun (2004), the post-traumatic growth process after trauma should be viewed as originating from the elaboration and contextualization of the event in the individual's life and representation of reality.

Balance and Harmony Across Life Domains

In a recent theoretical paper, Sirgy and Wu (2009) have proposed to expand the threefold orientation to happiness model proposed by Seligman (2002), by adding to it the contribution of balance to well-being. They define balance as a state "reflecting satisfaction or fulfilment in several important domains with little or no negative affect in other domains" (p. 185). According to Sirgy and Wu, in order to satisfy the full spectrum of human survival and growth needs, people have to be involved and actively invest their attention and resources in multiple life domains. Balance contributes to subjective well-being because of the satisfaction limit that people can derive from a single domain. Different life domains tend to focus on different human developmental needs. Moreover, an excessive investment on one or few life domains can be detrimental to well-being in other domains. The person could feel unable to devote the desired amount of time and resources to them, thus experiencing negative feelings and dissatisfaction in these neglected domains. A typical example is the widespread problem of the over-investment of psychological and material resources in work, to the detriment of family or leisure activities (Haworth, 1997).

Data collected in seven Western countries by an international team (Delle Fave, Brdar, Freire, Vella-Brodrick, & Wissing, 2010) confirmed the importance of harmony/balance as a component of well-being. When asked to provide their own definition of happiness, participants often referred to the achievement of a balance between different needs, commitments, and aspirations, using the term "harmony" to describe this condition. However, this conceptualization of harmony does not primarily convey the interpersonal nuance often associated with it (Early, 1997; Ferriss, 2002; Ho & Chan, 2009; Morling & Fiske, 1999; Muñoz Sastre, 1998). It reflects more specifically the perception of inner peace, self-acceptance, and serenity; a condition of balance and evenness that was best formalized by philosophical traditions in Asian cultures. In the Chinese language, the term used for harmony includes such meanings as "gentle", "mild", "peace", "quiet in mind and peaceful in disposition". Yan Ying (fourth century BC, quoted by Chenyang, 2008) additionally defined harmony as mixing different things and balancing opposite elements into a whole, like in cooking and making music. From a different cultural and philosophical perspective, the Greek tradition provided similar definitions of harmony, as in the Stoics' ideal of evenness of judgment and detachment, in Plato's description of the just man – which relies on the balance between reason, spirit, and appetites – and in Epicure's concept of *ataraxia* – freedom from worries or anxiety through the ability of maintaining balance and serenity in both enjoyable and challenging times (Chenyang, 2008).

The importance of cross-domain balance clearly emerged in the WHO's definition of quality of life as a multi-componential construct (WHOQOL Group, 1994). The focus on individual's perception of different life domains allows for identifying areas of potential change or development, as well as domain-specific difficulties, resources, and strengths (WHOQOL Group, 2004).

Another study (Wu, 2009) investigated the relationship between life satisfaction and the tendency to shift the importance of life domains according to the perceived have – want discrepancy, more specifically by upgrading the domains with small have – want discrepancy. Shifting tendency resulted to be positively and significantly correlated with both global life satisfaction and average domain satisfaction.

These findings are consistent with other studies, highlighting the complex interplay between different life domains in contributing to the general QOL ratings. In particular, impairments or limitations in one domain do not significantly modify the general QOL level, which is relatively stable (Cummins, 2000). For example, no significant differences were detected in the QOL ratings between people with chronic diseases and healthy participants (Arnold et al., 2004). Adaptation, as well as the shifting tendency can contribute to this process.

The relationship between overall quality of life and well-being across life domains was also detected in a study conducted among four groups of immigrants in Italy, characterized by different country of origin, years of stay in the host country, legal immigrant status, SES, and acculturation pattern (Delle Fave, & Bassi, 2009). Participants were invited to report their daily opportunities for optimal experience – the engaging and rewarding state of deep concentration and absorption in the ongoing activity first described by Csikszentmihalyi (1975). Findings detected group differences according to the level of socio-cultural adjustment, identified with higher SES, lower cultural distance between the homeland and the hosting country, more qualified job, and availability of social and family network providing support (Ataca & Berry, 2002; Zlobina, Basabe, Paez, & Furnham, 2006). In particular, groups with better socio-cultural adjustment reported both an easier access to optimal experiences in daily life and a greater variety of associated activity domains.

Cultural Diversity

There is overwhelming evidence of major cross-cultural differences in the definition and evaluation of both well-being and psychopathology (Diener, Oishi, & Lucas, 2003; Massimini & Delle Fave, 2000; Marsella & Yamada, 2007; Park, Peterson, &

Seligman, 2006). This is not surprising: cultures shape individuals' behaviour and conception of what a good life is, both providing a meaning-making system for daily events and interactions and fostering or limiting opportunities for goal setting, personal growth, and self-expression (Ryan & Deci, 2001; Uchida, Norasakkunkit, & Kitayama, 2004).

Before or besides being individual constructs, meanings and goals derive from the cultural context and its value system (Smith, Christopher, Delle Fave, & Bhawuk, 2002). Cultural differences substantially concern the weight and the meaning attributed to collective norms, daily activities, and social roles (Massimini & Delle Fave, 2000; Triandis, 1994). For example, most human communities attribute importance to formal education. However, both the degree of relevance and the meaning of education can vary across cultures. Specific activities or behaviours do not necessarily have the same meaning or function in different cultures: therefore, we should not expect them to have an invariant relation to well-being or individual development (Deci & Ryan, 2000).

Until now, well-being research has been grounded in the Western tradition, with its individualistic features shared by a minority of nations (Triandis, 1995). However, all human cultures are concerned with well-being (Kiran Kumar, 2004; Oishi, 2000). A broader, less culture-bound interpretation frame could promote a better understanding of the cross-cultural variations in definition, operationalization, and evaluation of the related constructs. For instance, research showed that the higher levels of SWB reported by European Americans compared with Eastern Asians are clearly grounded in cultural expectations and conceptualizations (Kitayama, Markus, & Kyurokawa, 2000; Kitayama, Snibbe, Markus, & Suzuki, 2004; Rao, Paranjpe, & Dalal, 2008; Suh, 2000).

Following the seminal work about self-construal by Markus and Kitayama (1991), and on the basis of previous research (Miller, 1984; Shweder & Bourne, 1984), several studies showed that members of cultures promoting independence build mental representations of their surroundings through the identification of their specific components, focus on individual dispositions in evaluating events or behaviours, and attribute power and authority to the individual. In contrast, people belonging to cultures promoting interdependence tend to represent their environment holistically, evaluate behaviour according to situational factors and attribute power to the group. Members of independent cultures are more motivated by contexts allowing personal agency and autonomy, while members of interdependent cultures are more motivated by contexts allowing for collective agency (Hernandez & Iyengar, 2001; Menon, Morris, Chiu, & Hong, 1999; Peng & Nisbett, 1999; Shweder, 2003).

All these elements should be taken into account in the psychotherapy process. From the perspective of positive psychology, the promotion of well-being should comprise the cultural competence of the patients, which is their optimal functioning contextualized in their daily cultural environment (Leong & Wong, 2003). In non-Western cultures people with behavioural limitations derived from various disabilities and chronic pathological conditions are often more integrated in society. Together with social cohesion and low levels of individualism, lack of facilities and specialized institutions paradoxically facilitate their active participation in the community life (Agarwal, 1995; Brown et al., 1998; Tanaka-Matsumi, & Draguns, 1997). In multi-cultural societies, minority citizens often interact with at least two social environments in their daily life: the host culture and the local community and family network from their own culture. The fitness of a given strength or coping strategy to both contexts should not be taken for granted. The process of accultur- ation, which comprises socio-cultural adjustment (Ward, 2001; Ward & Kennedy, 1994) and psychological adaptation, can unfold through different patterns: assimila- tion, separation, integration, and marginalization (Berry, 1997). These four patterns represent different degrees of co-presence of elements of the two cultures in the behaviour, experience, value system, and world outlook of the person. It is impor- tant to explore which acculturation pattern is prominent in the person's life, in order to implement those resources which are actually needed in their social context. For example, MacLachan and Carr (1994) have highlighted that in some cultures attributing the cause of mental disorders to social or supernatural causes, rather than to biological ones, can facilitate the patient's acceptance within the native com- munity. At the same time, it is important to avoid prejudices, a priori attributing to the person from a different country culture-related stereotypical behaviours and representations of reality and of the therapeutic process. Besides empathy, which is a crucial component of the psychotherapeutic relation, openness and curiosity towards the client's expectations and acculturation pattern are essential dimensions of the therapists' attitude. They also represent basic prerequisites to build an effec- tive intervention and to broaden their human and professional knowledge of other ways to interpret reality and to pursue well-being.

Goals and Meanings

Considering the complex pathways through which individual development unfolds, we have to acknowledge that good life is not necessarily related to good feelings. As reported by scholars from different disciplines (Bruni & Porta, 2006; Peterson, Park, & Sweeney, 2008; Ryff & Keyes, 1995; Sen, 1992), people can commit themselves to the pursuit of goals that they perceive as valuable, but that can under- mine their quality of life in the short term. As suggested by several studies, the kind of goals individuals set and pursue sheds light on their level of perceived self-concordance and self-determination in goal orientation (Gong & Chang, 2007; Sheldon et al., 2004). In a set of cross-cultural studies investigating optimal expe- riences and their relationship with future goals, participants mostly stressed the intrinsic value over the immediate reward derived from their goals. Pursuing fulfil- ment in energy consuming and challenging jobs (Delle Fave & Massimini, 2003a); investing resources in parental care to promote children's well-being (Delle Fave & Massimini, 2004); cultivating psychological complexity through high-concentration and engaging activities like volunteering, prayer, and meditation (Coppa & Delle Fave, 2007) joined participants within the shared perspective of self-selected goals.

This perspective, however, can be referred to the overarching dimension of meaning-making (Emmons, 2005). Through meaning-making humans organize their experience moment by moment (Kegan, 1994), integrating events and information into their own life history and developmental trajectory (Singer, 2004). Moreover, meaning-making is a dynamic process: throughout their lives, individuals ceaselessly revise their experiences, attribute new meanings to them, expand or narrow their own meaning system. In periods of uncertainty or change and in the adjustment to stressful events, high levels of meaning-making can counterbalance low levels of subjective well-being (Park, 2005; Park & Folkman, 1997; Shmotkin, 2005; Shmotkin, Berkovich, & Cohen, 2006). A meaning-centred coping strategy promotes adjustment and well-being in stressful situations, such as chronic disease (Emmons, Colby, & Kaiser, 1998; Folkman & Greer, 2000). In Antonovsky's construct of Sense of Coherence (SOC; Antonovsky, 1987), the attribution of meaning to life is related to the capacity to establish a coherence among different sensorial stimuli, referring them to a unitary and shared shape, or Gestalt (Amrikhan & Greaves, 2003). Several studies have highlighted that meaningfulness supports SOC even in situations characterized by low controllability or manageability. For example, the high levels of SOC reported by people with degenerative diseases are related to meaningfulness, rather than to the objectively low potential for controllability of the situation (Flannery & Flannery, 1990).

Meanings primarily stem from culture, allowing individuals to transcend their own limited self towards a wider vision of reality. Faith and religion have been specifically investigated from this perspective (Koenig, McCullough, & Larson, 2001; Sperry & Shafranske, 2005). In their turn, individuals are connected to the cultural meaningful world through processes of internalization and externalization (Vaalsiner, 2007). Individual experience of the world "transforms collective-cultural meanings into a personal-cultural system of sense" (Vaalsiner, 2007, p. 62), which undergoes a personal reconstruction and can be externalized through behaviours, goals, and strivings.

To this purpose, a distinction should be made between the long-term meaning-making process and meaning of daily activities within this lifelong perspective. Studies conducted in Western countries showed that a great majority of people spend a relevant portion of their daily time in low-challenge, low-meaning activities. Besides maintenance tasks, that are anyway related to basic needs, this is the case of unstructured leisure activities, such as buying and consuming goods, watching TV, surfing in Internet, and idling (Iso-Ahola, 1997; Larson & Verma, 1999). The quality of experience people associate to these activities is prominently negative. Boredom and apathy prevail, as well as low levels of physical and mental health (Delle Fave & Massimini, 2005b; Iso-Ahola, 1997). Intervention should take into account this problem, which is one of the prerequisites to engage in deviant behaviours or in substance abuse (Delle Fave & Massimini, 2003b; Larson, 2000) and can be related to the more general condition of languishing (Keyes, 2007).

Finally, individuals can intentionally attribute meaning to activities that are not valued or approved by the cultural context. By the way, this phenomenon is not limited to criminals, people suffering of marginalization, or substance addicts. In this case, a conflict can arise between the individual's meaning-making process and social rules and norms. The consistency or discrepancy between meanings that the individual and the cultural environment attribute to a given activity or domain is a critical issue in psychotherapy, because it involves not only the developmental pathway of the patient, but also the ethical principles and responsibility of the therapist.

Agency and Responsibility

Agency represents a central construct within the framework of positive psychology. It has been conceptualized in various ways, but some of them are specifically relevant to positive intervention (Bassi, Sartori, & Delle Fave, 2010). According to Bandura's socio-cognitive theory, there is a deep connection between human agency and social structure (Bandura, 2001). Social systems are the products of human activity which organize, guide, and regulate human behaviour. The most distinctly human core property of agency is the metacognitive ability to reflect upon oneself and the adequacy of one's thoughts and actions. The sense of agency emerges from intentional behaviour and high self-efficacy beliefs (Bandura, 1997). Social cognitive theory distinguishes between three modes of agency: individual, proxy, and collective agency, which are strictly related in everyday functioning. Personal agency is exercised individually. However, in many spheres of functioning, people do not have direct control over conditions that affect their lives. They exercise socially mediated agency, or proxy agency, through their influence on others who have resources, knowledge, and act on their behalf. Finally, many of the things people look for are achievable only by working together through interdependent effort. In the exercise of collective agency, they pool their knowledge, skills, and resources, and act in concert to shape their future (Bandura, 2006).

From a motivational and developmental perspective, self-determination theory (Deci & Ryan, 2000) describes human agency as a process that refers to those motivated behaviours emanating from one's integrated self. To be agentic is to be self-determined, and thus to be autonomous. The prototype of autonomous activity, from which agency emerges as an integrated process, is the intrinsically motivated behaviour, which is performed out of interest and requires no separable consequence, no external or intrapsychic promises or threats. Intrinsic motivation entails curiosity, exploration, spontaneity, and interest. Intrinsically motivated behaviours are performed when individuals are free from demands and constraints, and when the context fosters volition and self-determination

The economist Amartya Sen (1992) highlighted the connection between agency, intentionality, and responsibility. The sense of agency represents the property according to which relevant and meaningful actions take into account the relation between the person, the social context, and other people's needs. This approach emphasizes the mobilization of resources, the development and implementation of abilities and skills, self-determined behaviour, the building of social competencies and interpersonal relations, the pursuit of aims and activities which are meaningful for the individual and the society. This also implies that people can actively and voluntarily commit themselves to activities, goals, or relations that are considered as important, but that do not necessarily lead to individual benefits and pleasure. Individuals can invest psychic and material resources into activities which are relevant for the community, sometimes sacrificing – totally or partially – their own personal functioning (free time, relaxation, material goods, comforts).

As concerns application to psychotherapy, the construct of agency has two implications. First, it is of paramount importance to promote patients' awareness and active participation in the process of change, in all its components: from adherence to treatments to the adoption of a healthier lifestyle (Gregor, Zvolensky, Leen-Feldner, Yartz, & Feldner, 2006; Kipling, Forgas, & Von Hippel, 2005), from the cultivation of skills and competences to the active understanding and reinterpretation of stressful events and of their psychological consequences. Second, if we exclude the most extreme conditions, the person always has a more or less wide range of alternative activities to be engaged in during her life. A process of active selection takes place at the psychological level, leading individuals to preferentially select and pursue in their daily life activities, interests, meanings and goals (Csikszentmihalyi & Massimini, 1985; Massimini & Delle Fave, 2000). However, the evolution trend supported by psychological selection does not necessarily lead to an improvement of behaviour and quality of life. The ultimate result depends upon the type of activities and goals individuals pursue in their life. Development means growing complexity: to bring positive effects, change has to promote internal order and integration of the individual, and at the same time constructive information exchange with the environment. The outcome of an authentic development at the psychological level includes high levels of both personal and social well-being (Keyes, 1998), the latter comprising social integration as well as commitment to the improvement of the culture and of the quality of life of the others. An example of agency and responsibility promotion is the activity of CBR centres (Community Based Rehabilitation centres), whose inspiring principle is that the sustainable development of a social system has to start from the efforts of the community members, from the local awareness of priorities and from intervention strategies coherent and well suited to the local cultural background (Atkinson, Rolim Medeiros, Lima Oliveira, & Dias de Almeida, 2000). CBR centres run intervention programs in the domains of employment, welfare distribution, health care and prevention, disability, and education. Their main resources are the competence and know-how of community members, their agency and responsibility, in terms of both personal involvement and financial support of the programs.

Individual and collective agency and responsibility can be mobilized in stressful situations. Quarantelli (1985) reported that community wide behavioural data, such as the number of psychiatric hospitalizations, drug use, and police reports decreased following a devastating tornado. One of the features of growth is its interpersonal dimension. "Growthful" interactions should be facilitated to promote well-being of individual and of their communities (Joseph & Linley, 2006). Further research should be conducted on this topic in the psychotherapy perspective.

Being Versus Doing

Lanza del Vasto, a writer, philosopher, and follower of Gandhi's movement for non-violence, made a distinction between living and functioning, underlying the superiority of the former (1944). Psychotherapists should carefully consider this issue, especially within the approach of positive psychology. The term *optimal functioning* is often used in this context. However, it is quite easy to use it interchangeably with "optimal doing". Western societies are obsessed with performance, productivity and efficiency. People are often overwhelmed by the kind of social pressures and expectations coming from work, family, and relationships. Rogers (1963), who first attempted to provide a systematic description of the fully functioning person, referred to qualities such as self-acceptance, awareness of one's strengths and weaknesses, experience of life as a process, perception of purpose and meaning in life, authenticity, openness to change, and trust in relationships and cooperation. Similarly, Maslow (1970) defined self-actualization as being what a person is able to be. In their pioneer cross-cultural classification of value orientations, Kluckhohn and Stroedbeck (1961) used the term "being in becoming", referring to the development and integration of personality. This emphasis on identity building is sometimes forgotten in psychotherapy. Patients are often focused on practical, domain-related problems, and they look for quick and effective solutions to modify the situation and remove the problem. However, as widely discussed in stress and coping research, the problem-centred coping is not always viable and valuable as a pathway towards well-being. Not all situations can be changed or controlled. Many events happen despite and beyond human intentionality and expectations. As concerns therapists, they are often focused on prescriptions, be they tablets or lists of exercises that the patients have to perform between sessions. This attitude entails a twofold problem: it adds burden to the patients' already overloaded lives, and it prevents from achieving the ultimate goal of the intervention. Echoing the Greek philosopher Epictetus, one should first decide what he/she wants to be, and then act consequently.

Eudaimonia and Hedonia

Issues such as the building of human strength in different psychotherapeutic strategies and the characteristics of subjective well-being have become increasingly important in psychological research (Diener, Suh, Lucas, & Smith, 1999; Gillham & Seligman, 1999). According to the eudaimonic perspective, well-being consists of fulfilling one's potential in a process of self-realization. Under this umbrella some clinical researchers described concepts such as fully functioning person, meaningfulness, self-actualization, and vitality. From a different perspective, the hedonic approach to well-being focuses on subjective happiness, experiencing positive emotions versus negative emotions, and satisfaction in various domains of life (Diener et al., 1999; Gillham & Seligman, 1999). These two approaches are quite different but they complement each other in the construction of optimal well-being (Ryan & Deci, 2001). However, in psychotherapy research the eudaimonic view has found much more feasibility because it concerns human potential and personal strength (Ryff & Singer, 1996). In particular, Ryff's model of psychological well-being, encompassing autonomy, personal growth, environmental mastery, purpose in life, positive relations and self-acceptance has been found to fit specific impairments of patients with affective disorders (Fava et al., 2001; Rafanelli et al., 2002; Rafanelli et al., 2000; Ruini et al., 2002). It was thus chosen as a theoretical underpinning for a novel psychotherapeutic strategy aimed at increasing eudaimonic well-being: Well-Bing Therapy (WBT) (Fava, 1999), that will be described in detail in the next section.

Building Positive Mental Health: The Cement

After this synthetic overview of the issues that are worth analysing in positive psychotherapy interventions, we now provide some hints on evaluation instruments and clinical protocols that can be fruitfully utilized besides the traditional ones. In the clinical work, well-established and validated quantitative instruments are available to therapists, especially for the purpose of diagnosis. Most of these tools are designed to evaluate pathological symptoms, and they can be used longitudinally for monitoring changes and evidencing benefits of the therapy. The positive approach to clinical intervention has brought to the attention of professionals a wide range of new instruments that provide information on well-being and development. Since for many positive psychology constructs we are still in the identification and definition phase of research, only few of these instruments have been presently standardized and are available for professionals' clinical use.

The most popular scales assessing well-being dimensions have been extensively used with non-clinical populations, and their potential as clinical resources has still to be verified. This is true of the Satisfaction with Life Scale (SWLS; Diener, Emmons, Larsen, & Griffin, 1985), scales assessing post-traumatic growth (Joseph & Linley, 2006), the Values in Action Inventory of Strengths (VIA-IS; Peterson & Seligman, 2004), scales assessing gratitude (Emmons & McCullough, 2003), meaning (Schlegel, Hicks, Arndt, & King, 2009; Steger, Frazier, Oishi, & Kaler, 2006), values and goals (Sheldon & Kasser, 2001). Nevertheless, their potential as diagnostic tools primarily consists in their effectiveness in revealing to both client and therapist resources upon which to build the foundations of a treatment strategy (Seligman & Peterson, 2003).

Other instruments can be useful in the clinical practice. Among scales, WHOQOL-100 – briefly referred to in the section about balance across life domains – provides details on the quality of life perceived in the daily activities and contexts. A short form is also available, the WHOQOL-Bref (Skevington, Lofty, & O'connell, 2004). Findings obtained from large cross-cultural samples showed that perceived quality of life is a good predictor of future health outcomes, such as relapses and survival rates, without the need to adopt objective measures (Idler & Benyamini, 1997; Ried, Tueth, Handberg, & Nyanteh, 2006).

The Symptom Questionnaire (SQ) (Kellner, 1987) is as self-rating scale for assessing distress (anxiety, depression, somatic symptoms, and hostility) and well-being (relaxation, contentment, physical well-being, and friendliness). It has extensively been used in clinical studies, including psychotherapy research and drug trials. Well-being scales have frequently been found to be more sensitive in detecting differences between experimental and control conditions (Kellner, 1987).

Positive psychotherapy can also derive useful information from several qualitative instruments designed for research and intervention. For example, written narratives of external and inner events and emotions have proved to be beneficial for mental and physical health (Morrow & Nolen-Hoeksema, 1990; Niederhoffer & Pennebaker, 2002; Pennebaker, 1997; Stanton et al., 2000).

Finally, experience sampling procedures can be an effective tool for evaluating the course of treatment. For example, the experience sampling method (ESM; Csikszentmihalyi & Larson, 1987; Hektner, Schmidt, & Csikszentmihalyi, 2007) provides glimpses into the real life and habits of individuals thanks to the on-line repeated self-reports that people fill out during 1-week session, describing their behaviour and experience in the daily context. This information is otherwise difficult to detect through single administration instruments and during therapy sessions. In the ESM participants directly describe themselves while interacting with their environment, be it social, material, or natural. They report their experience during activities ranging from biologically driven behaviours, such as eating and resting, to more complex and culture-related tasks, such as solving a mathematical problem, reading a book, driving a car, and watching TV.

ESM can document the daily patterns of clinical change and the behavioural and experiential features of these changes (Hektner et al., 2007). In particular, studies were conducted on the transition process of long-time heroin addicts who were adjusting to life in a residential community treatment centre (Ravenna, Hölzl, Kirchler, Palmonari, & Costarelli, 2002), and on craving during methadone therapy (deVos, Van Wilgenburg, Van den Brink, Kaplan, & DeVries, 1996). Depressed individuals were followed to assess the effects of pharmacotherapy on daily mood fluctuation and behaviour (Barge-Schaapveld & Nicolson, 2002). ESM was also used in a comparative study to evaluate the treatment of panic disorders through CBT therapy based on traditional clinical sessions conducted by a therapist, and through a computer-assisted therapy partially replacing the sessions (Newman, Kenardy, Herman, & Taylor, 1997). Norton and colleagues (2003) explored with ESM the daily life of their bulimic patients. In a case study of a woman with panic disorder and agoraphobia, Delle Fave and Massimini (1992) integrated the use of ESM into ongoing psychotherapy.

However, the only instrument which presently has a clear and thoroughly tested clinical use is Ryff's Psychological Well-Being Scales. They are used within a specific psychotherapy for enhancing well-being (Well-Being Therapy, WBT) developed by Fava (1999) and tested in controlled trials, both alone (e.g. Fava, Rafanelli, Cazzaro, Conti, & Grandi, 1998a) and in addition to CBT (e.g. Fava et al., 2004, 2005). Well-Being Therapy is based on Ryff's (1989) six dimensions of psychological well-being (PWB). The final goal of the therapist is to lead the patient from an impaired level to an optimal level in the six dimensions of psychological well-being (Fava, 1999; Fava & Ruini, 2003).

Well-Being Therapy and Its Applications

WBT is a short-term treatment designed to extend over 8–12 sessions, which may take place every week or every other week. The duration of each session may range from 30 to 50 min. WBT emphasizes self-observation (Emmelkamp, 1974), with the use of a structured diary. It is directive, oriented on current problems which hinder sustained psychological well-being, and is based on an educational model (Fava, 1999; Fava & Ruini, 2003). It is structured so that early treatment emphasizes developing skills and capacity to sustain attention to aspects of daily experience/emotions that are positive, and subsequent sessions emphasize the promotion of psychological well-being.

WBT has been employed in several clinical studies. Other studies are currently in progress. In some cases WBT has been used alone. In other cases, it has been added to cognitive therapy using a sequential combination (first psychotherapy addressed the abatement psychological distress and subsequently the promotion of well-being). In some other cases it has been added to pharmacotherapy or behavioural treatment based on exposure. The effectiveness of well-being therapy has been tested through controlled investigation in a wide range of disorders. First of all, WBT proved to be effective in reducing the residual symptoms of affective disorders in the long term, similarly to CBT (Fava et al., 1998a). However, the comparison of two groups of patients randomly assigned to either a well-being therapy or cognitive behavioural treatment of residual symptoms showed a significant advantage of well-being therapy over cognitive behavioural strategies immediately after treatment. Well-being therapy was associated also with a significant increase in PWB, particularly in the Personal Growth scale. The small number of subjects suggested caution in interpreting this difference and the need for further studies with larger samples of patients with specific affective disorders. However, these preliminary results pointed to the feasibility of well-being therapy in the residual stage of affective disorders.

WBT was also used for the treatment of generalized anxiety disorder (GAD) (Fava et al., 2005). Significant advantages of the WBT-CBT sequential combination over CBT were observed, both in terms of symptom reduction and psychological well-being improvement. These results suggested the feasibility and clinical advantages of adding WBT to the treatment of GAD. A possible explanation for these findings is that self-monitoring of episodes of well-being may lead to a more comprehensive identification of automatic thoughts than that entailed by the customary monitoring of episodes of distress in cognitive therapy (Beck & Emery, 1985), and may thus result in a more effective cognitive restructuring. These results lend support to a sequential use of treatment components for achieving a more sustained recovery. The clinical description of a young patient with GAD, who successfully underwent this sequential treatment (CBT/WBT), has been recently published (Ruini & Fava, 2009).

A cognitive behavioural package including WBT, cognitive behavioural treatment of residual symptoms, and lifestyle modification was applied to recurrent depression and its effects were compared to classical CBT treatment (Fava, Rafanelli, Grandi, Conti, & Belluardo, 1998b). The combination of CBT and WBT produced a significantly lower level of residual symptoms after drug discontinuation, a significantly lower relapse rate at a 2-year and 6-year follow-up (Fava et al., 2004).

WBT's effectiveness was also tested in the attempt to identify strategies to improve medication effects during maintenance antidepressant treatment. The return of depressive symptoms during these treatments is a common and vexing clinical phenomenon (Baldessarini, Ghaemi, & Viguera, 2002; Bockting et al., 2008; Papakostas, Perlis, Seifert & Fava, 2007), and the efficacy of pharmacological strategies has proven limited (Schmidt, Fava, Zhang, Gonzales, Raute, & Judge, 2002, Chouinard & Chouinard, 2008). To examine whether an intervention that included well-being therapy might improve maintenance of medication effects, a strategy based on dose increase was compared with a sequential combination of cognitive-behaviour and well-being therapy with continuation of antidepressant drugs at the same dosage (Fava, Ruini, Rafanelli, & Grandi, 2002). All the patients treated only with antidepressants relapsed by 1-year follow-up while only one of the patients treated with psychotherapy did. The specific contribution of WBT, however, cannot be discerned from this type of study. Tolerance to antidepressant treatment has been associated with activation of the hypothalamic-pituitary-adrenal (HPA) axis (Fava, 2003). In a single case report, well-being therapy induced a normalization of the HPA axis (Sonino & Fava, 2003). It is thus conceivable that well-being therapy may, through this mechanism, restore and maintain remission with antidepressant drugs when response fails or is about to fail.

WBT could also be used in the treatment of post-traumatic stress disorder (Cottraux et al., 2008; Schnyder, 2005; Van Emmerik, Kamphuis, & Emmelkamp, 2008). Two cases were reported (Belaise, Fava, & Marks, 2005) in which patients improved, even though their central trauma was discussed only in the initial history-taking session. The findings from these two cases should of course be interpreted with caution (the patients may have remitted spontaneously), but are of interest because they indicate an alternative route to overcoming trauma and developing resilience. A randomized controlled trial is now in order.

Finally, WBT has been recently modified to be applied with children and adolescents, both in clinical and educative settings. These are pilot experiences which require confirmation with further research; however, their results are very promising. WBT school interventions were performed both in middle (Ruini, Belaise, Brombin, Caffo, & Fava, 2006; Tomba et al., 2010) and high schools (Ruini et al., 2009) demonstrating a significant effectiveness in promoting psychological well-being – particularly personal growth – compared to an attention placebo condition. WBT school interventions were found to be effective also in decreasing distress – particularly anxiety and somatization – and this effect persisted at 1-year follow-up. Other studies investigated WBT effects in reducing symptoms and in improving skills and competencies in children with mood, anxiety, and conduct disorders (Albieri, Visani, Offidani, Ottolini, & Ruini, 2009). Child WBT was associated in all patients with a decrease in symptomatology (particularly anxiety and somatization) and an improvement in psychological well-being (particularly autonomy and interpersonal functioning). In two of our four patients, WBT was associated also with improvements in school performance (Caffo, Belaise, & Forresi, 2008). These results are promising but further research with controlled design is needed.

To summarize, WBT has been originally developed as a strategy for promoting psychological well-being which was still impaired after standard pharmacological or psychotherapeutic treatments. It was based on the assumption that these impairments may vary from one illness to another, from patient to patient, and even from episode to another of the same illness in the same patient. This individualized approach characterizes the treatment protocol which requires careful self-monitoring before any cognitive restructuring takes place. As a result WBT may be used to address specific areas of concern in the course of treatment, in sequential combination with other approaches of pharmacological and psychological nature. The model is realistic, instead of idealistic, but more in line with the emerging evidence on the unsatisfactory degree of remission that one course of treatment entails and need of addressing several areas of concern in the treatment of patients with mood and anxiety disorders (Fava, Tomba, & Grandi, 2007). It is quite difficult to apply WBT in an acutely ill patient (e.g. in a major depressive episode), since the amount of negative thoughts may be at that stage overwhelming. WBT appears to be more suitable for addressing psychological issues that other therapies have left unexplored. However, these conclusions are, at present, tentative and may be modified by further studies and clinical experience. In the same vein, most studies have involved clinical individual WBT. Group format WBT has been applied only in educational settings. However, it is conceivable that the group format may be a future line of development of this strategy.

Building Positive Mental Health: Carpenters and End Users

Any process of change and growth, in the physical and in the psychological domains, requires the alliance between the two main characters: the therapist and the client. Rogers (1967) considered crucial for alliance promotion three components of the therapist's attitude: empathy, coherence, and unconditioned openness towards the client. More recently, research focused on additional cognitive dimensions, such as the shared definition of treatment goals, and client's perception of the relevance and adequacy of the proposed therapeutic pathway (Roth & Fonagy, 1996). The achievement of a strong alliance is even more important for a positive health psychology treatment, because of its innovative aspects. In particular, the expectations of the patients can be apparently frustrated by the therapist's attention to strengths rather than problems, to patient's blessings and responsibility rather than to stressors and victimization. A major challenge for the positive therapist is to balance the emphasis on resources with the acknowledgement of negative aspects. This balance can differ according to client's attitude, request, objective condition, and social support. A thorough exploration of the alliance building in positive psychotherapy is a priority for future research.

In spite of the cautions and open issues described in the previous pages, the spreading of positive therapy can have a tremendous impact on society. Instead of providing people with relief from symptoms, therapists will be able to offer support to growth and thriving through the exercise of personal agency, competences, and commitment (Duckworth, Steen, & Seligman, 2005). Such a change of perspective can mobilize resources at various levels: not only the clients would benefit from it, but also their families and their community. Supporting individuals in becoming aware of their strengths, in developing a more optimistic attributional style, in pursuing meaningful goals, personal growth, and self-expression can contribute to enhance their active participation in society. As shown in several studies, flourishing people are usually friendlier, more optimistic, more effective in work, more concerned with others' well-being, more sensitive to social issues (Keyes, 2007). Making people flourishing through positive psychology-based intervention is a valuable instrument to increase the well-being of communities.

Like in any psychotherapeutic process, clients in positive theraphy settings can learn about the mind, cognitive processes, and emotional regulation. They can become aware of their own cognitions, and they may begin to appreciate the interplay between perceptions, interpretations, evaluations, attributions, expectations, and emotions (Overholser, 2004). They can move from thinking about strategies for developing positive emotions or overcoming negative thoughts to experiencing them through mindfulness and awareness (Teasdale, 1999). When these intrinsic assets of the therapy process additionally involve the ability to experience growth, agency, self-efficacy, resilience, and meaning, individual development becomes the unfolding of the true human nature, as Aristotle meant when he defined eudaimonia.

References

Agarwal, A. (1995). Mass-media and health promotion in Indian villages. *Psychology and Developing Societies, 7*, 217–236.

Albieri, E., Visani, D., Offidani, E., Ottolini, F., & Ruini, C. (2009). Well-being therapy in children with emotional and behavioral disturbances: A pilot investigation. *Psychotherapy and Psychosomatics, 78*, 387–390.

Amrikhan, J. H., & Greaves, H. (2003). Sense of coherence and stress: The mechanics of a healthy disposition. *Psychology and Health, 18*, 31–62.

Antonovsky, A. (1987). *Unraveling the mystery of health: How people manage stress and stay well*. San Francisco: Jossey Bass.

Arnold, R., Ranchor, A., Sanderman, R., Kempen, G. I. J. M., Ormel, J., & Suurmeijer, T. P. B. M. (2004). The relative contribution of domains of quality of life to overall quality of life for different chronic diseases. *Quality of Life Research, 13*, 883–896.

Ataca, B., & Berry, J. W. (2002). Psychological, sociocultural and marital adaptation of Turkish immigrant couples in Canada. *International Journal of Psychology, 37*, 13–26.

Atkinson, S., Rolim Medeiros, R. L., Lima Oliveira, P. H., & Dias de Almeida, R. (2000). Going down to the local: Incorporating social organisation and political culture into assessments of decentralised health care. *Social Science and Medicine, 51*, 619–636.

Baldessarini, R. J., Ghaemi, S. N., & Viguera, A. C. (2002). Tolerance in antidepressant treatment. *Psychotherapy and Psychosomatics, 71*, 177–179.

Bandura, A. (1997). *Self-efficacy: The exercise of control*. New York: Freeman.

Bandura, A. (2001). Social cognitive theory: An agentic perspective. *Annual Review of Psychology, 52*, 1–26.

Bandura, A. (2006). Toward a psychology of human agency. *Perspectives in Psychological Science*, *1*, 164–180.

Barge-Schaapveld, D. Q., & Nicolson, N. A. (2002). Effects of antidepressant treatment on the quality of daily life: An experience sampling study. *Journal of Clinical Psychiatry*, *63*, 477–485.

Bassi, M., Sartori, R. D. G., & Delle Fave, A. (2010). The monitoring of experience and agency in daily life: A study with Italian adolescents. In M. Balconi (Ed.), *The neuropsychology of agency* (pp. 81–106). Milano: Springer Verlag Italia.

Beck, A. T., & Emery, G. (1985). *Anxiety disorder and Phobia*. New York: Basic Book.

Belaise, C., Fava, G. A., & Marks, I. M. (2005). Alternatives to debriefing and modifications to cognitive behavior therapy for posttraumatic stress disorder. *Psychotherapy and Psychosomatics*, *74*, 212–217.

Berry, J. W. (1997). Immigration, acculturation and adaptation. *Applied Psychology: An International Review*, *46*, 5–34.

Bockting, C. L. H., ten Doesschate, M. C., Spijker, J., Spinhoven, P., Koeter, M. W. J., & Schene, A. H., & the Delta Study Group. (2008). Continuation and maintenance use of antidepressants in recurrent depression. *Psychotherapy and Psychosomatics*, *77*, 17–26.

Brown, A. S., Varma, V. K., Malhotra, S., Jiloha, R. C., Conover, S. A., & Susser, E. S. (1998). Course of acute affective disorders in a developing country setting. *Journal of Nervous and Mental Disease*, *186*, 207–213.

Bruni, L., & Porta, P. L. (Eds.). (2006). *Economics and happiness: Framing the analysis*. Oxford: Oxford University Press.

Caffo, E., Belaise, C., & Forresi, B. (2008). Promotiong resilience and psychological well-being in vulnerable life stages. *Psychotherapy and Psychosomatics*, *77*, 331–336.

Chenyang, L. (2008). The ideal of harmony in ancient Chinese and Greek philosophy. *Dao*, *7*, 81–98.

Chouinard, G., & Chouinard, V. (2008). Atypical antipsychotics. *Psychotherapy and Psychosomatics*, *77*, 69–77.

Coppa, R., & Delle Fave, A. (2007). Religione ed esperienza ottimale: Una prospettiva eudaimonica. In A. Delle Fave (Ed.), *La condivisione del benessere. Il contributo della psicologia positiva* (pp. 77–98). Milano: Franco Angeli.

Cottraux, J., Note, I., Yao, S. H., de Meg-Guillard, C., Bonasse, F., Djamoussian, D., et al. (2008). Randomized controlled comparison of cognitive behavior therapy with Rogerian supportive therapy in chronic post-traumatic stress disorder. *Psychotherapy and Psychosomatics*, *77*, 101–110.

Csikszentmihalyi, M. (1975). *Beyond boredom and anxiety*. San Francisco: Jossey Bass.

Csikszentmihalyi, M., & Larson, R. W. (1987). Validity and reliability of the experience sampling method. *Journal of Nervous and Mental Disease*, *175*, 526–536.

Csikszentmihalyi, M., & Massimini, F. (1985). On the psychological selection of bio-cultural information. *New Ideas in Psychology*, *3*, 115–138.

Cummins, R. A. (2000). Objective and subjective quality of life: An interactive model. *Social Indicators Research*, *52*, 55–72.

Danna, K., & Griffin, R. (1999). Health and well-being the workplace: A review and synthesis of the literature. *Journal of management*, *25*, 357–384.

Deci, E. L., & Ryan, R. M. (2000). The "what" and "why" of goal pursuits: Human needs and the self-determination of behavior. *Psychological Inquiry*, *11*, 227–268.

Delle Fave, A. (2007). Individual development and community empowerment: Suggestions from studies on optimal experience. In J. Haworth & G. Hart (Eds.), *Well-being: Individual, community, and societal perspectives* (pp. 41–56). London: Palgrave McMillan.

Delle Fave, A., & Bassi, M. (2009). Sharing optimal experiences and promoting good community life in a multicultural society. *Journal of Positive Psychology*, *4*, 280–289.

Delle Fave, A., Brdar, I., Freire, T., Vella-Brodrick, D., & Wissing, M. P. (2010). The eudaimonic and hedonic components of happiness: Qualitative and quantitative findings. *Social Indicators Research*. DOI 10.1007/s11205-010-9632-5.

Delle Fave, A., & Massimini, F. (1992). Experience sampling method and the measurement of clinical change: A case of anxiety disorder. In M. W. deVries (Ed.), *The experience of psychopathology* (pp. 280–289). New York: Cambridge University Press.

Delle Fave, A., & Massimini, F. (2003a). Optimal experience in work and leisure among teachers and physicians: Individual and bio-cultural implications. *Leisure Studies, 22,* 323–342.

Delle Fave, A., & Massimini, F. (2003b). Drug addiction: The paradox of mimetic optimal experience. In J. Henry (Ed.), *European positive psychology proceedings* (pp. 31–38). Leicester, UK: British Psychological Society.

Delle Fave, A., & Massimini, F. (2004). Parenthood and the quality of experience in daily life: A longitudinal study. *Social Indicators Research, 67,* 75–106.

Delle Fave, A., & Massimini, F. (2005a). The relevance of subjective wellbeing to social policies: Optimal experience and tailored intervention. In F. Huppert, B. Keverne, & N. Baylis (Eds.), *The science of wellbeing* (pp. 379–404). Oxford: Oxford University Press.

Delle Fave, A., & Massimini, F. (2005b). The investigation of optimal experience and apathy: Developmental and psychosocial implications. *European Psychologist, 10,* 264–274.

del Vasto, L. (1944/1984). *Principi e precetti del ritorno all'evidenza.* Torino: Gribaudi.

deVos, J. W., Van Wilgenburg, H., Van den Brink, W., Kaplan, C. D., & DeVries, M. W. (1996). Patterns of craving and pharmacokinetics in long-term opiate addicts in methadone maintenance therapy. *Addiction Research, 3,* 285–295.

Diener, E., Emmons, R., Larsen, R. J., & Griffin, S. (1985). *The satisfaction with life scale. Journal of Personality Assessment, 49*(1), 71–75.

Diener, E., Oishi, S., & Lucas, R. (2003). Personality, culture, and subjective well-being: Emotional and cognitive evaluations of life. *Annual Review of Psychology, 54,* 403–425.

Diener, E., Suh, E. M., Lucas, R. E., & Smith, H. L. (1999). Subjective well-being: Three decades of progress. *Psychological Bulletin, 125,* 276–302.

Donaldson, S., Berger, D., & Pezdek, K. (2006). *Applied psychology: New frontiers and rewarding careers.* Mahwah, NJ: Erlbaum.

Duckworth, A. L., Steen, T. A., & Seligman, M. E. P. (2005). Positive psychology in clinical practice. *Annual Review of Clinical Psychology, 1,* 629–651.

Early, P. C. (1997). *Face, harmony and social structure: An analysis of organizational behaviour across cultures.* New York: Oxford University Press.

Emmelkamp, P. M. G. (1974). Self-observation versus flooding in the treatment of agoraphobia. *Behaviour Research and Therapy, 12,* 229–237.

Emmons, R. A. (2005). Striving for the sacred: Personal goals, life meaning, and religion. *Journal of Social Issues, 61,* 731–745.

Emmons, R. A., Colby, P. M., & Kaiser, H. A. (1998). When losses lead to gains: Personal goals and the recovery of meaning. In P. T. P. Wong & P. S. Fry (Eds.), *The human quest for meaning* (pp. 163–178). Mahwah, NJ: Erlbaum.

Emmons, R. A., & McCullough, M. E. (2003). Counting blessings versus burdens: An experimental investigation of gratitude and subjective well-being in daily life. *Journal of Personality and Social Psychology, 84,* 377–389.

Fava, G. A. (1999). Well-being therapy. *Psychotherapy and Psychosomatics, 68,* 171–178.

Fava, G. A. (2003). Can long-term treatment with antidepressant drugs worsen the course of depression? *Journal of Clinical Psychiatry, 64,* 123–133.

Fava, G. A., Rafanelli, C., Cazzaro, M., Conti, S., & Grandi, S. (1998a). Well-being therapy. A novel psychotherapeutic approach for residual symptoms of affective disorders. *Psychological Medicine, 28,* 475–480.

Fava, G. A., Rafanelli, C., Grandi, S., Conti, S., & Belluardo, P. (1998b). Prevention of recurrent depression with cognitive behavioral therapy. *Archives of General Psychiatry, 55,* 816–820.

Fava, G. A., Rafanelli, C., Ottolini, F., Ruini, C., Cazzaro, M., & Grandi, S. (2001). Psychological well-being and residual symptoms in remitted patients with panic disorder and agoraphobia. *Journal of Affective Disorders, 31,* 899–905.

Fava, G. A., & Ruini, C. (2003). Development and characteristics of a well-being enhancing psychotherapeutic strategy: Well-being therapy. *Journal of Behavior Therapy and Experimental Psychiatry, 34,* 45–63.

Fava, G. A., Ruini, C., Rafanelli, C., Finos, L., Conti, S., & Grandi, S. (2004). Six year outcome of cognitive behavior therapy for prevention of recurrent depression. *American Journal of Psychiatry, 161,* 1872–1876.

Fava, G. A., Ruini, C., Rafanelli, C., Finos, L., Salmaso, L., Mangelli, L., et al. (2005). Well-being therapy of generalized anxiety disorder. *Psychotherapy and Psychosomatics, 74,* 26–30.

Fava, G. A., Ruini, C., Rafanelli, C., & Grandi, S. (2002). Cognitive behavior approach to loss of clinical effect during long-term antidepressant treatment. *American Journal of Psychiatry, 159,* 2094–2095.

Fava, G. A., Tomba, E., & Grandi, S. (2007). The road to recovery from depression. *Psychotherapy and Psychosomatics, 76,* 260–265.

Ferriss, A. L. (2002). Does material well-being affect non-material well-being? *Social Indicators Research, 60,* 275–280.

Flannery, R. B., & Flannery, G. J. (1990). Sense of coherence, life stress, and psychological distress: A longitudinal study of intervening variables. *Social Science and Medicine, 25,* 173–178.

Folkman, S., & Greer, S. (2000). Promoting psychological well-being in the face of serious illness: When theory, research and practice inform each other. *Psycho-Oncology, 9,* 11–19.

Gillham, J. E., & Seligman, M. E. P. (1999). Footstep on the road to a positive psychology. *Behaviour Research and Therapy, 37,* 5163–5173.

Gong, Y., & Chang, S. (2007). The relationships of cross-cultural adjustment with dispositional learning orientation and goal setting. *Journal of Cross-Cultural Psychology, 38,* 19–25.

Greene, B. A., & Miller, R. B. (1996). Influences on achievement: Goals, perceived ability, and cognitive engagement. *Contemporary Educational Psychology, 21,* 181–192.

Gregor, K., Zvolensky, M., Leen-Feldner, E., Yartz, A., & Feldner, M. (2006). Perceived health, a test of incremental validity in relation to smoking outcome expectancies, motivation to smoke and desire to quit smoking. *Cognitive Behaviour Therapy, 35,* 28–42.

Haworth, J. T. (1997). Embodiment and quality of life. In J. T. Haworth (Ed.), *Work, leisure, and well-being* (pp. 103–116). London: Routledge.

Hektner, J., Schmidt, J., & Csikszentmihalyi, M. (2007). *Experience sampling method. Measuring the quality of everyday life.* New York: Sage.

Hernandez, M., & Iyengar, S. S. (2001). What drives whom? A cultural perspective on human agency. *Social Cognition, 19,* 269–294.

Higgins, E. T., & Trope, Y. (1990). Activity engagement theory: Implications of multiply identifiable input for intrinsic motivation. In T. E. Higgins & R. M. Sorrentino (Eds.), *Handbook of motivation and cognition: Foundations of social behaviour* (Vol. 2, pp. 229–264). New York: Guilford Press.

Ho, S. S. M., & Chan, R. S. Y. (2009). Social harmony in Hong Kong: Level, determinants and policy implications. *Social Indicators Research, 91,* 37–58.

Idler, E., & Benyamini, Y. (1997). Self-rated health and mortality: A review of twenty-seven community studies. *Journal of Health and Social Behavior, 38,* 21–37.

Ingstad, B. (1999). The myth of disability in developing nations. *The Lancet, 354,* 757–758.

Iso-Ahola, S. E. (1997). A psychological analysis of leisure and health. In J. T. Haworth (Ed.), *Work, leisure, and well-being* (pp. 131–144). London: Routledge.

Joseph, S., & Linley, A. (2006). Growth following adversity: Theoretical perspectives and implications for clinical practice. *Clinical Psychology Review, 26,* 1041–1053.

Karasek, R., & Theorell, T. (1990). *Healthy work: Stress, productivity, and the reconstruction of working life.* New York: Basic Books.

Kegan, R. (1994). *In over our heads.* New York: Cambridge University Press.

Kellner, R. (1987). A symptom questionnaire. *Journal of Clinical Psychiatry, 48,* 269–274.

Keyes, C. L. M. (1998). Social well-being. *Social Psychology Quarterly, 61,* 121–140.

Keyes, C. L. M. (2003). Complete mental health: An agenda for the 21st century. In C. L. M. Keyes & J. Haidt (Eds.), *Flourishing: Positive psychology and the life well-lived* (pp. 293–312). Washington, DC: American Psychological Association.

Keyes, C. L. M. (2007). Promoting and protecting mental health as flourishing: A complementary strategy for improving national mental health. *American Psychologist, 62*(2), 95–108.

Kipling W., Forgas J., Von Hippel W. (Eds.) (2005). *The social outcast: Ostracism, social exclusion, rejection, and bullying.* New York: Psychology Press.

Kiran Kumar, S. K. (2004). Perspectives on well-being in the Indian tradition. *Journal of Indian Psychology, 22*, 63–72.

Kitayama, S., Markus, H. R., & Kyurokawa, M. (2000). Culture, emotion and well-being: Good feelings in Japan and the United States. *Cognition and Emotion, 14*, 93–124.

Kitayama, S., Snibbe, A. C., Markus, H. R., & Suzuki, T. (2004). Is there any "free" choice? Self and dissonance in two cultures. *Psychological Science, 15*, 527–533.

Kluckhohn, R. R., & Stroedbeck, F. L. (1961). *Variations in value orientation.* Evanston, IL: Row Paterson.

Koenig, H. G., McCullough, M., & Larson, D. B. (2001). *Handbook of religion and health.* New York: Oxford University Press.

Larson, R. W. (2000). Toward a psychology of positive youth development. *American Psychologist, 55*, 170–183.

Larson, R. W., & Verma, S. (1999). How children and adolescents spend time across the world: Work, play, and developmental opportunities. *Psychological Bulletin, 125*, 701–736.

Leong, F. T. L., & Wong, P. T. P. (2003). Optimal human functioning from cross-cultural perspectives: Cultural competence as an organizing framework. In B. Walsh (Ed.), *Counseling psychology and optimal human functioning* (pp. 123–150). Mahwah, NJ: Erlbaum.

Linley P. A., Joseph S. (Eds.) (2004). *Positive psychology in practice.* London: Wiley.

MacLachan, M., & Carr, S. C. (1994). From dissonance to tolerance: Toward managing health in tropical cultures. *Psychology and Developing Societies, 6*, 119–129.

Maddux, J. E. (2008). Positive psychology and the illness ideology: Toward a positive clinical psychology. *Applied Psychology: An International Review, 57*(Suppl 1), 54–70.

Markus, H. R., & Kitayama, S. (1991). Culture and the self: Implications for cognition, emotion, and motivation. *Psychological Review, 98*, 224–253.

Marsella, A. J., & Yamada, A. M. (2007). Culture and psychopathology: Foundations, issues, and directions. In S. Kitayama & D. Cohen (Eds.), *Handbook of cultural psychology* (pp. 797–820). New York: Guilford Press.

Maslach, C. (1982). *Burnout: The cost of caring.* Englewood Cliffs, NJ: Prentice-Hall.

Maslach, C., Schaufeli, W., & Leiter, M. (2001). Job burnout. *Annual Review of Psychology, 52*, 397–422.

Maslow, A. (1970). *Motivation and personality* (2nd ed.). New York: Harper.

Massimini, F., & Delle Fave, A. (2000). Individual development in a bio-cultural perspective. *American Psychologist, 55*, 24–33.

Menon, T., Morris, M. W., Chiu, C. Y., & Hong, Y. Y. (1999). Culture and construal of agency: Attribution to individual versus group dispositions. *Journal of Personality and Social Psychology, 76*, 701–717.

Miller, J. G. (1984). Culture and the development of the everyday social explanation. *Journal of Personality and Social Psychology, 46*, 961–978.

Morling, B., & Fiske, S. T. (1999). Defining and measuring harmony control. *Journal of Research in Personality, 33*, 379–414.

Morrow, J., & Nolen-Hoeksema, S. (1990). Effects of responses to depression on the remediation of depressive affect. *Journal of Personality and Social Psychology, 58*, 519–527.

Muñoz Sastre, M. T. (1998). Lay conceptions of well-being and rules used in well-being judgements among young, middle-aged, and elderly adults. *Social Indicators Research, 47*, 203–231.

Newman, M. G., Kenardy, J., Herman, S., & Taylor, C. B. (1997). Comparison of palmtop-computer-assisted brief cognitive-behavioral treatment to cognitive-behavioral treatment for panic disorder. *Journal of Consulting and Clinical Psychology, 65,* 178–183.

Niederhoffer, K. G., & Pennebaker, J. W. (2002). Sharing one's story. On the benefits of writing or talking about emotional experience. In C. R. Snyder & S. J. Lopez (Eds.), *Handbook of positive psychology* (pp. 573–583). New York: Oxford University Press.

Norton, M., Wonderlich, S. A., Myers, T., Mitchell, J. E., & Crosby, R. D. (2003). The use of palmtop computers in the treatment of bulimia nervosa. *European Eating Disorders Review, 11,* 231–242.

Oishi, S. (2000). Goals as cornerstones of subjective well-being: Linking individuals and cultures. In E. Diener, & E. M. Suh (Eds.), *Culture and subjective well-being* (pp. 87–112). Cambridge, MA: MIT Press.

Overholser, J. C. (2004). Contemporary psychotherapy: Moving beyond a therapeutic dialogue. *Journal of Contemporary Psychotherapy, 4,* 365–374.

Papakostas, G. I., Perlis, R. H., Seifert, C., & Fava, M. (2007). Antidepressant dose reduction and the risk of relapse in major depressive disorder. *Psychotherapy and Psychosomatics, 76,* 266–270.

Park, C. (2005). Religion as a meaning-making framework in coping with life stress. *Journal of Social Issues, 61,* 707–729.

Park, C., & Folkman, S. (1997). The role of meaning in the context of stress and coping. *Review of General Psychology, 1,* 115–144.

Park, N., Peterson, C., & Seligman, M. E. P. (2006). Character strengths in fifty-four nations and the fifty US states. *Journal of Positive Psychology, 1,* 118–129.

Parker, S. (1997). Work and leisure futures: Trends and scenarios. In J. T. Haworth (Ed.), *Work, leisure, and well-being* (pp. 180–191). London: Routledge.

Peng, K., & Nisbett, R. E. (1999). Culture, dialectics, and reasoning about contradiction. *American Psychologist, 54,* 741–754.

Pennebaker, J. W. (1997). *Opening up: The healing power of expressing emotions.* New York: Guilford Press.

Peterson, C., Park, N., & Sweeney, P. J. (2008). Group well-being: Morale from a positive psychology perspective. *Applied Psychology, 57,* 19–36.

Peterson, C., & Seligman, M. E. P. (2004). *Character strengths and virtues: A classification and handbook.* Washington, DC: American Psychological Association.

Quarantelli, E. L. (1985). An assessment of conflicting views on mental health. The consequences of traumatic events. In C. R. Figley (Ed.), *Trauma and its wake* (pp. 173–215). New York: Brunner/Mazel.

Rafanelli, C., Conti, S., Mangelli, L., Ruini, C., Ottolini, F., Fabbri, S., et al. (2002). Psychological well-being and residual symptoms in patients with affective disorders. II. *Rivista di Psichiatria, 37,* 179–183.

Rafanelli, C., Park, S. K., Ruini, C., Ottolini, F., Cazzaro, M., & Fava, G. A. (2000). Rating well-being and distress. *Stress Medicine, 16,* 55–61.

Rao, R., Paranjpe, A., & Dalal, A. K. (2008). *Handbook of Indian psychology.* New Delhi: Cambridge University Press India.

Ravenna, M., Hölzl, E., Kirchler, E., Palmonari, A., & Costarelli, S. (2002). Drug addicts in therapy—Changes in life space in the course of one year. *Journal of Community and Applied Social Psychology, 12,* 353–368.

Ried, L., Tueth, M., Handberg, E., & Nyanteh, H. (2006). Validating a self-report measure of global subjective well-being to predict adverse clinical outcomes. *Quality of Life Research, 15,* 675–686.

Rifkin, J. (1995). The end of work as we know it. *Demos, 5,* 17–30.

Rogers, C. (1963). The actualizing tendency in relation to "motives" and to consciousness. In M. R. Jones (Ed.), *Nebraska symposium on motivation, 11* (pp. 1–24). Lincoln, NE: University of Nebraska Press.

Rogers, C. (1967). *On becoming a person: A therapist's view of psychotherapy*. London: Constable.

Rojek, C. (1995). *Decentring leisure*. London: Sage.

Roth, A., & Fonagy, P. (1996). *What works for whom? A critical review of psychotherapy research*. London: Guilford.

Ruini, C., Belaise, C., Brombin, C., Caffo, E., & Fava, G. A. (2006). Well-being therapy in school settings: A pilot study. *Psychotherapy and Psychosomatics, 75*, 331–336.

Ruini, C., & Fava, G. A. (2009). Well-being therapy for generalized anxiety disorder. *Journal of Clinical Psychology, 65*, 510–519.

Ruini, C., Ottolini, F., Tomba, E., Belaise, C., Albieri, E., Visani, D., et al. (2009). School intervention for promoting psychological well-being in adolescence. *Journal of Behavior Therapy and Experimental Psychiatry, 40*, 522–532.

Ruini, C., Rafnelli, C., Conti, S., Ottolini, F., Fabbri, S., Tossani, E., et al. (2002). Psychological well-being and residual symptoms in patients with affective disorders. I. *Rivista di Psichiatria, 37*, 171–178.

Ryan, R. M., & Deci, E. L. (2001). On happiness and human potentials: A review of research on hedonic and eudaimonic well-being. *Annual Review of Psychology, 2*, 141–166.

Ryff, C. D. (1989). Happiness is everything, or is it? Explorations on the meaning of psychological well-being. *Journal of Personality and Social Psychology, 6*, 1069–1081.

Ryff, C. D., & Keyes, C. L. M. (1995). The structure of psychological well-being revisited. *Journal of Personality and Social Psychology, 69*, 719–727.

Ryff, C. D., & Singer, B. (1996). Psychological well-being: Meaning, measurement, and implications for psychotherapy research. *Psychotherapy and Psychosomatics, 65*, 14–23.

Saravanan, B., Manigandam, C., Macaden, A., Tharion, G., & Bhattacharji, S. (2001). Re-examining the psychology of spinal cord injury: A meaning centered approach from a cultural perspective. *Spinal Cord, 39*, 323–326.

Schaufeli, W., & Bakker, A. (2004). Job demands, job resources, and their relationship with burnout and engagement: A multi-sample study. *Journal of Organizational Behaviour, 25*, 293–315.

Schlegel, R. J., Hicks, J. A., Arndt, J., & King, L. A. (2009). Thine own self: True self-concept accessibility and meaning in life. *Journal of Personality and Social Psychology, 96*, 473–490.

Schmidt, M. E., Fava, M., Zhang, S., Gonzales, J., Raute, N. J., Judge, R. (2002). Treatment approaches to major depressive disorder relapse. *Psychotherapy and Psychosomatics, 71*, 190–194.

Schnyder, U. (2005). Why new psychotherapies for post-traumatic stress disorder? *Psychotherapy and Psychosomatics, 74*, 199–201.

Seligman, M. E. P. (2002). *Authentic happiness: Using the new positive psychology to realize your potential for lasting fulfillment*. New York: Free Press.

Seligman, M. E. P., & Peterson, C. (2003). Positive clinical psychology. In L. G. Aspinwall & U. M. Staudinger (Eds.), *A psychology of human strengths: Fundamental questions and future directions for a positive psychology* (pp. 305–317). Washington, DC: American Psychological. Association.

Sen, A. (1992). *Inequality reexamined*. Oxford: Oxford University Press.

Sheldon, K. M., Elliot, A. J., Ryan, R. M., Chirkov, V., Kim, Y., Wu, C., et al. (2004). Self-concordance and subjective well-being in four cultures. *Journal of Cross-Cultural Psychology, 35*, 209–223.

Sheldon, K. M., & Kasser, T. (2001). Goals, congruence, and positive well-being: New empirical support for humanistic theories. *Journal of Humanistic Psychology, 41*, 30–50.

Shmotkin, D. (2005). Happiness in face of adversity: Reformulating the dynamic and modular bases of subjective well-being. *Review of General Psychology, 9*, 291–325.

Shmotkin, D., Berkovich, M., & Cohen, K. (2006). Combining happiness and suffering in a retrospective view of anchor periods in life: A differential approach to subjective well-being. *Social Indicators Research, 77*, 139–169.

Shweder, R. A. (2003). *Why do men barbeque? Recipes for cultural psychology*. Cambridge, MA: Harvard University Press.

Shweder, R. A., & Bourne, A. J. (1984). Does the concept of the person vary cross-culturally? In R. A. Shweder & R. A. LeVine (Eds.), *Culture theory: Essay on mind, self, and emotion* (pp. 158–199). Cambridge, UK: Cambridge University Press.

Singer, J. A. (2004). Narrative identity and meaning making across the adult life span: An introduction. *Journal of Personality, 72*, 438–459.

Sirgy, M. J., & Wu, J. (2009). The pleasant life, the engaged life, and the meaningful life: What about the balanced life? *Journal of Happiness Studies, 10*, 183–196.

Sivanathan, N., Arnold, K., Turner, N., & Barling, J. (2004). Leading well: Transformational leadership and well-being. In P. A. Linley & S. Joseph (Eds.), *Positive psychology in practice* (pp. 241–255). New York: Wiley.

Skevington, S., Lofty, M., & O'connell, K. (2004). The World Health Organization's WHOQOL-BREF quality of life assessment: Psychometric properties and results of the international field trial. A report from the WHOQOL group. *Quality of Life Research, 13*, 299–310.

Smith, K. D., Christopher, J. C., Delle Fave, A., & Bhawuk, D. P. S. (2002). Post-Newtonian metatheories in the natural sciences and in cross-cultural psychology. In P. Boski, F. J. R. van de Vijver, & A. M. Chodynicka (a cura di), *New directions in cross-cultural psychology* (pp. 107–125). Warsaw: Wydawnictwo Intytutu Psychologii PAN.

Sonino, N., & Fava, G. A. (2003). Tolerance to antidepressant treatment may be overcome by ketoconazole. *Journal of Psychiatric Research, 37*, 171–173.

Sperry K., & Shafranske E. P. (Eds.). (2005). *Spiritually oriented psychotherapy*. Washington, DC: American Psychological Association.

Stanton, A. L., Danoff-Burg, S., Cameron, C. L., Bishop, M., Collins, C. A., Kirk, S. B., et al. (2000). Emotionally expressive coping predicts psychological and physical adjustment to breast cancer. *Journal of Consulting and Clinical Psychology, 68*, 875–882.

Stebbins, R. A. (1997). Serious leisure and well-being. In J. T. Haworth (Ed.), *Work, leisure, and well-being* (pp. 117–130). London: Routledge.

Steger, M. F., Frazier, P., Oishi, S., & Kaler, M. (2006). The meaning of life questionnaire: Assessing the presence of and search for meaning in life. *Journal of Counseling Psychology, 53*, 80–93.

Suh, E. M. (2000). Self, the hyphen between culture and subjective well-being. In E. Diener, & E. M. Suh (Eds.), *Culture and subjective well-being* (pp. 63–86). Cambridge, MA: MIT Press.

Tanaka-Matsumi, J., & Draguns, J. (1997). Culture and psychopathology. In Berry, J. W., Segall, M. H., & Kagitçibasi, C. (Eds.), *Handbook of cross-cultural Psychology. Vol.3: Social behavior and applications* (pp. 449–492). Needam Heights, MA: Allyn and Bacon.

Teasdale, J. D. (1999). Metacognition, mindfulness and the modification of mood disorders. *Clinical Psychology and Psychotherapy, 6*, 146–155.

Tedeschi, R. G., & Calhoun, L. G. (2004). Post-traumatic growth: Conceptual foundations and empirical evidence. *Psychological Inquiry, 15*, 1–18.

Tomba, E., Belaise, C., Ottolini, F., Ruini, C., Bravi, A., Albieri, E., et al. (2010). Differential effects of well-being promoting and anxiety management strategies in a non clinical school setting. *Journal of Anxiety Disorders, 24*, 326–333.

Triandis, H. C. (1994). *Culture and social behaviour*. New York: McGraw-Hill.

Triandis, H. C. (1995). *Individualism and collectivism*. Boulder, CO: Westview.

Uchida, Y., Norasakkunkit, V., & Kitayama, S. (2004). Cultural constructions of happiness: Theory and empirical evidence. *Journal of Happiness Studies, 5*, 223–239.

Üstün, T. B., Chatterji, S., Bickenbach, J. E., Trotter II, R. T., Room, R., Rehm, J., & Saxena, S. (Eds.). (2001). *Disability and culture. Universalism and diversity*. Göttingen: Hogrefe and Huber Publishers.

Vaalsiner, J. (2007). Personal culture and conduct of value. *Journal of Social, Evolutionary, and Cultural Psychology, 1*, 59–65.

Van Emmerik, A. A. P., Kamphuis, J. H., & Emmelkamp, P. M. G. (2008). Treating acute stress disorder and posttraumatic stress disorder with cognitive behavioral therapy and structured writing therapy. *Psychotherapy and Psychosomatics, 77*, 93–100.

WHOQOL Group. (1994). Development of the WHOQOL: Rationale and current status. *International Journal of Mental Health, 23*, 24–56.

WHOQOL Group. (2004). Can we identify the poorest quality of life? Assessing the importance of quality of life using the WHOQOL-100. *Quality of Life Research, 13*, 23–34.

Ward, C. (2001). The A, B, Cs of acculturation. In D. Matsumoto (Ed.), *The handbook of culture and psychology* (pp. 411–445). Oxford: Oxford University Press.

Ward, C., & Kennedy, A. (1994). Acculturation strategies, psychological adjustment, and socio-cultural competence during cross-cultural transitions. *International Journal of Intercultural Relations, 18*, 329–343.

Warr, P. (1999). Well-being and the workplace. In D. Kahneman, E. Diener, & N. Schwarz (Eds.), *Well-being: The foundations of hedonic psychology* (pp. 392–412). New York: Russell Sage Foundation.

World Health Organization. (2004). *Promoting mental health: Concepts, emerging evidence, practice.* Summary report. Geneva: WHO.

Wu, C. (2009). Enhancing quality of life by shifting importance perception among life domains. *Journal of Happiness Studies, 10*, 37–47.

Zlobina, A., Basabe, N., Paez, D., & Furnham, A. (2006). Sociocultural adjustment of immigrants: Universal and group predictors. *International Journal of Intercultural Relations, 30*, 195–211.

Chapter 16
Recreate or Create? Leisure as an Arena for Recovery and Change

Joar Vittersø

A good life requires not only the possibility, but the realization of leisure. At least that was what Aristotle believed, and following Plato and other thinkers in Ancient Greece, he had a significant place for leisure in his scheme of thought (Kelly, 1990). In the Aristotlean approach, freedom from ordinary labor was necessary to build character. To actualize one's potentials a person needs freedom to engage in fulfilling activities, which generates not only pleasure but also virtue in a person. A strong emphasis on change toward self-fulfillment is normally connected with Aristotle's theory of developing virtues and character, since he defined all motion as the actualization of potentials. Hence, he seems to have argued that change is needed for humans to reach their respective goods or ends (Gewirth, 1998).

Today, the Greek ideal is confronted with views from a Protestant work ethic, which devaluates leisure and consider it as either useless or, at best, as time humans (unfortunately) need to recover from work, school, or other obligations (e.g., Haworth, 1997). The focus on leisure as recovery has partly to do with an increased number of job stressors and the feeling many people have of being overworked, which, among other things, stems from increased job demands following the high level of efficiency of modern work life (e.g., Evans, Gideon, & Barley, 2004; Schor, 1993). Besides the increased attention toward the restorative function of recreation, another reason why the virtues elements of leisure is downplayed in modern times, is that work life for many people represents an opportunity for self-fulfillment, or at least that is what many of us like to believe (Gardner, Csikszentmihalyi, & Damon, 2001). We do not need to spend our leisure time for self-fulfillment if we have appropriate growth opportunities at work.

The two main dimensions of leisure, i.e., recovery and change (often referred to as personal growth), are well known to students of positive psychology. For instance, Ryan and Deci (2001) argue that research on well-being has been derived from either a focus on happiness in terms of pleasure attainment (the hedonic approach) or from a focus on meaning and self-realization that defines well-being in terms of the degree to which a person is fully functioning (the eudaimonic approach).

J. Vittersø (✉)
University of Tromsø, Tromsø, Norway
e-mail: joar.vitterso@uit.no

R. Biswas-Diener (ed.), *Positive Psychology as Social Change*,
DOI 10.1007/978-90-481-9938-9_16, © Springer Science+Business Media B.V. 2011

The usefulness of making a distinction between two ways of being happy has been discussed elsewhere (see Kashdan, Biswas-Diener, & King, 2008, and the papers commenting upon this target article) and will not be elaborated in the current chapter. The taxonomy is mentioned to help readers connect the recovery aspect of leisure (reflecting, as further clarified below, many characteristics attributed to hedonic well-being) and the change aspect of leisure (reflecting many characteristics attributed to eudaimonic well-being) to the general literature of positive psychology.

I will deal with some particular tensions between recovery and change in a subsequent section. To prepare the reader for that debate, I will first comment briefly on some definitional issues regarding leisure, recovery, and change, and also give a general review of how leisure may connect with positive emotions and life satisfaction. To anticipate, the chapter concludes that leisure is an important source of emotional well-being that also contributes substantially to life satisfaction and overall happiness.[1]

In contrast to some popular theories in positive psychology, the assumption of the current chapter follows those of the theory of Functional Well-Being (e.g.,Vittersø, Søholt, Hetland, Thorsen, & Røysamb, 2010; Vittersø, 2010), claiming that change and personal growth are rarely experienced as pleasant. To clarify this point, a distinction is made between feeling states such as pleasure and happiness on the one hand, and feeling states such as engagement and interest on the other. Engagement is often a non-pleasant state of approach motivation, enabling the experiencer to execute the behavior needed to reach an important goal, even if giving it up would be more pleasant at the moment. In principle, leisure time offers the best opportunities for balancing the pleasures of recovery and goal fulfillment with the engagement needed to override the lack of pleasure that normally accompanies the process of personal growth and the development of skills.

Defining Leisure, Recovery, and Change

Following Csikszentmihalyi and LeFevre (1989), leisure can roughly be sorted into one of three categories of definitions. First, it may be defined as any time that is free, which usually means any time left free from obligations. A second way of defining leisure is to relate it to a specific activity that is freely chosen, such as playing bridge or tennis. Finally, a third category of definitions is based on the subjective experience of the individual, which means time that provides intrinsically rewarding experiences. Some researchers also make a distinction between leisure and recreation, saving the former for an overall human phenomenon in its own right rather than a leftover after work or school. Recreation, on the other hand, may be

---

[1] I treat life satisfaction and overall happiness as synonyms in this chapter because they both reflect a general evaluation of the degree to which life as a whole is favorable. I do, however, stress the distinction between satisfaction and happiness as an overall evaluation versus satisfaction and happiness as feeling states experienced in concrete situations. At the level of state experiences, I also consider satisfaction to be a feeling.

considered as more specific, more organized, and more related to restoration of mind and body (Kelly, 1990). I acknowledge that the difference between the two concepts sometimes is meaningful and important, but will nevertheless use the two terms interchangeable in the current chapter.

Any of the three groups of definitions make leisure relevant for positive psychology in two principal ways. First, the mere existence of leisure in a person's life is conductive to positive experiences and life satisfaction. This perspective is reviewed in the first section below. Another way in which leisure involves positive psychology concerns the very key elements of a good life. Leisure presents itself as a suitable case study for the investigation of mechanisms that generally are involved in human well-being. By understanding that which makes particular leisure activities valuable, studies of recreation may enable the field to learn more about how quality of life may be improved. A separate section of this chapter will investigate these elements of leisure, focusing in particular on opportunities for recovery and positive change.

Recovery is, in the current chapter, simply taken to mean a return to a homeostatic set point (e.g., Berntson & Cacioppo, 2000) or a mental baseline (Bonanno, 2009). It is assumed that recovery is experienced as pleasant and satisfactory, and that the regulation of homeostatic recovery basically is hedonically driven (e.g., Cabanac, 2010). The principle of hedonic regulation will be further detailed in the subsequent section entitled "Leisure and positive change."

Change normally refers to reorganization of the structure of a system (Valsiner, 1997), and can turn in a desired or an undesired direction. For example, in the terminology of life span psychology, Staudinger and Lindenberger refer to the former as a developmental gain, and the latter as a developmental loss (Staudinger & Lindenberger, 2003). In positive psychology, the idea of changes in human beings will first and foremost be associated with desirable or positive developments. Although the term "change" is seldom used or defined in psychology, synonyms or related concepts such as personal growth, self-actualization, flourishing, positively functioning, intrinsically motivated or fulfilling one's potentials or capabilities are commonly in use in the literature (Aspinwall & Staudinger, 2003; Dweck, 2000; Keyes & Haidt, 2003; Lane, 1996; Magnusson & Mahoney, 2003; Ryan, Huta, & Deci, 2008; Ryff, 1989; Vittersø, 2004; Waterman, Schwartz, & Conti, 2008). Few, if any, of these concepts are clearly defined and the term change will consequently be used very approximately in the present text basically as a synonym for the (equally unclear) concept of personal growth.

The Effects of Leisure on Well-Being

Early studies tended to show that the kinds of activities that affect people's mood in a positive direction first and foremost are leisure activities (Argyle, 2001). For example, Lewinshon and Sotlib (1973) discovered that the most pleasant activities listed by the participants in their study were all leisure activities, and recent and more sophisticated studies have corroborated this finding. Tkach and Lyubomirsky

(2006) reported that engaging in leisure activities was among the most success-ful strategies for increasing happiness, and Lu and Argyle (1994) describe how British adults with serious leisure commitments were happier than those without. Similar findings are reported elsewhere (e.g., Iwasaki, 2007; Laukka, 2007). In com-paring amateurs and professionals during a singing lesson, Grape and colleagues (Grape, Sandgren, Hansson, Ericson, & Theorell, 2003) found that only the ama-teurs reported increased emotional well-being when self-reports before and after the singing lesson were compared. Hence, it may be that it is the recreational setting in itself that adds to well-being, and not the activity as such.

Introducing the Day Reconstruction Method (DRM), which assesses how people spend their time and how they do experience the various activities and settings of their lives, Kahneman and his colleagues (Kahneman, Krueger, Schkade, Schwarz, & Stone, 2004) observed that leisure activities—such as watching TV, relaxing, eating, exercising, and spending time with friends—were by far more enjoyable than activities performed during work hours.

In a follow-up study, these authors (Kahneman, Krueger, Schkade, Schwarz, & Stone, 2006) illustrate another way in which leisure affects life satisfaction. In their sample, rich people spent more hours working than the poor, and since work activ-ities are more boring than leisure activities, these authors suggest that a suppressor effect is operating on the connection that is commonly found between life satisfac-tion and personal wealth (see e.g., Biswas-Diener, 2009; Lucas & Schimmack, 2009; Schyns, 2003). The nature of this suppressor effect is as follows. Higher income correlates positively with both life satisfaction and working hours. However, work-ing hours contribute negatively to emotional well-being, which in turn affects life satisfaction negatively. The studies from the Kahneman group also remind us how socioeconomic status affects attitudes toward, and use of, leisure time. Sociological approaches to leisure have a lot to say about the cultural premises for leisure opportunities and leisure experiences depend on cultural and societal structures (de Grazia, 1962; Haworth, 1997; Linder, 1970; Veblen, 1953).

The literature discussed above does not speak to the issue of causation. It is not necessarily the leisure activities themselves that enhance positive feelings and well-being. There are, however, some studies that demonstrate a causal relation between leisure and life satisfaction. For example, Reich and Zuatra (1981) asked students to engage in either two or twelve pleasant activities for a month. Compared with a con-trol group, both the activity groups reported increase quality of life. In a panel study among the elderly Searle and his colleagues (Searle, Mahon, Iso-Ahola, Sdrolias, & van Dyck, 1998) found an immediate effect of a leisure education intervention on measures of generalized locus of control and life satisfaction. However, after 18 weeks the effect on life satisfaction was no longer sustained.

Particular Leisure Activities

Does the influence from leisure to well-being depend on the kind of activity one is committed to? To answer the question, a useful distinction between active and passive leisure may be introduced, because active leisure is commonly reported to be more rewarding than the latter (Csikszentmihalyi, 1997; Tkach & Lyubomirsky, 2006). However, in their first DRM study, Kahneman and his group (Kahneman et al., 2004) found that among the ten activities that ranked highest on positive emotions, only exercise—ranking 6th on the positive emotion list—could be categorized as active leisure. The other nine were in descending ranking: intimate relations, socializing, relaxing, praying, eating, watching TV, shopping, preparing food, and being on the phone.

Csikszentmihalyi and LeFevre (1989) found a socioeconomic gradient in the relation between subjective experiences and active versus passive leisure. In their study, managers reported higher motivation in active leisure (operationalized as flow), in contrast to blue-collar workers, who were more motivated by passive (or non-flow) leisure.

An interesting mix of both active and passive leisure is present in the category of outdoor recreation. According to Ittelson and colleagues (Ittelson, Franck, & O'Hanlon, 1976), the most salient characteristic of an outdoor experience is the active process in which the individual can carry out his or her activities with a maximum of satisfaction. On the other hand, a series of studies have also documented the stress-reducing and restorative effects of natural environment and outdoor recreation. For instance, Ulrich, Dimberg and Driver (1991) found that physiological stress recovery was faster and more complete when participants were exposed to natural rather than urban environments, and he argues that a biologically prepared readiness for preferring natural environments may account for these findings. The restorative effect of nature environments has been confirmed in several studies (e.g., Hartig & Evans, 1993; Herzog, Black, Fountaine, & Knotts, 1997; Laumann, Garling, & Stormark, 2003; Parsons, 1991; Strumse, 1996; Tarrant, 1996; Ulrich, 1983; Wells & Evans, 2003). Outdoor recreation has further been shown to facilitate an impressive collection of well-being outcomes and other indicators of positive functioning (e.g., Herzog et al., 1997; Plante, Cage, Clements, & Stover, 2006; Tarrant & Green, 1999; Weinstein, Przybylski, & Ryan, 2009). For example, various forms of nature involvement consistently emerged as important spill-over effects on employees' job satisfaction (Kaplan, Bardwell, Ford, & Kaplan, 1996).

The Attention Restoration Theory (ART), developed by Stephen and Rachel Kaplan (Kaplan, 1995; R. Kaplan & Kaplan, 1989), holds that natural environments restore mental processes after fatigue caused by long-lasting directed attention. Restoration occurs with a distance from the causes of fatigue (*being away*), given a harmonious match between one's purposes and inclinations (*compatibility*). Two other elements of nature encounters that are considered beneficial by the ART are the interest driven and effortless attention (*fascination*) evoked in rich and coherently ordered environment (*extent*). It has been suggested that the first two benefits of ART encapsulate the recovery element of leisure, while the latter two sum up the change element, or at least the growth opportunities that follow from serious reflection upon unresolved personal problems or larger questions such as the meaning of life (see Herzog et al., 1997).

Leisure and Positive Change

Important ideas in the recreation literature, such as flow theory and the ART, appear to account for how recovery and change processes may occur simultaneously in leisure activities. Csikszentmihalyi has, for instance, argued that people cannot enjoy what they are doing unless they get better at it, and the process of getting better is the reason why flow is a force for growth (M Csikszentmihalyi & Csikszentmihalyi, 1988, p. 262). However, recent literature on the development of skills suggests that Csikszentmihalyi's assumption may be wrong (e.g., Ross, 2006). Actually, Csikszentmihalyi's own reasoning may challenge the simultaneously hypothesis, since he has claimed (Csikszentmihalyi, 1996) that humans are motivated by two contradictory sets of instructions. The first set of instructions is a conservative tendency made up of instincts for self-preservation, self-aggrandizement, and saving energy. In the context of leisure research, I believe these instructions are related to recovery. The second set of instructions reflects an expansive tendency made up of instincts for exploring, for enjoying novelty and risk. I believe these instructions speak to the process of positive change.

A closer look at relevant leisure studies reveals some possible explanations as to why recovery and change elements have been mixed-up in some parts of the literature. For example, leisure activities may be divided into different phases (Hammitt, 1980), and recovery needs not take place in the same phases as change (Hull, Stewart, & Yi, 1992). In a detailed analysis of the dynamics of a physical exercise, Hall and colleagues (Hall, Ekkekakis, & Petruzzello, 2002) found a substantial element of negative emotions during the most intense and strenuous phases of the event, even if it was dominated by pleasant feelings both before and after the intense phases. Moreover, a comparison of the post-exercise measures with the pre-exercise measures indicated significant affective benefits after the working out was finished. In the Hull et al. study, the phases that are most important for developing physical strengths had a transient but substantial negative impact on affect, whereas the relaxation phases after the exercise were experienced as more positive than the preparation phase before the intense exercise had begun.

Another reason why recovery and change may appear to co-occur in the leisure activities relates to the widespread classification of emotions as either positive or negative. A huge part of the recreation studies makes use of this dichotomization and, as a consequence, ends up with representing all the different positive feeling states that take place during a leisure event in one single variable. I believe this practice constitutes a problem, both for the recreation research (Vittersø, Vorkinn, Vistad, & Vaagland, 2000) and for the study of human well-being in general (Vittersø, Oelmann, & Wang, 2009). A "grab-bag" variable of positive emotion will mix together variance from feeling states that are very different hence it may prevent the researcher from discovering the elusive dynamics of recreation experiences, and from identifying the causes and effects of both recovery and change.

To illustrate how distinct positive emotions relate differently to recovery and change elements of leisure activities, Bjerke, Kaltenborn, and Vittersø (2006) tested the assumptions in ART using separate measures for relaxation, pleasure, and interestingness. The results revealed that relaxation was positively correlated with the ART component of *compatibility* but negatively correlated with the ART element of *fascination*. The data further showed that compatibility was correlated with feelings of pleasure, whereas fascination was mainly correlated with interestingness. Furthermore, in a field-experiment analyzing the effect of noise on leisure experiences, I and my colleagues found that noise from a snowmobile significantly reduced the quality of the leisure experience of cross-country skiers. The noise was particularly harmful to the relaxation part of the participants' feeling profiles, and it was to a significantly lesser degree harmful to the joyful part of their experiences (Vittersø, Chipeniuk, Vistad, & Skår, 2004).

Is the Development of Skills Pleasant?

The idea that an undifferentiated pleasure state is the companion of change and personal growth is widespread (Csikszentmihalyi, 1992; Fredrickson, Cohn, Coffey, Pek, & Finkel, 2008; Myers & Diener, 1995; Ryan & Deci, 2001; Watson, 2002), and may have been inspired by analogies to children, and how humans in the earliest phases of life develop skills and abilities in a playful mood (Denney, 1982). However, for adults to acquire the skills needed to perform an unfamiliar leisure activity, a process quite different from children's play is needed. Typically, when a grown-up is introduced to a new leisure activity, he or she will focus on generating proper actions while avoiding serious mistakes. After a period of training, normally less than 50 h, an acceptable level of proficiency has been attained, in which performance appears smoother and nasty mistakes occur more seldom. At this point, performance has basically become automated and individuals are able to carry out the leisure activity with minimal effort, and often with a substantial level of satisfaction (Ericsson, 2006).

The correlation between low effort and high satisfaction is intriguing and goes against the classic view that leisure is both pleasurable and character-building at the same time. The simultaneously hypothesis contradicts several mainstream theories in positive psychology as well. Consider, for example, the broaden-and-build theory (Fredrickson, 1998; Fredrickson & Cohn, 2008), which makes two central claims. First, all positive emotions are assumed to broaden people's momentary thought–action repertoires (the broaden hypothesis). Second, temporary and transient experiences of positive emotions over time build enduring personal resources (the build hypothesis). However, the idea that all positive emotions entail both broaden and build elements contradicts influential theories of emotions. For instance, neurobiological theories of emotions commonly divide positive emotions into appetitive emotions and consummatory emotions (e.g., Kringelbach & Berridge, 2010), each of which have a distinct phenomenology and different functions. It occurs to me that the appetitive emotions may be related to growth, change, and hence the building element of Fredrickson's theory, whereas the consummatory emotions are more likely related to concepts such as recovery (Kaplan, 1995), savoring (Bryant & Veroff, 2006) and also the broadening of attention (Carver, 2003).

Much empirical and theoretical evidence go against the notion that pleasure is connected with change and developing personal resources. According to the mere-exposure effect, it is familiarity, not novelty, that produces pleasure (Zajonc, 1968). More recent research have backed up this claim, discovering that easy-to-process stimuli produce higher activity over the zygomaticus region of the brain, which is an indicator of pleasant affect (Winkielman & Cacioppo, 2001). Similarly, the discovery of a neurological "liking system" as different from a neurological "wanting system" (Berridge, 1999) provides further support for the proposal of separating consummatory and appetitive emotion states. Hence, a recent literature review concluded that there appears to be at least two distinct classes of positive emotions represented in the brain, with separate but overlapping neuroanatomical substrates. The two correspond with the consummatory and appetitive taxonomy (Burgdorf & Panksepp, 2006).

A relevant illustration of why pleasure is not likely to build skills and personal resources appears if we combine the fluency thesis (Winkielman, Schwarz, Fazendeiro, & Reber, 2003), with an analysis of the processes that are performed during typical leisure activities. To start with Winkielman pleasure is supposed by him to be the emotional result for individuals dealing with easy tasks, during which the information processing runs fluently. Pleasure is typically found to occur in non-demanding situations dominated by familiarity, typicality, and symmetry; it denotes faster and less complex processing. In other words, pleasure may result from the dynamics of automated behavior simply because stimuli that are processed by high speed, low resource demand, and high accuracy will in itself produce pleasure.

As documented by Hill and Schneider (2006), automated activities are highly enjoyable, but they do not lead to improvements in skills or capabilities. This perspective contrasts a fundamental notion in flow theory, which claims that unless people get better at what they are doing, they ca not enjoy doing it any longer (Csikszentmihalyi & Csikszentmihalyi, 1988, p. 262). If automated skills are not only those most commonly employed in leisure activities, but also those that make leisure satisfactory and intrinsically enjoyable for adults, the idea that the joyfulness of flow acts as a magnet to learning (Csikszentmihalyi, 1997, p. 33) may be in trouble. As an alternative, Ericsson argues that the characteristics of flow are inconsistent with the demands of what he calls deliberate practice (Ericsson, 1996, p. 25). By deliberate practice, Ericsson refers to a set of nuts and bolts that seems necessary for effective learning to take place. The most important elements in deliberate practice are concentrated attention toward a well-defined task with an adequate difficulty level for the particular individual, informative feedback, opportunities for repetition, and corrections of errors (Ericsson, 1996, pp. 20–21). Based on the extensive studies of the acquisition of expert performance (e.g., Ericsson, Charness, Feltovich, & Hoffman, 2006), one is tempted to ask if the efforts needed for change and personal growth are stripped for, rather than filled with, enjoyment.

According to the idea of pleasure as a common currency (Cabanac, 1992), this is a reasonable argument. The concept implies that when people must choose among competing behaviors, pleasure is the priority scale against which they make priorities. Cabanac suggests that behavior is selected by subjects who maximize their pleasures and minimize their displeasures, and that homeostatic stability rather than change provides the pleasure that they seek. In support of this assumption, Cabanac has conducted a series of experiments showing how thermal comfort regulates the amount of physical effort people are willing to carry out at a given temperature. For example, in one of his studies (Cabanac, 1992) self-reported pleasantness was used to establish the optimal room temperature for given level of physical activity (running on a treadmill with a certain resistance). A similar procedure established the optimal level of physical activity for a given room temperature. In the second phase of this experiment new participants were asked to either regulate the slope of the treadmill, given a constant room temperature, or to regulate the room temperature, given a constant slope on the treadmill. In either case the participants regulated the slope (or temperature) in almost perfect accordance with the prediction of the common currency hypothesis. An impressive 97% of the variance in the theoretical variable of pleasure maximization was explained by the actual behavior of the participants in this experiment.

Cabanac's studies suggest that when given a free choice, humans put in the effort needed to keep their physiology in homeostatic balance, but not more. The question is whether this assumption is in conflict with widely used theories in positive psychology, explaining that pleasant emotions motivate growth rather than stability? After all, the premise of flow theory (Csikszentmihalyi, 2009), broaden-and-build theory (Fredrickson & Cohn, 2008), self-determination theory (Deci & Ryan, 2000), and other theories is the idea that, given a varied number of prerequisites, it simply feels good to build one's potential. In other words, a general message from positive psychology is that personal growth and the development of skills is intrinsically pleasant. However, if these assumptions are correct, why are sedentary lifestyles and unhealthy behaviors blooming in western societies? Given that the process of personal growth is intrinsically pleasant, why do we need intervention programs and other kinds of external stimulation to keep up a healthy lifestyle? After all, such programs are not needed to make us watch TV or eat chocolate.

However, we are not spending all our spare time eating snacks and watching TV. There is, after all, a lot of effortful and active leisure going on. One reason why active leisure is attractive even if it may be short on pleasure compared to passive leisure may be attributed to engagement and interest. According to the functional model of well-being (FWB; Vittersø, 2010), engagement means being in a mode in which the urge of an immediate return to homeostatic balance is pushed back. The function of engagement is supposed to promote willingness to continue an ongoing activity even if it does not feel pleasant to keep on. Hence, in the context of the leisure approach taken in this chapter, to postpone a return to homeostatic balance means to postpone behavior leading to recovery. Accordingly, the best opportunities for personal growth are created when immediate returns to homeostatic set-points are delayed. In other words, positive change occurs at the expense of recovery.

There are instances in which engagement is highly correlated with pleasure. Sometimes engagement/interest correlates substantially with pleasure/satisfaction, but sometimes this correlation disappears (e.g., Higgins, 2006; Iran-Nejad, 1987; Silvia, 2006; Vitterø, Overwien, & Martinsen, 2009). One factor that may affect the association between engagement and pleasure is personal experience and the importance of the activity relative to the personal goals and striving for the individuals under study. For example, Hsaiao and Thayer (1998) reported that experienced exercisers noted enjoyment as the main motivator for working out, whereas the beginners were motivated by health and aesthetic reasons. If it takes engagement to become an experienced athlete, it seems reasonable to speculate that the experienced exercisers could have been more engaged than the inexperienced exercisers, and that engagement was the moderator of the association between activity and the reported pleasure. Some support of the engagement as moderator hypothesis was found in a study conducted by me and one of my students (Vitterø & Søholt, 2010). We found that trait engagement as measured a month before a long outdoor hike predicted the reported pleasantness during the event, and that state pleasantness strongly predicted motivation for doing a similar hike in the future. Trait pleasantness did not predict state pleasantness during the hike.

Future Research

Passive leisure is normally reported to be more pleasant than active leisure (Kahneman et al., 2004). Nevertheless, effortful and extremely active leisure is sometimes reported to be the most intense and enjoyable of all the activities humans can think of (Csikszentmihalyi, 1975). This contradiction suggests that positive psychology still has a way to go before the dynamics between good feelings and good functioning is properly understood. For example, flow theory suggests, as does the model of FWB, that engagement is a prerequisite for optimal experiences. However, flow theory suggests that five other prerequisites also help promote flow experiences, and these are: high challenges and skills; clear and proximal goals; immediate feedback; and highly focused attention (Schmidt, Shernoff, & Csikszentmihalyi, 2007). It is not clear though, which of these elements that are necessary and/or sufficient for flow to occur. Moneta and Csikszentmihalyi have for instance suggested that the balance between challenges and skills is the only determinant of all possible subjective experiences (1999, p. 606). This is not very likely, since most evidence suggest that the balance between challenges and skills hardly explains more than 5–10% of the variance in subjective experiences. Hence we obviously need to clarify what skill development feels like and what role the balance between challenges and skills really have.

Similarly, the development of personal potentials may not necessarily be following the same paths as the development of skills and expertise. For example, the Self-Determination Theory (Deci & Ryan, 2000) suggests that intrinsically motivated people are not bound by the hedonic motivation that is regulated by the set-point of an equilibrium. Rather, they are naturally inclined to engage in activities that interest them and to act in the direction of increased psychological differentiation and integration. Given the right circumstances, people move toward personal and interpersonal coherence whether this behavior leads to satisfaction of homeostatic needs or not. The issue of whether the psychological differentiation and integration can develop without tedious repetitions, intense concentration or the effortful pushing of one's physical capacities is not known, and should capture more research interest in the years to come.

Finally, when it comes to the broaden-and-build theory, more studies are needed to clarify the issue of whether all the positive emotions actually contribute to both broadening attention and building skills. In the FWB approach, interest and engagement contribute to building skills, but they narrow down attention. According the FWB, skills develop when attention is limited and highly focused. Future research may decide which of the two hypotheses that turns out to be most reasonable.

Conclusions

A huge number of studies has shown that leisure activities are important for people's overall quality of life. Positive emotions are normally increased during leisure activities. These positive experiences tend to last beyond the moment and spill over to general evaluation of life as a whole, although the leisure activities must be maintained in order to keep its effect on well-being alive over longer periods of time.

Given the right context and motivational states, leisure may offer opportunities for both recovery and positive change. However, the history of leisure has revealed that recreation has been used both well and not so well. The free men of the Ancient Greece took advantage of their leisure time to develop the forerunners of modern science, and Csikszentmihalyi has suggests that the world would have been a dull place if our ancestors had used their free time simply for passive entertainment or restorative purposes, instead of finding opportunities to explore beauty and knowledge (Csikszentmihalyi, 1997). On the other hand, the populace of the Roman Empire was offered "bread and circus" in their spare time, and ball games have been used by kings and emperor to distract a starving population. A 100 years ago, middle-class housewives wasted the opportunity for a tremendous increase in possible leisure time for an almost obsessive concern for housekeeping. Practically, all time freed up due to new technologies and housekeeping aids in the first half of the twentieth century was eaten up by higher standards of housework, and the question is whether this was a prudent investment of time (Schor, 1993).

Today, much time is devoted to working long hours and watching more TV (Harvey & Mukhopadhyay, 2007). The promise of positive psychology is to gain more knowledge of the consequences of active and passive leisure, to learn about the dynamics of leisure as recovery and leisure as growth works, and last but not least, to better understand how the balances between work and leisure affects happiness and opportunities for bringing our lives to flourishing completion.

References

Argyle, M. (2001). *The psychology of happiness* (2nd ed.). Hove: Routledge.

Aspinwall, L. G., & Staudinger, U. M. (Eds.). (2003). *A psychology of human strengths: Fundamental questions and future directions for a positive psychology.* Washington: American Psychological Association.

Berntson, G. G., & Cacioppo, J. T. (2000). From homeostasis to allodynamic regulation. In J. T. Cacioppo, L. G. Tassinary, & G. G. Berntson (Eds.), *Handbook of psychophysiology* (pp. 459–481). Cambridge, UK: Cambridge University Press.

Berridge, K. C. (1999). Pleasure, pain, desire and dread: Hidden core processes of emotion. In D. Kahneman, E. Diener, & N. Schwarz (Eds.), *Well-being: The foundations of hedonic psychology* (pp. 527–559). New York: Russell Sage Foundation.

Biswas-Diener, R. (2009). *Material wealth and subjective well-being.* Unpublished doctoral thesis, University of Tromsø.

Bjerke, T., Kaltenborn, B., & Vittersø, J. (2006). Cabin life: Restorative and affective aspects. In N. McIntyre, D. Williams, & K. McHugh (Eds.), *Multiple dwellings and tourism: Negotiating place, home and identity* (pp. 87–102). Wallingford, UK: CABI.

Bonanno, G. A. (2009). *The other side of sadness. What the new science of bereavement tells us about life after loss.* New York: Basic Books.

Bryant, F. B., & Veroff, J. (2006). *Savoring; A new model of positive experience.* Mahwah, NJ: Lawrence Erlbaum.

Burgdorf, J., & Panksepp, J. (2006). The neurobiology of positive emotions. *Neuroscience & Biobehavioral Reviews, 30,* 173–187.

Cabanac, M. (1992). Pleasure. The common currency. *Journal of Theoretical Biology, 155,* 173–200.

Cabanac, M. (2010). The dialectics of pleasure. In M. L. Kringelbach & K. C. Berridge (Eds.), *Pleasures of the brain* (pp. 113–124). Oxford: Oxford University Press.

Carver, C. S. (2003). Pleasure as a sign you can attend to something else: Placing positive feelings within a general model of affect. *Cognition and Emotion, 17,* 241–261.

Csikszentmihalyi, M. (1975). *Beyond boredom and anxiety.* San Francisco: Jossey-Bass.

Csikszentmihalyi, M. (1992). *Flow. The psychology of happiness.* London: Rider.

Csikszentmihalyi, M. (1996). *Creativity: Flow and the psychology of discovery and invention.* New York: Harper Collins.

Csikszentmihalyi, M. (1997). *Finding flow. The psychology of engagement with everyday life.* New York: Basic Books.

Csikszentmihalyi, M. (2009). Flow. In S. J. Lopez (Ed.), *The encyclopedia of positive psychology* (Vol. I, pp. 394–400). Malden, MA: Wiley-Blackwell.

Csikszentmihalyi, M., & Csikszentmihalyi, I. S. (Eds.). (1988). *Optimal experience. Psychological studies of flow in consciousness.* Cambridge: Cambridge University Press.

Csikszentmihalyi, M., & LeFevre, J. (1989). Optimal experience in work and leisure. *Journal of Personal and Social Psychology, 56,* 815–822.

Deci, E. L., & Ryan, R. M. (2000). The "what" and "why" of goal pursuits: Human needs and the self-determination of behavior. *Psychological Inquiry, 11,* 227–268.

de Grazia, S. (1962). *Of time, work, and leisure.* New York: The Twentieth Century Fund.

Denney, N. W. (1982). Aging and cognitive changes. In B. B. Wolman (Ed.), *Handbook of developmental psychology* (pp. 807–827). Englewood Cliffs, NJ: Prentice Hill.

Dweck, C. S. (2000). *Self-theories: Their role in motivation, personality, and development.* Hove: Psychology Press.

Ericsson, K. A. (1996). The acquisition of expert performance: An introduction to some of issues. In K. A. Ericsson (Ed.), *The road to excellence. The acquisition of expert performance in the arts and sciences, sports, and games* (pp. 1–50). Mahwah, NJ: Lawrence Erlbaum.

Ericsson, K. A. (2006). The influence of experience and deliberate practice on the development of superior expert performance. In K. A. Ericsson, N. Charness, P. J. Feltovich, &

R. R. Hoffman (Eds.), *The Cambridge handbook of expertise and expert performance* (pp. 683–703). New York: Cambridge University Press.

Ericsson, K. A., Charness, N., Feltovich, P. J., & Hoffman, R. R. (Eds.). (2006). *The Cambridge handbook of expertise and expert performance*. New York: Cambridge University Press.

Evans, J. A., Gideon, K., & Barley, S. R. (2004). Beach time, bridge time, and billable hours: The temporal structure of technical contracting. *Administrative Science Quarterly, 49*, 1–38.

Fredrickson, B. (1998). What good are positive emotions? *Review of General Psychology, 2*, 300–319.

Fredrickson, B. L., & Cohn, M. A. (2008). Positive emotions. In M. Lewis, J. M. Haviland-Jones, & L. F. Barrett (Eds.), *Handbook of emotions* (3rd ed., pp. 777–796). London: The Guilford Press.

Fredrickson, B. L., Cohn, M. A., Coffey, K., Pek, J., & Finkel, S. M. (2008). Open hearts build lives: Positive emotions, induced through meditation, build consequential personal resources. *Journal of Personality and Social Psychology, 95*, 1045–1062.

Gardner, H., Csikszentmihalyi, M., & Damon, W. (2001). *Good work. When excellence and ethics meet*. New York: Basic Books.

Gewirth, A. (1998). *Self-fulfillment*. Princeton, NJ: Princeton University Press.

Grape, C., Sandgren, M., Hansson, L.-O., Ericson, M., & Theorell, T. (2003). Does singing promote well-being? An empirical study of professional and amateur singers during a singing lesson. *Integrative Physiological and Behavioral Science, 38*, 65–74.

Hall, E. E., Ekkekakis, P., & Petruzzello, S. J. (2002). The affective beneficence of vigorous exercise revisited. *British Journal of Health Psychology, 7*, 47–67.

Hammitt, W. E. (1980). Outdoor recreation: Is it a multi-phase experience? *Journal of Leisure Research, 12*(2), 107–115.

Hartig, T., & Evans, G. W. (1993). Psychological foundations of nature experience. In T. Gärling & R. G. Golledge (Eds.), *Behavior and Environment. Psychological and Geographical Approaches*. London: Elsevier.

Harvey, A. S., & Mukhopadhyay, A. K. (2007). When twenty-four hours is not enough: Time poverty of working parents. *Social Indicators Research, 82*, 55–77.

Haworth, J. T. (1997). *Work, leisure and well-being*. London: Routledge.

Herzog, T. R., Black, A. M., Fountaine, K. A., & Knotts, D. J. (1997). Reflection and attentional recovery as distinctive benefits of restorative environments. *Journal of Environmental Psychology, 17*, 165–170.

Higgins, E. T. (2006). Value from hedonic experience *and* engagement. *Psychological Review, 113*, 439–460.

Hill, N. M., & Schneider, W. (2006). Brain changes in the development of expertise: Neuroanatomical and neurophysiological evidence about skill-based adaptations. In K. A. Ericsson, N. Charness, P. J. Feltovich, & R. R. Hoffman (Eds.), *The Cambridge handbook of expertise and expert performance* (pp. 653–681). New York: Cambridge University Press.

Hsaiao, E. T., & Thayer, R. E. (1998). Exercising for mood regulation: The importance of experience. *Personality and Individual Differences, 24*, 829–836.

Hull, R. B., Stewart, W. P., & Yi, K. Y. (1992). Experience patterns: Capturing the dynamic nature of recreation experience. *Journal of Leisure Research, 24*, 253–268.

Iran-Nejad, A. (1987). Cognitive and affective causes of interest and liking. *Journal of Educational Psychology, 79*, 120–130.

Ittelson, W. H., Franck, K. A., & O'Hanlon, T. J. (1976). The nature of environmental experience. In S. Wapner, S. B. Cohen, & B. Kaplan (Eds.), *Experiencing the environment* (pp. 187–206). New York: Plenum Press.

Iwasaki, Y. (2007). Leisure and quality of life in an international and multicultural context: What are major pathways linking leisure to quality of life. *Social Indicators Research, 82*, 233–264.

Kahneman, D., Krueger, A. B., Schkade, D., Schwarz, N., & Stone, A. (2004). A survey method for characterizing daily life experience: The day reconstruction method. *Science, 305*, 1776–1780.

Kahneman, D., Krueger, A. B., Schkade, D., Schwarz, N., & Stone, A. (2006). Would you be happier if you were richer? A focusing illusion. *Science, 312*, 1908–1910.

Kaplan, S. (1995). The restorative benefits of nature: Toward an integrative framework. *Journal of Environmental Psychology, 15*, 169–182.

Kaplan, R., Bardwell, L. V., Ford, H. A., & Kaplan, S. (1996). The corporate back-40: Employee benefit of wildlife enhancement effort on corporate land. *Human Dimensions of Wildlife, 1*, 1–13.

Kaplan, R., & Kaplan, S. (1989). *The experience of nature.* Cambridge: Cambridge University Press.

Kashdan, T. B., Biswas-Diener, R., & King, L. A. (2008). Reconsidering happiness: The costs of distinguishing between hedonics and eudaimonia. *The Journal of Positive Psychology, 3*, 219–233.

Kelly, J. R. (1990). *Leisure.* Englewood Cliffs, NJ: Prentice Hall.

Keyes, C., & Haidt, J. (Eds.). (2003). *Flourishing: Positive psychology and the life well-lived.* Washingdon, DC: American Psychological Association.

Kringelbach, M. L., & Berridge, K. C. (Eds.). (2010). *Pleasures of the brain.* Oxford: Oxford University Press.

Lane, R. E. (1996). Quality of life and quality of persons: A new role for government? In A. Offer (Ed.), *In pursuit of the quality of life* (pp. 256–293). Oxford: Oxford University Press.

Laukka, P. (2007). Uses of music and psychological well-being among the elderly. *Journal of Happiness Studies, 8*, 215–241.

Laumann, K., Garling, T., & Stormark, K. M. (2003). Selective attention and heart rate responses to natural and urban environments. *Journal of Environmental Psychology, 23*, 125–134.

Lewinshon, G., & Sotlib, I. H. (1973). Pleasant activities and depression. *Journal of Consulting and Clinical Psychology, 41*, 261–268.

Linder, S. B. (1970). *The harried leisure class.* New York: Columbia University Press.

Lu, L., & Argyle, M. (1994). Leisure satisfaction and happiness as a function of leisure activity. *Kaohsiung Journal of Medical Science, 10*, 89–96.

Lucas, R. E., & Schimmack, U. (2009). Income and well-being: How big is the gap between the rich and the poor? *Journal of Research in Personality, 43*, 75–78.

Magnusson, D., & Mahoney, J. L. (2003). A holistic person approach for research on positive development. In L. G. Aspinwall & U. M. Staudinger (Eds.), *A psychology of human strengths. Fundamental questions and directions for a positive psychology* (pp. 227–243). Washington, DC: American Psychological Association.

Moneta, G., & Csikszentmihalyi, M. (1999). Models of concentration in natural environments: A comparative approach based on streams of experiential data. *Social Behavior and Personality, 27*, 603–638.

Myers, D. G., & Diener, E. (1995). Who is happy? *Psychological Science, 6*, 10–19.

Parsons, R. (1991). The potential influences of environmental perception on human health. *Journal of Environmental Psychology, 11*, 1–23.

Plante, T. G., Cage, C., Clements, S., & Stover, A. (2006). Psychological benefits of exercise paired with virtual reality: Outdoor exercise energizes whereas indoor virtual exercise relaxes. *International Journal of Stress Management, 13*, 108–117.

Reich, J. W., & Zuatra, A. (1981). Life events and personal causation. *Journal of Personality and Social Psychology, 41*, 1002–1012.

Ross, P. E. (2006). The expert mind. *Scientific American, 295*, 64–71.

Ryan, R. M., & Deci, E. D. (2001). On happiness and human potentials: A review of research on hedonic and eudaimonic well-being. *Annual Review of Psychology, 52*, 141–166.

Ryan, R. M., Huta, V., & Deci, E. L. (2008). Living well: A self-determination theory perspective in eudaimonia. *Journal of Happiness Studies, 9*, 139–170.

Ryff, C. D. (1989). Happiness is everything, or is it? Explorations on the meaning of psychological well-being. *Journal of Personality and Social Psychology, 57*, 1069–1081.

Schmidt, J. A., Shernoff, D. J., & Csikszentmihalyi, M. (2007). Individual and situational factors related to the experience of flow in adolescence. A multilevel approach. In A. D. Ong & M. H. M. van Dulmen (Eds.), *Oxford handbook of methods in positive psychology* (pp. 542–558). Oxford, UK: Oxford University Press.

Schor, J. (1993). *The overworked American. The unexpected decline of leisure*. New York: Basic Books.

Schyns, P. (2003). *Income and life satisfaction. A cross-national and longitudinal study*. Unpublished doctoral thesis, Erasmus University Rotterdam.

Searle, M. S., Mahon, M. J., Iso-Ahola, S. E., Sdrolias, H. A., & van Dyck, J. (1998). Examining the long term effects of leisure education on a sense of independence and psychological well-being among the elderly. *Journal of Leisure Research, 30*, 331–340.

Silvia, P. J. (2006). *Exploring the psychology of interest*. New York: Oxford University Press.

Staudinger, U. M., & Lindenberger, U. (2003). Why read another book on human development? Understanding human development takes a metatheory and multiple disciplines. In U. M. Staudinger & U. Lindenberger (Eds.), *Understanding human development. Dialogues with lifespan psychology* (pp. 1–13). Dordrecht: Kluwer Academic Publishers.

Strumse, E. (1996). *The psychology of aesthetics: Explaining visual preferences for agrarian landscapes in Western Norway*. Unpublished Doctoral Dissertation, Bergen.

Tarrant, M. A. (1996). Attending to past outdoor recreation experiences: Symptom reporting and changes in affect. *Journal of Leisure Research, 28*, 1–17.

Tarrant, M. A., & Green, G. T. (1999). Outdoor recreation and the predictive validity of environmental attitudes. *Leisure Sciences, 21*, 17–30.

Tkach, C., & Lyubomirsky, S. (2006). How do people pursue happiness? Relating personality, happiness-increasing strategies, and well-being. *Journal of Happiness Studies, 7*, 183–225.

Ulrich, R. S. (1983). Aesthetic and affective responses to natural environment. In I. Altman & J. F. Wohlwill (Eds.), *Behavior and the natural environment*. London: Plenum Press.

Ulrich, R. S., Dimberg, U., & Driver, B. F. (1991). Psychophysiological indicators of leisure benefits. In B. L. Driver, P. J. Brown, & G. L. Peterson (Eds.), *Benefits of leisure* (pp. 72–89). State College, PA: Venture Publishing, Inc.

Valsiner, J. (1997). *Culture and the development of children's actions. A theory of human development* (2nd ed.). New York: John Wiley & Sons.

Veblen, T. (1953). *The theory of the leisure class* (2nd ed.). New York: New American Library.

Vittersø, J. (2004). Subjective well-being versus self-actualization: Using the flow-simplex to promote a conceptual clarification of subjective quality of life. *Social Indicators Research, 65*, 299–331.

Vittersø, J., Chipeniuk, R., Vistad, O. I., & Skår, M. (2004). Recreational conflict is affective: The case of cross-country skiers and snowmobiles. *Leisure Sciences, 26*, 227–243.

Vittersø, J., Oelmann, H., & Wang, A. L. (2009). Life satisfaction is not a balanced estimator of the good life. Evidence from reaction time measures and self-reported emotions. *Journal of Happiness Studies, 10*, 1–17.

Vittersø, J., Overwien, P., & Martinsen, E. (2009). Pleasure and interest are differentially affected by replaying versus analyzing a happy life moment. *The Journal of Positive Psychology, 4*, 14–20.

Vittersø, J., & Søholt, Y. (2010). The interplay between emotions and motivation in outdoor recreation. Manuscript in preparation.

Vittersø, J., Søholt, Y., Hetland, A., Thorsen, I. A., & Røysamb, E. (2010). Was Hercules happy? Some answers from a functional model of human well-being. *Social Indicators Research, 95*, 1–18.

Vittersø, J., Vorkinn, M., Vistad, O. I., & Vaagland, J. (2000). Tourist experiences and attractions. *Annals of Tourism Research, 27*, 432–450.

Vittersø, J. (2010). Functional well-being: Happiness as feelings, evaluations and functioning. In I. Boniwell & S. David (Eds.), *The Oxford handbook of happiness*. Oxford: Oxford University Press.

Waterman, A. S., Schwartz, S. J., & Conti, R. (2008). The implications of two concepts of happiness (Hedonic enjoyment and eudaimonia) for the understanding of intrinsic motivation. *Journal of Happiness Studies, 9*, 41–79.

Watson, D. (2002). Positive affectivity: The disposition to experience pleasurable emotional states. In C. R. Snyder & S. J. Lopez (Eds.), *Handbook of positive psychology* (pp. 106–119). Oxford: Oxford University Press.

Weinstein, N., Przybylski, A., & Ryan, R. (2009). Can nature make us more caring? Effects of immersion in nature on intrinsic aspirations and generosity. *Personality and Social Psychology Bulletin, 35*, 1315–1329.

Wells, N. M., & Evans, G. W. (2003). Nearby nature: A buffer of life stress among rural children. *Environment and Behavior, 35*, 311–330.

Winkielman, P., & Cacioppo, J. T. (2001). Mind at ease puts a smile on the face: Psychophysiological evidence that processing facilitation elicits positive affect. *Journal of Personality and Social Psychology, 81*, 989–1000.

Winkielman, P., Schwarz, N., Fazendeiro, T. A., & Reber, R. (2003). The hedonic marking of processing fluency: Implications for evaluative judgement. In J. Musch & K. C. Klauer (Eds.), *The psychology of evaluation. Affective processes in cognition and emotion* (pp. 189–217). Mahwah, NJ: Lawrence Erlbaum.

Zajonc, R. B. (1968). Attitudinal effects of mere exposure. *Journal of Personality and Social Psychology (Monograph Supplement), 9*, 2–27.

Chapter 17
Positive Computing

Tomas Sander

Introduction

In his opening speech at the International Positive Psychology Association (IPPA) Conference in June 2009, Martin Seligman, founder of Positive Psychology, formulated a formidable challenge: By the year 2051, 51% of the world population should be flourishing. This is an ambitious goal given that even in the richer, "happier" Western world only 2 in 10 people are considered to be genuinely psychologically flourishing, according to some studies (e.g., Keyes, 2009; Huppert & So, 2009).

A necessary condition for achieving the 51% goal is that Positive Psychology develops a delivery model for its well-being enhancing interventions that scales up globally. Meeting the 51% goal will require a sea change in how we look at public policy (Diener, Lucas, Schimmack, & Helliwell, 2009) and at national accounts of well-being where raising those accounts is made a major policy goal. Research by positive psychologists, such as Sonja Lyubomirsky and Barbara Fredrickson, focusing on positive interventions, suggests that besides good policies there is also a significant role that individuals can play by changing their attitudes, beliefs, and behaviors (e.g., Lyubomirsky, 2008; Fredrickson, 2009) in order to lastingly raise their level of well-being. But how can these change processes of individuals be supported in a truly scalable fashion?

The main thesis of this position paper is that we should take a radically new look at information technology to uncover the possibilities it can play in contributing to the 51% goal. I will present several arguments for the proposition that information technology is uniquely positioned for assisting individuals with their flourishing in a way that is effective, scalable, and ethically responsible. Following the tradition of successful, galvanizing notions such as Positive Psychology and Positive Health, I propose to call the study of information technology from the perspective of human flourishing Positive Computing.

T. Sander (✉)
HP Labs, Princeton, NJ 08540, USA
e-mail: tomas.sander@hp.com

R. Biswas-Diener (ed.), *Positive Psychology as Social Change*,
DOI 10.1007/978-90-481-9938-9_17, © Springer Science+Business Media B.V. 2011

The question what "flourishing" or the "good life" is has been around for millennia and different answers have been given within religion, philosophy, and increasingly within psychology. To have a better understanding of the key term of "flourishing," we briefly review some of the contemporary conceptualizations of well-being that have been given within Positive Psychology:

- Diener et al. pioneered the model of subjective well-being (SWB), which is defined as a subjective sense of satisfaction with one's life, the presence of frequent positive affect, and only lower levels of negative affect (e.g., Diener, 1984, 1994). This approach is sometimes called the hedonic approach.
- Ryff's model of psychological well-being is an example of a conceptualization of well-being influenced by the idea of "self-actualization" (Ryff, 1989). Its six dimensions are: autonomy, environmental mastery, personal growth, positive relations with others, purpose in life, and self-acceptance. This model can complement a subjective well-being approach.
- Seligman speaks about "three pillars" of the good life (Seligman, 2002): the pleasant life, characterized through the presence of positive emotions, the engaged life, where one is engaged in satisfying activities and utilizes one's strengths and talents, and the meaningful life, in which one serves a purpose larger than oneself. He recently suggested adding positive relationships to this list.
- Sheldon et al. focus on how pursuing and achieving goals that are aligned with a person's core values and beliefs leads to personal growth (Sheldon & Elliot, 1999; Sheldon & Houser-Marko, 2001).
- Deci and Ryan stress the importance of the fulfillment of the basic psychological needs of autonomy, competence, and relatedness (a sense of belonging) for well-being (Deci & Ryan, 2000).
- Hayes et al. put the focus on actively moving toward one's important life goals and values, independent of whether that makes one feel good or bad in the moment (Hayes, Strosahl, & Wilson, 1999). Thus this approach downplays the role that positive hedonic tone plays for leading a fulfilling life.

Different researchers and individuals assign varying importance to the elements in this admittedly incomplete list. In addition, characterizations of the good life vary considerably across cultures (e.g., Markus & Kitayama, 1991). The first conclusion from this list is that there is no universal notion of what well-being or human flourishing "really" is. Fortunately, for the purpose of coming up with a good working definition for Positive Computing such an agreement is also not necessary. Much more important is that the list of goals is kept open for ongoing revision and is inclusive, so it can reflect and honor people's diverse perspectives. Otherwise a global acceptance and scale cannot be reached. The second conclusion is that the objective of enhancing flourishing provides computer scientists with a rich set of plausible sub-goals that are valuable to pursue and that will require quite different technical approaches. For the remainder of the chapter we use the term "flourishing" as a family resemblance term for the type of constructs in the list above and can now define:

> Positive Computing is the study and development of information and communication technology that is consciously designed to support people's psychological flourishing in a way that honors individuals' and communities' different ideas about the good life.

If technology can make good on the promise articulated in this chapter to significantly increase well-being in a scalable cost-effective way, this benefits individuals and societies enormously. Evidence to support this claim includes Lyubomirsky, King, and Diener's study that people higher in well-being are more successful in life domains such as health, income, work performance, and social relationships (Lyubomirsky, King, & Diener, 2005). Fredrickson has shown that positive emotions help people build psychological and social resources and enhance resilience (Fredrickson, 2009). Pressman and Cohen have found that higher well-being leads to increased longevity (Pressman & Cohen, 2005). Seligman argues that higher well-being predicts lack of depression and better physical health (Seligman, 2008).

The structure of the chapter is as follows. Section "How Computers Can Help Flourishing on a Global Scale" gives six reasons why information technology is an indispensable aid for flourishing. Section "Technological Capabilities Relevant to Positive Computing" presents key technology enablers for Positive Computing. Section "Dealing with Challenging Situations" looks at how Positive Computing can assist coping with adversities and challenges. Section "Addressing Ethical Concerns and Data Privacy" describes ethical and privacy challenges Positive Computing raises, and how one can approach them. Section "Concluding Remarks" concludes the chapter.

How Computers Can Help Flourishing on a Global Scale

This section describes six reasons for the key thesis of this chapter: Positive Computing can be effective in helping billions of people achieve greater psychological flourishing. Throughout the chapter additional examples and research results in support of these reasons will be mentioned.

1. **Anytime, anywhere access to powerful mobile phones.** What sets smartphones (like the iPhone) apart from anything that existed previously is that they are powerful computing devices *that are always with us*. Thus unlike a human coach to whom one has access for typically 1 hour a week they are able to deliver Positive Psychology applications in any situation and at any time, ideally when they are most beneficial.

2. **Computers can collect and act upon data relevant for flourishing.** These data include information about how we feel (our emotions), what we do (our behaviors), and with whom we do it (our relationships). These data can serve multiple functions. Inspection leads to more *self-awareness and insight* into how we live

our lives and can help us move in deeply valued directions. They can support *contextualization and customization* so that *the right Positive Psychology resource is delivered at the right time*. For example, if the data suggest the user is stressed, the computer can deliver a Positive Psychology resource right then and deliver a specific resource that is *right for the person* (some people prefer to relax by listening to a guided meditation, some by talking to a friend and some by taking a walk).

3. **Computers are persistent and can be highly persuasive.** Fredrickson and Lyubomirsky (e.g., Lyubomirsky, 2008; Fredrickson, 2009) have suggested that raising one's level of happiness is not accomplished by quick fixes but requires motivation, effort, and consistency comparable to an exercise program or diet. In support of ongoing lifestyle changes computers can send motivational information and reminders, track progress, and use many other powerful techniques to persuade users to take positive actions. Computers have already been successfully deployed for lifestyle change programs such as weight-loss and exercise (e.g., Denning et al., 2009; Consolvo et al., 2008b).

4. **Information Technology can create environments and experiences beneficial for flourishing.** Information and communication technology mediates much of what we do. Many people spend more time with their computer or phone than with any one person or other activity in their lives. Reality which is already often computer-mediated can thus be designed and "augmented" with flourishing in mind. Computers can assist in correcting negativity biases through the display of more accurate, balanced information about our day, our life, and our memories. An example from the work place involves the emotionally taxing job of call-center agents where it is common that a whole work day can go sour due to one bad call with a customer (Millard & Hole, 2008). After each call the agents release a token on how the call went and the software displays the aggregated information to them. As there are usually many more good calls than bad ones, this helps to put a bad call into perspective. Some psychologists have argued that in today's society for many (though not for all) situations our evolutionary motivated negativity biases do not serve us anymore. Information technology can extend our memory in a more balanced way and correct this bias where so desired.

5. **Scalability.** Computing technology meets massive scalability requirements. As examples, note that within a few years Facebook gathered more than 400 million users. In 2009 more than half of the world population owns a cell phone and more than three in four adults in the United States own a computer. Hardware prices continue to fall creating inexpensive access for more and more people in the years to come. This trend allows Positive Computing to contribute to the democratization of Positive Psychology in two ways. First, by making the fruits and insights of Positive Psychology available to a wide group of people and, second, by making it easier for people and communities to create and distribute their own version of Positive Psychology which may be different from what is done in its currently most prolific basis of research activities in the United States.

6. **Openness and participation.** Computer systems can be designed as open platforms, e.g., by providing open interfaces. These interfaces can be used by other programmers to build new applications on top of existing ones or to modify existing applications. This allows programmers from diverse backgrounds to participate in creating diverse Positive Computing applications that are appropriate for the communities they serve.

For the above reasons there is a remarkable opportunity for technology to support people in new and innovative ways that are not available in an offline world. In addition the principles of openness and scalability can drive a democratization of Positive Psychology by making its benefits available to more people and by allowing diverse communities to create their own versions of what flourishing means for them and how it should be supported.

There are also obstacles that need to be overcome to realize such a vision. Technologies consciously designed to monitor and influence deeply how we think, feel, and act are still radically novel and will for some trigger fears of a Big Brother and technology abuse. These concerns got to be taken seriously. At least some of them can be mitigated through the proper design of the technology itself, e.g., to protect user privacy. We revisit ethical and privacy concerns in more detail in section "Addressing Ethical Concerns and Data Privacy".

Another objection is that computers are unlikely to fully replace the wise, compassionate counsel of a personal coach, doctor or therapist. There may be some truth to this for a variety of reasons. Perhaps surprisingly, research by Nass et al. (e.g., Reeves & Nass, 1996) has shown that people *do* tend to treat computers as if they were social actors. People respond to computers socially and emotionally while being fully aware that computers are not human. For Positive Computing it would be a remarkable achievement if users justifiably regarded their computer as a resource comparable to a "supportive, caring friend, which acts in their best interests." Users already develop emotional relationships with personal technology a prime example being how many people "love" their smartphone. For helping professionals Positive Computing creates a remarkable opportunity to provide their clients with customized resources outside the weekly therapy session.

Technological Capabilities Relevant to Positive Computing

Collecting Data for Positive Applications

In this section we look at which data can be reasonably collected and utilized by Positive Computing applications.

- Location data: where a person is at a particular time (both from a built-in GPS and collecting data about the nearest cell phone tower)
- Movements, e.g., whether a person is standing or walking can be determined from the accelerometer included in some of today's smartphones.

- Analysis of voice in phone calls for symptoms of depression can be done using speech analysis software by Sung, Marci, and Pentland (2005), which can run on smartphones. It monitors voice for slowed speech and other patterns suggesting depression.
- Analysis of text (e.g., email or online postings) for moods and emotions using linguistic analysis software developed by Pennebaker, Francis, and Booth (2001).
- Collection of physical sensor data such as galvanic skin response (GSR), blood pressure, heart rate, and heart rate variability. These can give insight into levels of emotional arousal.
- Analyzing pressure on a mouse reveals levels of user frustration (Reynolds, 1999).
- The microphone of a phone can be used to detect whether a user is currently engaged in a conversation and might thus be helpful to determine an appropriate time to interrupt the user.
- Analyzing typing behavior for indicators of cognitive and physical stress (Vizer, 2009).
- A user's communication patterns, e.g., whom he calls or emails, for how long and how often.
- Calendar data indicating how a user spends his time.

Based on these data, it is first possible to detect (some) situations when a user is particularly in need of support or a boost in well-being, e.g., when he is stressed or depressed. Second, these data help determine when it is a good time to interrupt the user with by a Positive Computing application. (For example, at work it may not be appropriate, whereas at home it is.) User activity recognition from sensor data is an active area of research.

How to leverage these data in a way that enhances human flourishing is an exciting question for both computer scientists and forward-looking positive psychologists. In an interesting related project Pentland et al. argue enthusiastically for what they call "reality mining" (Pentland, Lazer, Brewer, & Heibeck, 2009): "Reality mining, which pulls together these crumbs using statistical analysis and machine learning methods, offers an increasingly comprehensive picture of our lives, both individually and collectively, with the potential of transforming our understanding of ourselves, our organizations, and our society in a fashion that was barely conceivable just a few years ago. It is for this reason that reality mining was recently identified by Technology Review as one of '10 emerging technologies that could change the world' (Technology Review, April 2008)." Examples for the benefits from reality mining are assessment and improvement in individual and community health, including some mental health applications such as screening for depression based on voice analysis and physical movement patterns (Sung et al., 2005). Pentland et al. take mostly a health-related perspective. Positive psychologists can look at these data afresh from their own novel perspective, i.e., how the data can be put to use to enhance flourishing for individuals and communities.

Affective Computing and the Personal Happiness Assistant (PHA)

Affective Computing is a research area started by Picard (1997), which investigates how computers can recognize, interpret, and express human emotions. Positive Computing can leverage many of these fascinating capabilities. However, Positive Computing does not reduce to Affective Computing as in addition to emotional approaches Positive Computing will also incorporate cognitive approaches (e.g., to enhance cognitive constructs such as optimism, hope, self-efficacy, curiosity) and interpersonal approaches to contribute to forming and maintaining higher quality relationships.

Applications of Affective Computing discussed by Picard include online learning software that recognizes when the student is frustrated and adapts its presentation accordingly, a digital disk jockey that selects songs appropriate to one's moods, giving interactive virtual agents the ability to express emotions and empathy in response to the user's emotions and moods (e.g., through facial expression and word choice), and for creating an "augmented memory system" in which a wearable, always-on camera captures video images of a user's life, and in which those that have been determined to be of emotional significance will automatically be kept while others are deleted.

Let us start with an example. Christian Nold, a British artist, has created "emotion maps" since the year 2000 (Nold, 2009). He provided individuals with a Galvanic Skin Response (GSR) sensor allowing to measure emotional arousal, and a Global Positioning System (GPS) device. Users wear these devices as they walk around their communities and the measured data are recorded. By overlaying the collected date on a geographical map (like Google Earth), Nold created an emotion map of the user's physical environment. Nold writes: "People who actually wore the device and tried it out while going for a walk, and then saw their own personal emotion map visualized afterward, were baffled and amazed." He also used this technique in a communal way where people share and combine their maps to create a joint map of their communal environment.

Popular, empirically validated interventions in Positive Psychology as comprehensive include "Three good things," "Keeping a gratitude journal," and "Savoring of past, present or future experiences" (see, e.g., Lyubomirsky, 2008; Fredrickson, 2009; Seligman, 2002 for an overview). They all point to the happiness increasing value that comes from consciously experiencing, remembering, and re-experiencing one's good moments, presumably by helping to develop a more optimistic outlook, counteracting hedonic adaptation through conscious appreciation, and through experiencing more positive affect when reliving good moments.

Many of today's mobile phones are GPS-enabled, and can connect wirelessly with external devices or sensors, for example, with a GSR sensor worn on the hand. For a discussion of cost-effective GSR sensors that are convenient to wear, have a good battery life see, and can wirelessly connect with a computer (see Fletcher, 2010).

Based on these technical building blocks and the related ideas, we can now envision a first example of what non-trivial Positive Psychology inspired technology might be. A "Personal Happiness Assistant (PHA)" application is part of a mobile phone. Its job is to record data about a person's emotional arousal and locations. The PHA automatically transmits arousal data to the user's PC, so the user can view them on a convenient size monitor. The PHA application displays the time and location for peak arousal situations (good and bad). The user can select and annotate good experiences with a short description of what the experience is about, add a photo or tag them with the positive emotion that was most dominant in that situation (joy, pride, enthusiasm, awe, etc.) Alternatively, he can tag the experience with a personal strength he was using.

The benefit of tagging experiences with positive emotions or strengths present is that they can be searched for later, e.g., with a query "show me all the experiences in the last months where I experienced a sense of pride." This is a convenient way to build up "positivity portfolios," which have been suggested by Pawelski and Fredrickson (Fredrickson, 2009).

The success of Positive Computing will be critically determined by the level of end-user acceptance it achieves. For this positive technology needs to be convenient and pleasurable to use. More automation, rather than manual processes will usually do better. For example data collection should run seamlessly in the background once turned on and the data should be automatically pushed onto a platform where they can be easily manipulated. A user should not have to change sensor batteries every few hours. When presented data should be of high quality with respect to the purpose for which they were collected. For the PHA example sensor data need to be cleaned from motion artifacts as the GSR sensor measures sweating which can also come from the physical exertion. To filter out motion artifacts accelerometer data from the smartphone have been used. Solid engineering is required to get all of this to work well, but there are no insurmountable theoretical limitations.

The PHA example also exemplifies the usefulness of having an open platform. Collecting basic data about emotions, memories, etc. will be a useful building block of many Positive Psychology applications and should thus be reusable. Developers will come up with many innovative ideas, e.g., how to share some of this information with friends or to upload it to a social networking site that computes joint "joy maps" of cities, etc.

The focus of the just described PHA is on identifying high arousal moments. This is still quite incomplete, given that there are many serene moments in a person's life that might be worth capturing as well. It is an interesting question how to capture serene moments of well-being in a user-friendly way. Computer scientists have investigated a variety of digital approaches for capturing memories that a solution may built upon (e.g., Hodges, 2006; Hoven & Eggen, 2008).

Note that the PHA also captures stressful moments in a person's life. We describe how those can be used to improve well-being in section "Dealing with Challenging Situations".

Persuading People to Take Positive Action

The PHA described above helps people to gain more insight about what they deeply enjoy. And that may naturally lead them to want *to do* more of that. Positive Psychology has assembled a general "catalogue" of activities that have been empirically shown to improve well-being (e.g., Lyubomirsky, 2008; Fredrickson, 2009; Seligman, 2002). This section explores how technology can assist people take "positive actions," such as:

- using one's strengths regularly and in novel ways
- compassionate acts
- writing 20 min about one's best self
- writing a gratitude journal
- active constructive responding to others
- spending more time with other people
- exercise
- savoring experiences
- loving-kindness meditation
- relaxation
- using one's skills
- playing

Successfully motivating positive actions over time helps overcome a major challenge of lifestyle change programs: It is hard to follow through on one's initial intentions on a consistent basis. For example taking an online strengths inventory reveals to an individual a bundle of personal strengths (*Clifton Strengthsfinder*; *VIA Inventory of Strengths*; *CAPP strengths assessment tool*), which is itself considered a helpful intervention. But how long does the effect of this intervention last? More benefit ensues, the strengths inventory manuals advice, if a person cultivates and applies his strengths over time. This of course becomes easy to forget and after a few weeks one may wonder: "What is it exactly that I am supposed to do? And what are my strengths again?"

To support an *ongoing growth process*, the PHA can support, say, working with two strengths a week, by sending in the morning an *SMS reminder* to the user about the currently worked on strength. The SMS message suggests a *concrete action* what the user can do with this strength today and thereby makes it *simple* for the user to take action, e.g.:

> Utilizing your strength "love of learning" helps you be energized and fulfilled. What can you learn more about today?

Later in the day an SMS message is sent requesting the user to text back a word or two what he actually learned something about as well as a rating how much he enjoyed it. These responses are stored in the user's "Strengths Bank" where they can be reviewed periodically and utilized to create further insight. If this messaging is done with varying, interesting, relevant content this is a major step toward motivating and supporting users who wish to actively cultivate their strengths *over an extended period of time.* See the work by Fogg and Allen (2009) for more suggestions on how to use SMS effectively for persuasive purposes. An additional benefit of using SMS technology is that it is available on almost all mobile phones in the United States.

Fogg and others created the field of "persuasive technology" which he defines as "any interactive computing system designed to change people's attitudes or behaviors" (Fogg, 2003). Coercion and deception are not considered persuasive technologies by Fogg. Persuasive technology researchers have already created a number of impressive applications within health coaching and to promote lifestyle changes such as eating better, boosting physical activity and quitting smoking. Computer simulations have been used to teach about HIV infection risks and computer games to teach young girls about social skills. Fogg and his students at the Stanford University Persuasive Technology Lab have also conducted work on how to create Facebook applications that spread "virally" and how to create persuasive online video (e.g., for YouTube).

A promising experiment for Positive Computing will be to pick target behaviors from the list of positive actions and to investigate if and how persuasion techniques can support their adoption. Many (though not all) positive actions have the attractive feature to be rewarding and enjoyable *at the very time they are performed.* To get a sense of the sophisticated persuasion techniques that have been used in persuasive applications, here is a list of examples (e.g., Fogg, 2003):

- reduction, where a desired action is simplified to make it easy for a user to perform it,
- tunneling, where a user is led through a pre-determined sequence of steps,
- tailoring, where the persuasion techniques are matched to the user, e.g., for education level, the user's interests, etc.
- social comparison: users like to benchmark themselves against others.
- normative influence: leveraging the desire of users to conform, e.g., by sharing a tracked behavior with the user's in-group.
- self-monitoring in a way that is not tedious.
- social learning: learning from how others do certain things.
- praise.
- reminders.
- reciprocity.
- operant conditioning through positive reinforcement: very popular in video games, however needs to be used carefully due its possible abuse for manipulation.
- presentation of information through virtual human actors, which can apply principles of mimicry, empathy and appropriate display of emotional responses to increase rapport with the user (Bailenson & Yee, 2005).

In conclusion persuasive technology will provide Positive Computing with a valuable set of capabilities to effectively influence users to change their behaviors.

Will all of Positive Computing be "persuasive"? That is unlikely given for example that flourishing comprises goals related to self-actualization, closer to insight, autonomous choices, and value congruent living. Technologies to support these processes will help us gain greater insight into ourselves and how we live our lives but are not "persuasive" per se.

Computers and Purpose in Life

Computer technology has traditionally been optimized for getting tasks done. Recently, Human Computer Interaction (HCI) researchers have started to take a much broader perspective by exploring how computers can support people in living congruently with their values and what is important to them (Karat, Karat, & Vergo, 2004). This thread of HCI research is highly relevant for Positive Computing. Arguably, if computer applications can be successfully designed to help people pursue their deepest values then computers do actively contribute to a value-congruent, maybe even purposeful life.

The HCI researcher Zimmerman wishes to design technology that helps people "to be who they want to be" (Zimmerman, 2009). For computer scientists and positive psychologists interested in flourishing this makes an excellent starting point. As one example, it led Zimmerman to a mobile application which supports busy Zen Buddhists in their spiritual practice. The application enables them to participate meaningfully at the meditation sessions of their Zen centers even when they cannot physically be present. The system provides a live audio connection, so the sound of the gong beginning and ending the meditation session is transmitted in real time. In addition, remote participants are visually represented at the Zen Center itself. This creates a sense of communal presence and practice. The application also allows practitioners to create shared experiences. Sangha members can take and post photos with their mobile phone related to a communally explored theme that then appear as wallpapers on other Sangha members' phones.

Hassenzahl is another HCI researcher (e.g., Hassenzahl & Tractinsky, 2006; Hassenzahl, 2008 who began to ask how technology can fulfill the three basic human needs of autonomy, competence, and relatedness formulated in Self-Determination Theory (Deci & Ryan, 2000). Hassenzahl did a study which showed that users already perceive that computers support autonomy and competence but do not significantly support relatedness.

It is plausible that computers can support the need for relatedness in substantial ways. The huge success of social networking sites that allows friends to stay in touch more easily is an obvious example. Less known, yet powerful and innovative technologies that can have an impact on relatedness have been created in the HCI research community, e.g., technologies for communicating presence. An example is a picture frame that lightens up when a remote lover touches her own version of the frame communicating that she is thinking of her partner at home (Chang, Resner, Koerner, Wang, & Ishii, 2001). Which forms of technology support for relatedness will turn out to be genuinely nourishing and fulfilling is an interesting open question.

The work of Zimmermann, Hassenzahl, and other innovative HCI researchers suggests a meaningful and promising inquiry for Positive Computing that is much broader than just building "well-being gadgets," like the Personal Happiness Assistant discussed earlier:

1. What are important candidates for values, human needs, goals, or activities relevant to flourishing?
2. Which of these candidates are already served well through technology and which ones are not?
3. How can existing computing technology that is used every day be improved to serve those needs better?
4. What novel technologies can be created to support underserved needs?

Dealing with Challenging Situations

Although the majority of Positive Psychology research focuses on strengthening positive aspects in people's lives, there are also benefits if computers can help people to deal better with the negative events, moods or thoughts in their life. From the perspective of Positive Psychology it improves important Positive Psychology constructs such as a person's positivity ratio, i.e., the ratio from positive to negative emotions (Lyubomirsky, 2008) as well as a person's resilience in the presence of adversity, which also provides some protection from depression (Martin, 1998; Reivich & Shatté, 2003). To make dealing with negative challenges an explicit part of Positive Computing broadens the appeal of Positive Computing to a much wider audience by extending it from those motivated by personal growth to those primarily interested in dealing better with their problems.

There are at least five things that computers can do to support users when negative events happen:

1. Provide *better insight into negative events and patterns* through the abilities of the computer to record them. The PHA we discussed can be such a tool to create more insight. As the PHA measures arousal it also captures negative situations. A user can use this data about negative events as basis for an analysis and decide if something needs to be changed.
2. *Alert users to the presence of stressful situations* in the moment they are occurring and thereby giving them the ability to respond immediately. An example is a GSR mouse (possibly enhanced with pressure sensors (Reynolds, 1999)) that can alert users if they are highly stressed at work.
3. *Make adequate resources available* to the user on demand. The term "resources" should be seen in its broadest sense. The resource library can include audio with guided meditations and calming music for an anxious user and helpful, targeted information for users facing common difficult situations, like an upcoming public speech and much more.

4. In case a stressful event is foreseeable, a user can be *primed with appropriate resources* upfront, for example, by reminding him of his list of strengths or inviting him to do a meditation 15 min before a challenging situation.
5. Assist users *to cope in real time when a challenging situation is happening.*

As an example for the ambitious 5th point a real breakthrough were achieved if a future PHA can successfully assist a user to dispute negative (automatic, or irrational) thoughts as pioneered in Cognitive Behavioral Therapy (CBT). The first generation online CBT systems are not yet able to enter into an intelligent dialog with the user. Indeed general language understanding and reasoning about complex or unexpected everyday events is currently out of reach for computers. Yet there are also promising developments such as work by Daily (2005) on creating natural affective dialogs with users that can potentially be leveraged for meaningful dialogs about emotionally difficult situations. Even in the absence of the ability of intelligent dialogs solving the much easier problem of displaying on demand targeted information to the user for countering maladaptive beliefs in common difficult situations would already be a major progress about what is available today.

A PHA which has recorded our best moments annotated with emotions, strengths, and other metadata can assist users directly in the disputation of common "cognitive distortions" such as "I am a failure." or "I am undesirable." A prominent CBT technique is to collect contrary evidence. In our case the PHA likely already has a collection of contrary evidence on file. Digital memories of situations annotated with the emotion "pride" can be presented to the user for review if they provide counterevidence to the thought of being a failure. Situations that have been annotated with emotions such as "love" and generally positive social situations likely contain counterevidence for self-labeling of the user as undesirable. Thus the PHA offers unique new possibilities, not possible in the offline world, to enter into a dialog with the user by identifying the user's issue and guiding him toward appropriate counterevidence from the PHA's knowledge base. This knowledge base ideally contains both user-generated and expert-generated content. In addition to challenging negative thoughts, a similar technical approach might be usable to develop other cognitive resources such as optimism and hope.

Addressing Ethical Concerns and Data Privacy

In this section we discuss privacy and ethical concerns that arise when designing Positive Computing technology. The simple Personal Happiness Assistant described above already demonstrates significant privacy challenges. Little is considered as sensitive and personal as our emotions. The ability to manage and control the impression we give to others is basic to our lives. Unintended disclosure of this information can have disastrous consequences for its owner. An additional adversarial use of this sort of technology is hinted at by the fact that GSR sensors are used in lie detectors (besides sensors measuring heart rate, blood pressure, and breathing rate). Picard discusses the lie detector concern (Picard, 1997) concluding that it is very hard to use this technology *against* the user's will. Users can fool these systems with some effort or training which gives reassurance. Nevertheless, disclosure of data that has been "objectively" collected about intimate details of our lives can greatly contradict our interests, e.g., when abused by the government, marketers, or our spouse. It is thus of utmost importance to put the data subject in full control of his own data, to educate him about risks and how to protect against them, and also to apply strong technical privacy and security protection measures (see, e.g., Spiekermann & Cranor, 2009, for background on how to engineer systems in a privacy protecting manner). These protection measures include the use of default encryption of collected records so that lost or stolen devices do not compromise a user's privacy, and the ability for users to entirely rewrite and "fake" their own records to give some protection in the presence of coercion to disclose them. Another applicable good privacy practice is to put policies in place that service providers keep user data only for a relatively short time and to have mechanisms to enforce this (e.g., by external audits). Otherwise the data are at risk of being subpoenaed in criminal or civil cases (e.g., divorce) or could be broken into. Typically, in the United States, legal protections for data kept on personal devices are higher than for data residing on the servers of some third-party providers. Another relevant privacy practice to reduce the risk from sharing of information is *minimization* of the information flow to what is needed for the task at hand, rather than sharing everything by default. For example uploading a daily emotional "average" to a social networking site is less risky then sharing detailed emotion maps and whereabouts. The latter data could be abused by marketers and stalkers. Even if obvious identifiers are removed from such data they may still remain unique and thereby remain at least in principle linkable to an individual (e.g., Narayanan & Shmatikov, 2008). Nevertheless, good techniques for pseudonymizing and aggregating data prior to sharing them with other parties or applications are necessary for good privacy. Another important protection mechanism will be the design of reasonable default and easily customizable policies for whom data are shared with (coach/therapist, friends, the public, Positive Psychology researchers, etc.)

Cloud service providers that are entrusted with Positive Computing related data have to make themselves accountable for implementing best security, privacy and data handling practices and provide tangible proof that demonstrates they are doing the right thing? Another key question is whether the legal regimes in various parts of the world adequately protect these data. Privacy laws in EU countries treat privacy as a human right and put strict limitations on how sensitive data (which include in the EU definition data about health, sexual orientation, union membership, etc) can be used. In other jurisdictions this is less clear.

Another type of a very practical privacy issue that arises when designing Positive Computing technologies is how to give users real-time feedback or alerts. Users may not wish this to be obvious to other people they are with. SMS messages can be a private channel to alert users. For an application in which a user tracks his exercise goals Consolvo et al. (2008a) created an aesthetically pleasing cell phone screen display based on the metaphor of a garden. The closer the user comes to reaching his goals, the more the garden is populated with flowers, bees, etc. Providing users access to an interface that tracks a variety of goals without revealing to outsiders what exactly is being tracked might provide an acceptable privacy compromise for only moderately concerned users.

There are other ethical concerns beyond privacy that designers need to be aware of. A technology that is meant to assist people in enhancing their autonomy has an extra responsibility to honor user autonomy and related ethical principles in its own interactions with the user. There has been a rich discussion on ethics in the persuasive technology community (Fogg, 2003; Berdichevsky & Neuenschwander, 1999; Atkinson, 2006; Davis, 2009) and many of the insights carry over to Positive Computing. First, a user needs to be made fully made aware of how the technology is intended to influence him and how it is working. This way he can make an informed decision whether he wants to use it. Second, the technology should not misinform about the data collected, results of an analysis and other information. We already mentioned the principle that technology which deeply interacts with how people live their lives needs to be carefully designed not to push values or behaviors on people that are not their own. Fogg recommends to conduct a "stakeholder analysis" as part of an ethically aware design process. Such an analysis should involve all the direct and sometimes also indirect users of the technology and consider their respective needs, benefits, and losses. (Indirect users of the PHA include other people, e.g., a partner, who might be affected by the use of the technology.)

Another ethical issue to look out for is whether technology introduces biases against certain groups of people. As a cartoonish example of an ethically question-able Positive Computing technology imagine, an application that advises people to surround themselves only with upbeat people on the theory that happiness has been shown to be "contagious." Then after a user has rated her acquaintances with respect to their perceived levels of happiness the application tracks and monitors whom the user calls, sends emails to and allocates calendar time with and attempts to influence the user to spend more time with the "happy" people and less time with the "unhappy" people. This application increases discrimination rather than reducing it and is at best a zero-sum game as it arguably reduces the happiness of the already unhappy group even further. A more "compassionate" win–win application would keep track that users on a regular basis share at least some of their time with people who are less fortunate then they are. (Positive Psychology has validated the many benefits that come from "giving" as well.)

In conclusion I believe that through a combination of technical and policy mea-sures privacy and security concerns can be sufficiently addressed possibly at the cost of limiting excessive data sharing. A design process which pays sufficient attention to the benefits for individual stakeholders and groups is likely to lead to Positive Computing applications that are useful to its primary users without harming or unduly disadvantaging others.

Concluding Remarks

This chapter suggests to study systematically how computing can assist human flourishing, i.e., Positive Computing. Clearly, the ideas are at an early stage, but as this chapter demonstrates there is already plenty of existing technology that can be adapted for raising psychological well-being. The overall goal of bringing about flourishing through technology provides an intriguing new perspective for looking at technology and its uses. It provides novel sub-goals to design for (say to raise a user's positivity ratio above a 3:1 threshold (Fredrickson, 2009) or to help correct negativity biases). For Positive Psychology researchers and computer scientists this creates exciting opportunities for collaboration. By combining their respective strengths, namely, the grounding of Positive Psychology in scientific methods and the ability of computer scientists to create powerful technologies, this will surely produce results that would not be possible by either group acting alone. If Positive Computing technology is made fun, exciting and engaging I have no doubt that this will be successful with consumers as well.

References

Atkinson, B. (2006). Captology: A critical review. *Proceedings of the First International Conference on Persuasive Technology*, 171–182.

Bailenson, J., & Yee, N. (2005). Digital chameleons: Automatic assimilation of nonverbal gestures in immersive virtual environments. *Psychological Science, 16*, 814–819.

Berdichevsky, D., & Neuenschwander, E. (1999). Toward an ethics of persuasive technology. *Communications of the ACM, 43*(5), 51–58.

CAPP strengths assessment tool. Retrieved from www.cappeu.com/realise2.htm

Chang, A., Resner, B., Koerner, B., Wang, X., & Ishii, H. (2001). *LumiTouch: An emotional communication device.* Proceedings from the CHI'01 Extended Abstracts on Human Factors in Computing Systems, Seattle, WA.

Clifton Strengthsfinder. Retrieved from www.strengthsfinder.com

Consolvo, S., Klasnja, P., McDonald, D. W., Avrahami, D., Froehlich, J., LeGrand, L., et al. (2008a). *Flowers or a robot army? Encouraging awareness & activity with personal, mobile displays.* Proceedings from the 10th international Conference on Ubiquitous Computing, Seoul, Korea.

Consolvo, S., McDonald, D. W., Toscos, T., Chen, M. Y., Froehlich, J., Harrison, B., et al. (2008b). *Activity sensing in the wild: A field trial of UbiFit garden.* Proceedings of the Conference on Human Factors & Computing Systems, Florence, Italy.

Daily, S. (2005). Digital story explication as it relates to emotional needs and learning. *Media Arts and Sciences.*

Davis, J. (2009). *Design methods for ethical persuasive computing.* Proceedings from the 4th International Conference on Persuasive Technology, Claremont, CA.

Deci, E., & Ryan, R. (2000). The "what" and "why" of goal pursuits: Human needs and the self-determination of behavior. *Psychological Inquiry, 11*, 227–268.

Denning, T., Andrew, A., Chaudhri, R., Hartung, C., Lester, J., Borriello, G., et al. (2009). *BALANCE: Towards a usable pervasive wellness application with accurate activity inference.* Proceedings of the 10th Workshop on Mobile Computing Systems and Applications, Santa Cruz, CA.

Diener, E. (1984). Subjective well-being. *Psychological Bulletin, 95*, 542–575.

Diener, E. (1994). Assessing subjective well-being: Progress and opportunities. *Social Indicators Research, 31*, 103–157.

Diener, E., Lucas, R., Schimmack, U., & Helliwell, J. (2009). *Well-being for public policy*. Oxford: Oxford University Press USA.

Fletcher, R., Dobson, K., Goodwin, M. S., Eydgahi, H., Wilder-Smith, O., Fernholz, D., et al. (2010). iCalm: Wearable sensor and network architecture for wirelessly communicating and logging autonomic activity. *IEEE Transactions on Information Technology in Biomedicine, 14*(2), 215–223.

Fogg, B. (2003). *Persuasive technology: Using computers to change what we think and do*. San Francisco: Morgan Kaufmann Publishers.

Fogg, B., & Allen, E. (2009). *10 uses of texting to improve health*. Proceedings from the 4th international Conference on Persuasive Technology, Claremont, CA.

Fredrickson, B. (2009). *Positivity: Groundbreaking research reveals how to embrace the hidden strength of positive emotions, overcome negativity, and thrive*. New York: Random House, Inc.

Hassenzahl, M. (2008). *User experience (UX): Towards an experiential perspective on product quality*. Proceedings from the 20th international Conference of the Association Francophone D'interaction Homme-Machine, Metz, France.

Hassenzahl, M., & Tractinsky, N. (2006). User experience – A research agenda. *Behaviour and Information Technology, 25*(2), 91–97.

Hayes, S., Strosahl, K., & Wilson, K. (1999). *Acceptance and commitment therapy: An experiential approach to behavior change*. New York: Guilford Press.

Hodges, S., Williams, L., Berry, E., Izadi, S., & Srinivasan, J. (2006). *Sensecam: A retrospective memory aid*. Proceedings of Ubicomp, Orange County, CA, 177–193.

Hoven, E., & Eggen, B. (2008). Informing augmented memory system design through autobiographical memory theory. *Personal and Ubiquitous Computing, 12*(6), 433–443.

Huppert, F. A., & So, T. T. C. (2009). *Measuring subjective well-being: An opportunity for NSOs?* Proceedings from OECD/ISQOLS Meeting, Florence, Italy.

Karat, J., Karat, C., & Vergo, J. (2004). Experiences people value: The new frontier of task analysis. In N. A. Stanton (Eds.), *The handbook of task analysis for human-computer interaction* (pp. 585–603). New York: Elsevier.

Keyes, C. L. K. (2009). *Toward a science of mental health*. Oxford: Oxford University Press USA.

Lyubomirsky, S. (2008). *The how of happiness: A scientific approach to getting the life you want*. New York: Penguin Group.

Lyubomirsky, S., King, L., & Diener, E. (2005). The benefits of frequent positive affect: Does happiness lead to success? *Psychological Bulletin, 131*, 803–855.

Markus, H., & Kitayama, S. (1991). Culture and the self: Implications for cognition, emotion, and motivation. *Psychological Review, 98*, 224–253.

Millard, N., & Hole, L. (2008). In the Moodie: Using 'affective widgets' to help contact centre advisors fight stress. *Affect and Emotion in Human-Computer Interaction: From Theory to Applications, 4868*, 186–193.

Narayanan, A., & Shmatikov, V. (2008). Robust de-anonymization of large sparse datasets. *Security and Privacy, 18*, 111–125.

Nold, C. (2009). *Emotional cartography – Technologies of the self*. Retrieved from http://emotionalcartography.net

Pennebaker, J., France, M., & Booth, R. (2001). *Linguistic inquiry and word count (liwc): Liwc2001*. Mahwah, NJ: Lawrence Erlbaum Associates.

Pentland, A., Lazer, D., Brewer, D., & Heibeck, T. (2009). *Using reality mining to improve public health and medicine*. Robert Wood Johnson Foundation [White Paper].

Picard, R. (1997). *Affective computing*. Cambridge: MIT.

Pressman, S., & Cohen, S. (2005). Does positive affect influence health? *Psychological Bulletin, 131*, 925–971.

Reeves, B., & Nass, C. (1996). *The media equation: How people treat computers, television, and new media like real people and places*. New York: Cambridge University Press.

Reivich, K., & Shatté, A. (2003). *The resilience factor: 7 keys to finding your inner strength and overcoming life's hurdles*. Noida: Random House.

Reynolds, C. (1999). *Measurement of frustration with computers*. Cambridge: MIT.

Ryff, C. (1989). Happiness is everything, or is it? Explorations on the meaning of psychological well-being. *Journal of Personality and Social Psychology, 57*, 1069–1081.

Seligman, M. (1998). *Learned optimism*. New York: Pocket Books.

Seligman, M. (2002). *Authentic happiness: Using the new positive psychology to realize your potential for lasting fulfillment*. New York: Simon and Schuster.

Seligman, M. (2008). Positive health. applied psychology. *An International Review, 57*, 3–18.

Sheldon, K., & Elliot, A. (1999). Goal striving, need-satisfaction, and longitudinal well-being: The self-concordance model. *Journal of Personality and Social Psychology, 76*, 482–497.

Sheldon, K., & Houser-Marko, L. (2001). Self-concordance, goal-attainment, and the pursuit of happiness: Can there be an upward spiral? *Journal of Personality and Social Psychology, 80*, 152–165.

Sung, A., Marci, C., & Pentland, A. (2005). Objective physiological and behavioral measure for tracking depression. *Technical Report, 595*, 1–20.

VIA inventory of strengths. Retrieved from www.viacharacter.org

Vizer, L. M. (2009). *Detecting cognitive and physical stress through typing behaviour*. Proceedings from the 27th International Conference Extended Abstracts on Human Factors in Computing Systems, Boston, MA.

Zimmerman, J. (2009). *Designing for the self: Making products that help people become the person they desire to be*. Boston: ACM Press.

Part VII
Change the World

Chapter 18
Changing the World: The Science of Transformative Action

Scott Sherman

It was considered the most dangerous place in America.

If terrorists could target one place in the nation, this would be it. Inside these gates, there was enough plutonium and uranium to kill tens of millions of people. Inside these gates, if you could breach the security, you would find the "most deadly devices ever invented" (Cameron & Lavine, 2006) by humankind.

Everywhere armed guards patrolled the property from watchtowers that resembled prison fortresses. Anti-aircraft guns shielded against a blitz from above. The walls were constructed several feet thick, so as to withstand invasions and attacks. Menacing razor wire fences kept out intruders, and security cameras kept watch over your every move.

To stop suicide bombers, powerful security measures had been installed. Sentries with submachine guns would halt you at the entrance and swab your car for explosive residues. There were more armed guards at the second stop, scanning your fingerprints to match them with government records. To enter through this second station, you needed to have top-secret clearance; the government would investigate the details from the last 10 years of your life.

After all, national security was at stake.

You had to get clearance through two more security stops, each one more intensive and thorough than the last. Guards with automatic weapons reviewed your entrance permits behind windows of bulletproof glass and 4-inch thick metal doors.

And if you finally made it inside, you would discover what had once been shrouded in secrecy:

This was the birthplace of every nuclear weapon America had ever produced.

This was Rocky Flats. For years, this place in Colorado had been clandestine and concealed. It was only 16 miles from Denver, but few residents of that city had any idea what was here.

They did not know that, every single day, the world's most lethal weapons were being produced in their backyards. These were plutonium pits—hollow spheres,

S. Sherman (✉)
Transformative Action Institute, Los Angeles, CA, USA
e-mail: ssherman@transformativeaction.org

R. Biswas-Diener (ed.), *Positive Psychology as Social Change*,
DOI 10.1007/978-90-481-9938-9_18, © Springer Science+Business Media B.V. 2011

some as small as grapefruits. But each one could destroy a major city. Each one had the explosive force of the bomb that razed Hiroshima. That bomb alone had killed 140,000 people.

But this description didn't even begin to hint at the deadly force of the Rocky Flats arsenal. The plutonium pits produced at Rocky Flats were far more destructive than the atomic blasts that had laid waste to Japanese cities. These pits were just the first step in a chain reaction; they would detonate a thermonuclear fire 600 times stronger than the A-bombs used in World War II (Obmascik, 2000). Each one unleashed a force equivalent to 18 billion pounds of TNT.

During the time of the Cold War, there were more than 70,000 of these nuclear triggers produced at Rocky Flats. Yet the weapons plant operated in total secrecy. Because of national security concerns, it was hidden from public sight. Few citizens and neighbors even knew about the danger in their backyard.

Until the accident.

In 1969, a small piece of plutonium spontaneously burst into flames. It ignited a firestorm that swept through the Rocky Flats complex, releasing radioactive materials into the skies above Denver. It was the largest industrial fire in the history of the United States, causing $200 million in damage. A subsequent investigation revealed that this was not the first mishap at the facility. There had been a history of nuclear accidents, undisclosed and unbeknownst to the public.

Thus began an ugly conflict and controversy that betrayed the deep ideological fissures in the nation.

On one side were the people who believed that this site was vital to national security. Most workers at Rocky Flats, for instance, took pride in performing their patriotic duty: They were defending the United States against nuclear attack. They were providing safety against the "evil empire" of the Soviet Union. By building thousands of nuclear weapons, they were deterring an enemy's assault on the country.

Indeed, this was during the Cold War, a time fraught with peril and fear. American schools instructed children how to duck and cover to protect themselves from atomic attacks. The Russian leader Nikita Kruschev had taunted the Western powers, threatening: "We will bury you!" In the Cuban missile crisis, the world had gone to the brink of thermonuclear war. To the defenders of Rocky Flats, it seemed obvious that they were on the front lines of protecting the nation. They were responsible for a strong national defense.

On the other side were citizens and activists who were worried about the government spending hundreds of billions of dollars on unnecessary weapons of mass destruction. They cited the problem of "overkill"—the fact that there were already enough nuclear weapons to destroy life on earth many times over. A single nuclear launch would invite massive retribution that would leave more than 100 million Americans dead, as well as billions more people across the planet. Prominent scientists warned of nuclear winter that could lead to the extinction of the human race, and the devastation of the planet. "Except for fools and madmen, everyone knows that nuclear war would be an unprecedented human catastrophe," wrote Carl Sagan (Sagan, 1983).

In the decade after the accident, tens of thousands of people came out to Rocky Flats to protest the proliferation of nuclear weapons. Hundreds were arrested as they put their bodies on the railroad tracks, trying to halt the transportation of nuclear materials.

In 1982, two Catholic nuns actually managed to infiltrate Rocky Flats, raising a flag that dubbed it a "Death Factory." They were dragged away by security guards just as they were hanging another sign, comparing Rocky Flats to Nazi concentration camps (Buffer, 2003).

But it was not just a nuclear holocaust that the activists feared. They also warned of the environmental consequences of a radioactive leak. This could be devastating to the earth, not to mention public health. The toxic and carcinogenic materials on this site were unprecedentedly high. Thirteen rooms at Rocky Flats had radioactive levels of "infinity"—that is, radioactivity levels so high that they went off the scale on measuring devices (Obmscik, 2000).

The workers at the plant felt under siege. As building manager Bob DeGrazio remembered, employees felt that they were "saving the world" from the danger of Soviet attacks. But instead of gratitude, he and his coworkers were met only with hatred. "We were called murderers," he recalled (Interview, January 2007).

This distrust pervaded everything. The people at Rocky Flats had a bunker mentality—as if they were fighting against the entire world, including their fellow Americans. They especially had a hostile, antagonistic relationship with Congress and federal agencies. The workers knew that they were not subject to government regulation or oversight. Because of national security concerns, they had the right to keep everything confidential. But the government, egged on by the citizens, wanted to investigate possible violations of environmental law. Given the secret history of radioactive leaks and accidents, legislators were concerned that hazardous wastes and nuclear disasters could poison millions of people throughout the American West.

To the staff at Rocky Flats, environmental laws were nuisances. As one manager recalled, the whole situation was "very combative. [We] saw the regulators and activist community as enemies" (Cameron & Lavine, 2006).

And little did they know that the enemies were about to attack.

In 1989, the federal government launched a raid. Dozens of FBI agents, armed with guns and search warrants, stormed the site. For the next 20 days, they occupied the buildings and shut down all operations.

Borrowing the terminology of a military invasion, they called their offensive "Operation Desert Glow." It was unprecedented for one government agency to declare war on another. But this was a criminal investigation. Members of the Justice Department joined in on the raid. They alleged massive violations of the law and crimes that could endanger people's lives.

Rocky Flats was a mess. The problems seemed too big and costly to solve within our lifetimes. The government estimated that it would take 70 years and $36 billion to clean up the dangerous residues of the nuclear weapons produced there. And these threats would not truly disappear for millennia; the half-life of plutonium was more than 24,000 years (Cameron & Lavine, 2006).

For the average citizen, this situation could seem overwhelming. Rocky Flats was a lightning rod for some of the most controversial, contentious issues of our time:

Terrorism.
National security.
Nuclear weapons.
Environmental catastrophe.
A massive threat to human health.

All sides in the drama were entrenched for a major battle. But how could anyone win? When the battle lines were so ugly and divisive, how could you solve a problem so enormous?

More than a decade ago, I set out to investigate the mystery of Rocky Flats, as well as hundreds of places like it—places where people seemed to confront insurmountable obstacles and enemies on all sides. These were some of the biggest problems that society faced: from economic woes to crises of public health and education. In sum, they were very much like the crises that we see in America today.

I wanted to know how ordinary citizens—people like you and me—could actually go out and change the world. How could we overcome the biggest problems that we face?

For years, I had heard people quote the dictum of Margaret Mead: "Never doubt that a small group of committed citizens can change the world. In fact, it's the only thing that ever has." But, as comforting as these words may have been, they didn't actually explain *how* citizens could make a difference. Was there a science to social change? Were there strategies that would reliably lead people to win?

Like President Obama, I had been a community organizer in my younger days. I had been engaged in actions where committed citizens were trying to take power over their own lives. I had seen countless people try to confront massive problems that faced them—from racism and violence to deadly chemicals that threatened to poison their children.

Many of these people were poor. Many were women. Most were people of color. All were individuals who had traditionally been excluded from the corridors of power.

Often they were fighting the most powerful forces in the world. Often they were battling the US President, the Congress, and multinational corporations. Often they were outspent 1,000 to 1.

And often they were winning.

This was an unsung story of modern-day heroism. It wasn't featured on the nightly news; nobody read about it in the daily papers. But there were dozens of successful cases of ordinary citizens, against all odds, solving the biggest problems that bedevil our society.

Of course, countless other citizens were unsuccessful. I had seen so many community struggles take years and years, only to end in loss and frustration. I had seen so many good-hearted people get burnt out. I had seen so many people feel overwhelmed and exhausted.

It was no wonder that most people felt powerless to make change. A national survey of American college students showed that millions subscribed to the pessimistic claim that, "realistically, an individual can do little to bring about major changes in our society" (Hurtado & Pryor, 2007).

It seemed to me that such cynicism was unwarranted. After all, there were so many heartwarming stories of individuals who had succeeded. There were countless organizers and activists with years of experience in social change—people who had fought hundreds of battles and passed down their lessons. There were training manuals and workshops, each one promising to reveal what led citizens to victory.

I was chagrinned to find, however, that there was little agreement about what actually worked. Changing the world was more art than science. Everyone had a pet theory about the best way to make a difference. Many times these theories seemed to contradict each other; many times, when I tried to put them into practice, they backfired.

There was no scientific research into how people actually could change the world. Nobody had analyzed the hundreds of case studies to find common factors that led to success and failure.

So until the time that research was done, there would continue to be lots of contradictory stories, false exhortations, and utopian words of advice. There would be many romantic, idealistic quotes (like the one by Margaret Mead) about people's power to make a difference. And, of course, there would be slogans.

I remember one time in California, when I watched a crowd of hundreds of individuals marching through the streets, chanting the familiar refrain: "The people, united, will never be defeated!"

A friend of mine, who was a stand-up comedienne, whispered to me jokingly: "I don't think it's actually true!

"Maybe we should change the slogan to be more accurate," she added, tongue-in-cheek. "Maybe we should march through the streets, chanting: 'The people, united, will sometimes win and sometimes lose!'"

While her point was humorous, it made me return to the fundamental question: When do people actually win, and when do people lose?

I decided to do the research myself. I went back to the university to study the science of social change. For nearly a decade, I conducted doctoral research into what actually worked when people tried to change the world.

I ended up reviewing hundreds of case studies of citizens working for public health, environmental protection, women's rights, racial justice, and social equality. I selected sixty for which I could find the most information. Then, for each of these cases, I coded for nearly 120 factors that might be correlated with success and failure.

And, at the end of 10 years, the results were surprising:

Almost everything that I believed to be true was wrong.

I had been taught that law would work.

But research proved this to be false.

In fact, after reviewing dozens of cases across the country, I found that legal strategies were one of the factors most strongly correlated with failure. When people went to court, they almost always lost.

Perhaps this shouldn't be surprising. After all, many of these citizens had little access to money or powerful attorneys; they couldn't afford the legal costs. "Poor people have access to the courts," quipped one judge in Texas, "in the same sense that Christians had access to the lions when they were dragged into a Roman arena" (Elias, 1990).

Moreover, people tended to feel like control was out of their hands once they placed their faith in attorneys. Even the best pro bono legal teams spoke in complicated jargon and Latin phrases that seemed baffling to the citizens.

But worst of all, the law only divided the parties further. The legal system was adversarial. Rather than bringing parties together toward a common solution, it tended to exacerbate differences. It polarized opponents and made enemies for life. Legal strategies were not going to succeed.

Fortunately, I had been taught that politics would work.

But the research proved this to be a myth as well.

The problem with politics was that it wasn't an equal playing field. If people got together to sign petitions and lobby legislators and speak at public hearings, their chances of victory were slim. After all, the opposing side had more money and more power; most importantly, it had more connections to the people in power. Lobbyists for corporations might dine with the decision makers in Washington; they played golf together and sent their children to the same private schools. Ordinary citizens stood little chance of getting their own voices heard, no matter how many voting campaigns or other political events they attended.

So if law didn't work and politics didn't work, perhaps science would be more successful. Especially in cases like Rocky Flats, where people felt like they were being poisoned, all they would have to do is show evidence of harm. They could get scientists from universities who would run epidemiological studies that proved the presence of dangerous radioactive isotopes. Then surely they would win.

The research appeared to dash this hope as well.

Scientific arguments were not triumphant because both sides could quote them. Where citizens showed scientific studies showing threats to human health, corporations and governments would counter with their own experts, who showed that a site was perfectly safe. Given conflicting evidence, it was hard for ordinary people to win.

At this point, you may wonder what was successful. Law didn't work; politics didn't work; and even science didn't work. Thus many groups decided to "fight the power."

They decided to target the enemy, to focus on one individual, and to humiliate that person until he conceded defeat.

They engaged in the art of war—an antagonistic, adversarial battle where they would take any means necessary to defeat their foe. They would play on people's rage; they would mobilize followers by stirring up their fears and their hatreds; they would win at other people's expense.

While these tactics may seem unduly harsh, they are actually the rules of engagement for most political battles in the United States. These cutthroat strategies are precisely the ones that Republicans often use against Democrats, and the ones that Democrats often use against Republicans.

And they, too, do not work.

I was astonished. My research had destroyed every myth about how to change the world. All the conventional wisdom was wrong.

Indeed, there was a simple reason that the most popular strategies—even the ones used by powerful politicians in major parties—were so unsuccessful in making a difference in the world.

These strategies resembled a never-ending feud, one in which both sides tried to cripple each other. Each time that they were vanquished by their foes, they would aim for vengeance and retribution against their enemies. Any victory was temporary. In the end, everyone was weakened. As Gandhi commented, "The philosophy of an eye for an eye leaves the whole world blind."

The entire idea of waging war against your enemies was dangerous. When people engaged in adversarial, antagonistic battles, they were doing little to solve their problems.

In fact, I realized that my whole research had been framed around the wrong question. I had originally been asking: How does David conquer Goliath? How do people overcome the world's largest corporations and governments?

But what I found was that the military metaphor blinded me from the truth: The way people succeeded was not adversarial at all. Instead of fighting the power, they *leveraged* the power of corporations and governments to work for a better future. As Lincoln once noted, the best way to eliminate your enemy is to make him your friend.

These winning strategies I have come to call "transformative action." In the rest of this chapter, I will give a brief overview of how transformative action works.

The first principle of transformative action—the first strategy for success—is exposing injustice.

Many of the biggest scandals of the last few decades were illegal or unethical acts taking place under the cover of secrecy. Think of Enron and its corporate fraud. Think of Bernie Madoff and his $50 billion-dollar Ponzi scheme. These deceptions could not have taken place had there been greater transparency and accountability. Instead, they were hidden from view. When people exposed each of these schemes, they collapsed.

Immoral and illegal practices can only thrive in secrecy, when they are well hidden from view. For example, corporations often release thousands of tons of illicit chemicals into the air and water; it is cheaper for them to do this illegal dumping, rather than disposing of the materials properly or retrofitting their facilities to produce less waste. They know that the government has limited capacity for enforcing environmental laws; the chances are that they won't get caught in their illegal behavior.

However, if individuals can shine the light of day upon these transgressions, then everyone can see the problem. The citizens are likely to stir the consciences of thousands of people; even their adversaries will be ashamed when their behavior is brought to light. The executives at these corporations know that their actions were wrong; that's why they tried to hide such illicit behavior from view. When such transgressions are brought to light, it can cause a public relations disaster for the company. The shareholders may suffer as well, as the stock drops.

Supreme Court Justice Louis Brandeis once noted that, "sunlight is the best disinfectant." In other words, it is only by shining light on problems in society that we can start to heal them. If left in the dark, corruption and deceit can infect everything.

Transformative action is about "speaking the truth to power." But it does not seek to demonize anyone; it's not about embarrassing, humiliating, or treating people like enemies who need to be destroyed. Instead it's about overcoming the problems of society, while uplifting all people.

In this sense, the first principle of transformative action builds upon the legacy of nonviolence pioneered by Mohandas Gandhi, Dorothy Day, Martin Luther King, Jr., Cesar Chavez, Aung Saan Suu Kyi, and other social change leaders of the twentieth century.

Nonviolent strategies have proven extraordinarily successful at exposing injustice and protesting social problems in the last 100 years. All around the world, the strategies of nonviolent social change have produced dramatic transformations that would have been thought impossible just a few decades ago.

The entire Soviet Union collapsed without a fight. Communism virtually vanished from Europe without violence. Meanwhile, brutal military dictatorships across South America were overturned peacefully and democratically by the nonviolent masses. From the Philippines to Liberia, nonviolent revolutions also toppled brutal regimes. Most recently, in South Africa, a nonviolent movement led by Bishop Desmond Tutu and Nelson Mandela managed to end the racist regime of apartheid. Even against Nazi Germany, nonviolence was successful in the few cases it was attempted.

"The historical results were massive," commented political scientists Ackerman and DuVall. "Tyrants were toppled, governments were overthrown, occupying armies were impeded, and political systems that withheld human rights were shattered. Entire societies were transformed, suddenly or gradually, by people using their nonviolent resistance to destroy their opponents' capacity to control events" (Ackerman & DuVall, 2000).

Yet the potential of nonviolence has hardly been explored. As peace activist David Dellinger said, the "theory and practice of nonviolence are roughly at the same stage of development as those of electricity in the early days of Marconi and Edison" (Nagler, 1982).

To call on the words of Gandhi:

> We are constantly being astonished these days at the amazing discoveries in the field of violence. But I maintain that far more undreamt of and seemingly impossible discoveries will be made in the field of nonviolence. (Easwaran, 1978, p. 50)

Indeed, Gandhi considered nonviolence itself to be a science. Yet, in his own lifetime, he was never able to scientifically prove how to transform hatred into goodwill or enemies into allies. Only in the last decade have scientists across the world made major breakthroughs in these areas...

Until recently, the science of psychology was devoted to what goes wrong with human beings. There was a diagnostic manual of nearly 1,000 pages that could help determine what mental illnesses and pathologies were afflicting humans. We knew much about depression, deviance, and disease. We could easily identify neurotic, psychotic, and sociopathic behavior. But we had little insight into humans at their best. Few scientists had studied excellence in our species.

This situation has been changing since the turn of the twenty-first century. Now there is burgeoning research into the field of positive psychology. Hundreds of studies have begun to identify what goes right with human beings: their strengths and character virtues—things like courage, love, compassion, kindness, and altruism.

These emerging scientific findings dovetail nicely with the second principle of transformative action: what we call "social aikido."

Social aikido is about the science of transforming negatives into positives. Just like the martial art of aikido, where you can turn the strength of your opponent into your advantage, this social phenomenon is about transforming enemies into allies and hatred into goodwill.

Why would goodwill be a superior strategy to hostility? Wouldn't it make sense that you should try to intimidate, harass, and humiliate your opponents until they become so weak that they succumb? This was certainly the traditional idea of how people win: You win by going to battle. You win by defeating the other side. This seems to make sense.

In fact, conflict theory mostly studied how one side could gain a victory over the other (Oberschall, 1997). It was based on the idea that some people would win, while other people would inevitably lose. As one leading sociologist defined it, "the aims of the (parties in a conflict) are to neutralize, injure, or eliminate rivals" (Coser, 1956).

Social aikido turns this idea on its head: It insists that the true goal is for *everyone* to win. The ideal situation is to "exalt all sides" (Easwaran, 1978). Instead of triumphing over their antagonists, citizens seek to eliminate the antagonisms all together.

Transformative action changes the struggle from one of "you versus me," to one where "you and I are working together against the common problems we share." From a very practical standpoint, it is clear why this strategy might prove more effective than traditional conflict strategies: When two parties are struggling against each other, they often pour a great amount of energy, time, money, and resources into defeating the opponent, rather than the problem itself. What results? The losing side is often bitter and resentful. It may have lost the battle, but it will probably seek revenge.

For example, most protest movements in the United States mobilize hundreds of grassroots activists and enraged citizens against the existing power structure. They denounce corporate leaders and government officials. They hold mock trials of their enemies, condemning them for "crimes against humanity." They burn their opponents in effigy and rally against their evils.

These strategies often prove ineffective for several reasons: First, they attack people, rather than attacking the problem. Second, they encounter tremendous resistance from the people being attacked. The government leaders and corporate executives invest a considerable amount of energy, time, and resources into battling back against the grassroots activists. There builds up an enormous amount of anger, resentment, ill will, and acrimony between the warring parties. Meanwhile, the problems themselves are rarely solved. The groups have been focusing all their attention on each other, rather than the problems that confront them.

A transformative movement seeks to change the perspective from a win–lose situation to a win–win situation. This is the basis of negotiation theory, consensus building, and alternative dispute resolution (Fisher & Ury, 1991). It is a powerful force for bringing people together. It seeks to transform the enemy into a friend. It is based on understanding and respect, rather than divisiveness and conflict.

Hundreds of scientific studies have supported the idea that people working together will be much more productive than people who are competing against each other. For instance, social psychologists David and Roger Johnson reviewed dozens of studies that had been conducted in North America on the effects of competition and cooperation. Most of the evidence showed that people performed better when they were united with others toward a common goal rather than when they were competing against opponents. Sixty-five studies found that working together leads to higher achievement and success in an activity than does competition. Only eight studies came to the opposite conclusion.

Indeed, after reviewing the extensive literature on the subject, researcher Alfie Kohn concluded that competition "drags us down, devastates us psychologically, poisons our relationships (and) interferes with our performance" (Kohn, 1986). In fact, the "superiority of cooperation held for all subject areas and all age groups" (Kohn, 1986). From business to education to social change, cooperative efforts seem to produce the best results.

The findings of conflict resolution theory confirm that cooperative strategies are the most effective. At the end of his life, Morton Deutsch, the leading scholar in the field, summarized the discoveries of his 50 years of studying conflict.

Studies repeatedly showed that people who use antagonistic and adversarial tactics are most likely to escalate the intensity of a conflict; the results of such strategies are increased hostility, suspicion, and distrust. They lead to a breakdown in communication and an atmosphere of threats and coercion. Overall, antagonistic tactics destroy relationships (Deutsch, 1985).

On the other hand, people who use cooperative strategies (similar to the principles of transformative action theory) tend to engage in constructive solutions to their problems.

According to all the evidence, the most profound and enduring positive changes in intergroup relations happen when groups are working together on a common goal. They are no longer fighting each other; they are now cooperating and uniting to achieve some greater victory that will leave all parties better off. The hostility and suspicion between the groups diminishes substantially; their communication improves; and, most importantly, they overcome the barriers and prejudices that had been dividing them.

But why is this so effective? This is where the lessons of positive psychology are so important. Researchers have studied the people who are most likely to be kind and altruistic. It turns out that happier people are more likely to help others in need.

This flies in the face of most conventional wisdom on social change. Saul Alinsky, the inspiration for community organizing, used to emphasize the need to "agitate" people and "rub their resentments raw." He figured that happy people would be complacent; they wouldn't care much about changing society. It's only people who were outraged and full of anger who would rise up in action.

And part of this is true: When people were outraged by some injustice, it was an effective way of rousing citizens who might ordinarily be apathetic. Citizens who had never been involved in politics would suddenly find themselves as leaders. Indeed, one of the principles of social movement theory is that "suddenly imposed grievances" are likely to cause a community to mobilize (McAdam, McCarthy, & Zald, 1988). A plan for a toxic waste incinerator is likely to mobilize angry opposition from the community. Citizens are likely to become upset, uniting against this perceived threat to their health and well-being.

Transformative action theory does not dispute the effectiveness of mobilizing people against injustice. Indeed, all of the major experiments of nonviolence—whether led by Gandhi, King, Chavez, or others—have come about in response to grave injustices such as exploitation or discrimination.

However, transformative action theory postulates that anger, while effective in mobilizing a social movement, will not be very effective at actually *solving* the problem. Anger hurts the individual; it breaks down social relations; it builds walls between people.

Overwhelming medical evidence shows the deleterious effects of anger. People who suffer from chronic hostility suffer a 5–7 time greater risk of dying before age 50; moreover, frequent feelings of frustration and rage can tremendously increase the chances of developing a life-threatening malady like heart attacks, strokes, cancer, depression, and anxiety (Novaco, 2000).

Moreover, anger leads to emotional distance and separation. It can harm people in many ways. Not only do people have less control over their behavior, they also invite dangers such as retaliation, social censure, and loss of supportive relationships. One medical expert described anger as "eruptive, destructive, unbridled, savage, venomous, burning, and consuming" (Novaco, 2000).

Of course, anger can also be seen as energizing and empowering. It can be seen as something valuable, especially in the face of injustice. As environmental activist Julia Butterfly Hill has written, "we have a right—and a responsibility—to be angry," when confronted with corporate malfeasance. "We have a right and responsibility to be angry when we see old-growth forests getting clearcut and toxic wastes being dumped in minority neighborhoods. We should *not* be victims, passively accepting injustice. Instead we should become indignant about injustice. But then we must convert that energy into something stronger. If we are angry when we act, it will destroy the situation and destroy us. Instead, we must transform our anger and transform the situation" (Hill, 2000a).

Hill continues: "I knew that to hate... was to be a part of that same violence I was trying to stop. . .. You see that a lot in activists. . .. The intense negative forces... wind up overcoming many of them. They get so absorbed by the hate and anger that they become hollow" (Hill, 2000b).

Martin Luther King, Jr. explained the same idea:

> In struggling for human dignity, the oppressed of the world must not allow themselves to become bitter or indulge in hate campaigns. To retaliate with hate or bitterness would do nothing but intensify the hate in the world. (King, 1986, p. 8)

For King, the central principle of nonviolence was love. This was not a sentimental, romantic notion. Instead, it meant goodwill toward all people—even those who were racist, even those who bombed his church and killed four little girls. King wanted to oppose people's actions, but not the people themselves. He wanted to get rid of the evil system, but "not the individual who happens to be misguided, who happens to be misled, who was taught wrong" (King, 1986).

Transformative strategies are never the result of anger or malice. Anger, rage, and hatred are forms of violence. True transformative action means not even harboring ill will toward your adversaries. This may sound difficult to do, but it is crucial for leading an effective movement. Late in his life, Gandhi commented:

> I have learnt through bitter experience the one supreme lesson to conserve my anger, and as heat conserved is transmuted into energy, even so our anger controlled can be transmuted into a power which can move the world. (Easwaran, 1978, p. 47)

But transformative action is more than just social aikido; it's more than simply fighting against injustice. There has to be a next step of constructing a better alternative. All the energy that is normally poured into anger should be channeled into constructive pursuits.

Typically, the most famous strategies of a nonviolent social change campaign are those that respond to injustice: marches, protests, boycotts, and acts of civil disobedience.

These are the techniques that the Civil Rights movement used very effectively throughout the South during the 1950s and 1960s. In cities such as Selma and Birmingham, they proved that these tactics could be very powerful in winning converts to their cause and in tearing down the structures of racism and injustice that scaffolded American society.

Yet King realized late in his life that responding to injustice was only the first step. It was a great victory to end discrimination in restaurants, but if African Americans did not have the money to purchase food in these restaurants, then their hard-won rights were meaningless.

In a similar vein, he once mused that:

> "If one is in search of a better job, it does not help to burn down the factory. If one needs more adequate education, shooting the principal will not help. ... (I)f housing is the goal, only building and construction will produce that end. To destroy anything, person or property, can't bring us closer to the goal we seek." (King, 1986, p. 58)

There needed to be a constructive program: a better alternative and vision for the future. This is the third principle of transformative action.

King was assassinated before he started on a constructive program. But this was already the direction that his thinking was taking in the last few years of his life. He was beginning to address problems of poverty and economic injustice; he was beginning to address the need for creating an entirely new society.

Ironically, it was Malcolm X who pointed out the psychology behind the constructive program. In his autobiography, he talked about the most important lesson he ever learned. His mentor, Elijah Muhammad, took two glasses of water. Into one of the glasses he poured some oil so that the water became viscous and dirty. The other glass remained clean, pure, and pristine. Never tell anyone that they have a dirty glass of water, he instructed Malcolm. They will resent you for pointing out their problems. They will go into denial. They will get upset. They may even end up fighting you.

A much better strategy is to hold up a clean glass of water and let the other person make a choice for himself (Haley, 1964).

After all, as transformative activist Sharif Abdullah, points out: "Protests are not effective in solving problems. They are good at *pointing out* problems, but they do nothing to resolve them.

"A person who spends his time fighting the power is really just acknowledging his own powerlessness. In effect, he is saying that he has no power to change conditions of his community; instead, he has to complain, scream, cajole, and coerce some other person to make some changes for him. A much better strategy is to acknowledge the power you already have to change conditions in your community" (Abdullah, 1993).

Abdullah contends that even the most impoverished people in communities fighting against toxic wastes have some power to make a difference in their community. The belief that they have no power is a jail that they have built for themselves. Indeed, Abdullah believes that people spend too much time protesting the conditions in which they live, rather than creating a constructive program around a better vision of the future.

"If I want to have the perfect chocolate chip cookies, I don't go out and protest the terrible cookies that are being made at the Keebler cookie factory," Abdullah comments. "Instead, I get a recipe, and I start making them for myself" (Abdullah, 1993). Similarly, if citizens want to create a better society, it does little good to spend their entire time protesting the old one. It's better to start creating the new society that they want to see.

In any constructive program, there must be positive, creative goals. Normally, revolutions are reacting to the problems of the past—trying to overthrow some unjust social order. But transformative revolutions look toward creating a better future. Essentially, they attempt to promote a vision of the ideal society.

Today there are literally thousands of people who are engaging in scientific experiments to create this better world. They are called social entrepreneurs.

Unlike traditional business entrepreneurs, who focus on making a profit, social entrepreneurs are using their expertise to solve the biggest problems facing society.

These are people like Katherine Chon. As a young girl, she read about the slavery in her history books. In college, she learned that slavery still exists in the modern world—that it is, in fact, the second largest criminal industry on the planet. Rather than drowning in despair or proclaiming that she was powerless, Chon helped start one of the most powerful and effective organizations in the world combating the trafficking of human beings. Her ultimate goal is to create a world without slavery.

Another social entrepreneur also got his start while he was still in college. Mark Hanis was a young man whose grandparents had survived the Holocaust. Like many Jews, he heard the vows that humanity would "never again" allow another genocide. Yet in college, he learned that there had been numerous campaigns of ethnic cleansing and mass murder since the time of the Nazis. In places like Cambodia, Serbia and Rwanda, the world stood by helplessly as millions of people were slaughtered. Hanis created an organization to end genocide in our times.

Still other social entrepreneurs are people like Majora Carter and Van Jones. They are creating an organization that seeks to address both the economic crisis and the ecological crisis at the same time. Their organization, Green for All, was dedicated to creating 5 million new jobs in environmental restoration and regeneration— jobs for impoverished people who otherwise would be drowning in the financial meltdown. They too have a powerful vision of the future.

All these social entrepreneurs were not just protesting the way that the world worked. They were taking power into their own hands to create a better future. As newscaster Scoop Nisker would say at the end of every depressing broadcast, "If you don't like the news, go make some of your own."

And so perhaps it would be a group of social entrepreneurs—unsung heroes and heroines—who would solve the problem of Rocky Flats.

Today the most dangerous place in the world has been transformed into a wildlife refuge.

The deadly weapons are gone. The machine guns, the prison-like fortresses, and the terrorist targets are history. The infinity rooms, where radioactive hazards measured off the charts, no longer exist.

Now deer, elk, and prairie dogs roam. Native flora and fauna are returning to the land, including species that had once been endangered and under threat of extinction. Even mountain lions have settled the refuge. One journalist described the land as "a hiker's dream" with rolling grasslands, deep valleys, and flourishing wildlife, set against a backdrop of snow-covered mountains (Kelly, 2005).

The solution is something that could not have been imagined in 1989, when the United States was still engaged in a Cold War against the Soviet Union. Now the entire communist threat is gone, transformed by a series of nonviolent revolutions. And the weapons facility that produced enough nuclear bombs to destroy the world has been transformed into fields of wildflowers.

It resembles nothing so much as the biblical image of beating swords into ploughshares. This is the world's first example of a nuclear weapons facility being shut down and transformed into peaceful purposes.

Most remarkably, the project was finished 60 years early, and more than $30 billion under budget. And it was cleaned to a standard that was 13 times more rigorous than the original federal regulations required.

How did they achieve such stunning results? This process had all the hallmarks of transformative action:

First of all, activists were successful in exposing the problem of injustice. For decades, the nuclear weapons facility had operated in complete secrecy. But a few courageous citizens voiced their concerns about pollution and contamination. At first they may have been dismissed. But their fears were soon vindicated. They were able to shine a light on serious violations of law—transgressions that could pose significant threats to human health.

But this was only the beginning. The real success of Rocky Flats came from a transformation of enemies into allies. All the parties that had previously distrusted each other—the workers, the government, and the local citizen activists—decided to work together toward a common vision.

Moreover, this vision was not simply about responding to problems, or just cleaning up the mess. It was a positive vision of a better future: a beautiful wildlife refuge where people could bike and hike, and where wildlife would flourish and thrive.

Of course, there are still critics of the Rocky Flats solution. One activist, LeRoy Moore of the Rocky Mountain Peace and Justice Center, does not believe that the site can ever be safe for humans. In his view, Rocky Flats will continue to be contaminated for thousands of years; even minimum levels of plutonium will pose a threat to human health.

But John Rampe, an environmental scientist, insists that the site is safe. Researchers have conducted hundreds of tests of the soil and wildlife to ensure that it is clean enough for families and children to visit. According to Rampe, the chances of anyone getting cancer from visiting the wildlife refuge are miniscule—approximately 1 in 200,000. And that level of risk would only come if people "made 100 visits a year, spending 2.5 h per visit for 30 years (Kelly, 2005).

The truth of the matter is that the site is remediated far better and faster than anyone could have ever imagined. If you would have told the protesters 20 years ago that the nuclear weapons facility would be transformed into a wildlife refuge, that enemies would have worked together, and that the culture of secrecy would have given way to transparency, they never would have believed it.

As Michigan Business Professor Kim Cameron attests, the real story of Rocky Flats is "the achievement of extraordinary success well beyond the expectations of almost any outside observer."

And this is the secret of success. When confronted by massive social problems, we need not give up hope. There is an actual science of how we solve them, and how we create the future.

As the futurist Buckminster Fuller once said, "You never change things by fighting the existing reality. To change something, build a new model that makes the existing model obsolete."

This is transformative action.

References

Abdullah, S. (1993). Interview by author, 2 July. Portland, Oregon.

Ackerman, P., & DuVall, J. (2000). Nonviolent power in the twentieth century. *PS: Political Science & Politics, 2*, 147–148.

Anger and resentment kill. (2000). Retrieved from http://www.angerviolence.com/health.html

Buffer, P. (2003, June). *Rocky flats history.* Retrieved from http://www.lm.doe.gov/documents/sites/co/rocky_flats/RockyFlats_HistoryBook_rev2.pdf

Cameron, K. S., & Lavine, M. (2006). *Making the impossible possible: Lessons from the cleanup of America's most dangerous nuclear weapons plant.* San Francisco: Berrett-Koehler.

Coser, L. (1956). *The functions of social conflict.* New York: The Free Press.

Deutsch, M. (1985). *Distributive justice: A social-psychological perspective.* New Haven, CT: Yale University Press.

Easwaran, E. (1978). *Gandhi the man.* Petaluma, CA: Niligri.

Elias, S. (1990). *Legal breakdown.* Berkeley, CA: Nolo Press.

Fisher, R., & Ury, W. (1991). *Getting to yes: Negotiating agreement without giving in.* New York: Penguin Books.

Haley, A. (1964). *The autobiography of Malcolm X.* New York: Castle Books.

Hill, J. (2000a). *The legacy of Luna.* San Francisco: Harper Collins.

Hill, J. (2000b). Speech to pioneers conference.

Hurtado, S., & Pryor, J. (2007). *The American freshman: National norms for fall 2006.* Los Angeles: Higher Education Research Institute, UCLA.

Interview with Bob Degrazio (2007, January). *Weapons to wildlife: The newsletter of the Rocky Flats Cold War Museum.*

Johnson, E. (1990). *The deadly emotions: The role of anger, hostility, and aggression in health and emotional well-being.* New York: Praeger.

Kelly, D. (2005, February 7). Dispatch from rocky flats: An idyllic scene polluted with controversy. *Los Angeles Times.*

King, M. (1986). *A testament of hope: The essential writings of Martin Luther King Jr.* San Francisco: Harper & Row.

Kohn, A. (1986). *No contest: The case against competition.* Boston: Houghton Mifflin.

McAdam, D., McCarthy, J., & Zald, M. (1988). *Social movements.* Newbury Park, CA: Sage Publications.

Nagler, M. (1982). *America without violence.* Covelo, CA: Island Press.

Niehoff, D. (1999). *The biology of violence: How understanding the brain, behavior, and environment can break the vicious circle of aggression.* New York: The Free Press.

Novaco, R. (1986). *Anger as a clinical and social problem.* Orlando, FL: Academic Press.

Novaco, R. (2000). *Anger.* Oxford: Oxford University Press.

Oberschall, A. (1997). *Social movements: Ideologies, interests, and identities*. London: Transaction Publishers.

Obmascik, M. (2000, June 25). Rocky Flats: The price of peace. *Denver Post*.

Sagan, C. (1983). *The nuclear winter*. Retrieved from http://www.cooperativeindividualism.org/sagan_nuclear_winter.html

Shekelle, R. (1983). Hostility, risk of coronary disease, and mortality. *Psychosomatic Medicine, 45*, 109–114.

Siegman, A., & Smith, T. (1994). *Anger, hostility, and the heart*. Hillside, NJ: Erlbaum.

Susskind, L., & Field, P. (1996). *Dealing with an angry public: The mutual gains approach to resolving disputes*. New York: The Free Press.

Williams, R. (1980). Type a behavior, hostility, and coronary arthrosclerosis. *Psychosomatic Medicine, 42*, 539–549.

Editor's Afterword

Editing a volume such as the one you are now holding in your hands is a privileged undertaking. I learned a tremendous amount reading these chapters – and a fair bit about editing. Someone once told me that it is only after you have taken a course that you are finally ready to take the course. This is certainly true of editing. Now that I have cut my teeth as an editor I feel as if I am truly ready to tackle a book like this! As the common lament goes: If only I had the opportunity to go back and do it again, knowing what I know now. . ...

The good news is that one of the lessons I learned is that an editor's afterword can be used as a professional catch-all to include additional information I feel is missing from this volume. In this case, I rely on the voices of prominent figures in positive psychology who did not contribute a chapter to this book. You have no idea how hard it is to pin down someone like Barb Fredrickson, whose speaking, teaching, and writing schedules are a juggling act of circus-act caliber. Academics tend to be busy, and my invitation to contribute to this book was met by several refusals, apologies, and consolations. I realized, however, that while many professionals may not have time to write an entire chapter virtually everyone has time to write a few words. To this end, I encouraged Fredrickson and other notables in the field of positive psychology to pass along brief commentaries.

I was particularly impressed with the commentaries of Todd Kashdan and Sonja Lyubomirsky, both of whom emphasized the personal responsibility of positive psychologists to affect the good that they study. Kashdan and Lyubomirsky both enjoy fast-paced research positions at highly respected universities. It would be easy enough for them to teach their courses, publish, and enjoy the public applause for their respective popular books. Instead, however, they openly advocate a wider definition of the role of researcher to include a more active role in public policy debates and improving societal institutions such as schools. It remains unclear to what extent political engagement might be seen as a compromise of scientific objectivity. Certainly, it is a potential tradeoff that every academic must weigh for himself or herself. Be that as it may, Kashdan and Lyubomirsky both make the case that academics must be willing, at the very least, to consider the issue. In their own words,

Todd Kashdan: Consider the litany of policy issues where psychology can inform best practice – education, healthcare, science and technology, international relationships, and preserving and enhancing the environment. More generally, from what we know about the mental biases of human beings, we can improve the decision making of individuals and groups. Our antiquated educational system is a prime example of the chasm between scientific knowledge and current practice. Currently, our schools require children to narrowly concentrate on discovering the *correct answer* to clearly defined questions formulated by other people. Unfortunately, this approach is divorced from what children confront in their daily lives – terrain where the problems often have yet to be formulated and the available information and possible answers are often ambiguous at best. Our children are being trained for the future by passively consuming information about what happened in the past. With this approach, our children are ill-prepared for practical and creative thinking. A more scientifically informed approach would focus on how to be mindfully aware of the unique nature of any given situation, how to tolerate ambiguity, and how to critically examine and synthesize diverse perspectives. This is not about being politically correct. This is about recognizing that our knowledge and perspective is limited. Among other biases, our preferences are driven by the status quo, immediate gratification, and comparisons to other people that are physically or socially nearby. For these reasons, only through multiple perspectives can we grasp the totality of an idea or issue. If we value productivity, creativity, motivation, and human welfare, then it is time for psychologists to leave the safety of their laboratories and enter the fray.

Sonja Lyubomirsky: Many people hold an idealistic portrait of the white-coat scientist – toiling over the lab bench, analyzing data, meeting in conference rooms with graduate students and post docs, and typing research reports. To me, the future of positive psychology cannot be divorced from its future as an empirical, hypothesis-testing-based science. But what is the point of that "pure" or "basic" science if it lodges itself in the laboratory, never ventures beyond the university classroom walls, or remains trapped in dense, abstruse journals? To be sure, many scientists do their work because they absolutely love the process of science – they labor just for the pure joy and pleasure and intellectual challenge. But we scientists are not paid to have this unadulterated joy satisfied. Ultimately, our salaries and research funding come from taxpayers and generous donations and students' fees. The fundamental goal of all of our committed efforts is to disseminate and interpret our theories and empirical findings to make a bona fide contribution to the world. Accomplishing this goal requires active and deliberate industry. And, fortunately, scientists (without lab coats) have found that doing good also happens to foster joy.

Barb Fredrickson took a somewhat different tack. Instead of commenting on the moral obligations of scientists she weighed in with an important message about the mechanism by which positive change might be brought to society. Not surprisingly for the originator of broaden and build theory, Fredrickson envisions positive emotion as having tremendous potential for creating a better world. What I like so much about this message is that most people consider emotion the domain of the individual. We often assume that our subjective emotional experiences reside deep within and are, by definition, a personal and unique phenomenon. Fredrickson argues just the opposite. Your happiness, as it were, becomes a social tonic to the extent that it directly affects those around you; and those around them. ...

Barb Fredrickson: Much positive psychology to date concerns individuals. This is certainly true of my own research focus, which centers on positive emotions. Studies from my and other labs have demonstrated that fleeting positive emotions – like joy, serenity, gratitude, and the like – expand the boundaries of awareness and initiate health-promoting biochemical cascades in ways that nourish personal development, little by little changing how people fare and who they become months down the road. It's vital to recognize, however, that emotions are contagious. Sophisticated social network analyses find that positive emotions are especially so, capable of "infecting" whole communities over time through both direct and indirect (e.g., your friend's friend's mother) social ties. What's good for the individual, then, turns out to be good for the collective. By cultivating positive emotions in ourselves, we not only unlock health-promoting processes within our own bodies and minds, but also, through our resultant actions and attitudes, we increase the odds that those around us find something to smile about, offering them a fresh dose of gratitude, joy, or amusement. With such ripple effects extending up to three degrees of separation, efforts aimed at social change can strategically target individuals situated within the hubs of their social networks. Interventions that increase their health and well-being are thus leveraged to increase the health and well-being of whole communities. With our ever-increasing globalization, positivity can even spread boundlessly across national borders, spreading peace and health, and building resilience to inevitable adversity and challenge. These collective positive psychology phenomena deserve greater empirical test in the decades to come.

Interestingly, two of the experts I contacted for this afterword spoke directly to the issue of positive uses of technology. As psychologists we often get wrapped up in the intriguing worlds of subjective construction, social influence and genetic determinants. Too rarely, in my opinion, do we acknowledge the importance of seemingly mundane daily activities like chatting on the phone, stopping at traffic signals, or online social networking. There is an increasing awareness that technology is a useful tool for delivering the innovations of positive psychology and for helping people to flourish. The commentaries offered by David Myers and Neal Mayerson dovetail nicely with the chapter on positive computing by Tomas Sander. In both cases, these men are not only important figures in positive psychology, but philanthropists who are harnessing technology for social change. I am inspired by Myers' attention to a population widely considered disabled and Mayerson's argument that technology can be harnessed to better engage people in positive psychology interventions.

David Myers: As a person with hearing loss, I have benefitted many times from how the United Kingdom (and the Nordic countries) provide assistive listening – via "hearing loops" that broadcast sound wirelessly via hearing aids and cochlear implants, which can serve as customized, in-the-ear loudspeakers. Most American venues, including theaters and worship places, instead offer assistive listening that is hearing aid incompatible (requiring one to locate, check out, and wear a special receiver and headset, which few people with hearing loss will do). After confirming that the technology works beautifully in my home (putting my TV loudspeakers right in my ears), I introduced this hearing aid compatible assistive listening to West Michigan, where it can now be found in hundreds of public venues, including all gate areas of Michigan's second largest airport. With a spirit of collective efficacy, fellow hearing advocates, informed by www.hearingloop.org and by two dozen articles in various hearing-related periodicals, are now introducing the technology to other communities. These include New York City, which has installed it in 488 subway information booths. In 2010 a national service club organization and the president of the American Academy of Audiology joined the advocacy. News stories appeared in media such as *Scientific American*. New companies have begun manufacturing and marketing this product. As more and more people appreciate this doubled hearing aid functionality, we are seeing how positive thinking and collective grit can enable social change and promote human flourishing and positive aging for those with hearing loss.

Neal Mayerson: Positive psychology is being applied by a variety of helping practitioners, from psychotherapists treating clinical disorders, to teachers in classrooms, to coaches helping people with a variety of subclinical problems of daily living and in pursuit of personal aspirations. Though practitioners are incorporating the "latest and greatest" from psychological science, most are still delivering their services via old methodologies that do not take full advantage of advanced communication technologies. These technologies, especially when combined with positive psychology, address one of the most vexing challenges in the helping professions – namely how to engage people in the helping process and keep them involved long enough to experience the benefits of the process.

This problem of engaging clients/patients in services for a long enough period of time to deliver an adequate treatment dosage is a well-documented dilemma for practitioners. People drop out of intervention programs prematurely at relatively high rates and for a variety of reasons, including cost of services, the inconvenience of pre-appointed times, and inadequate alliance building between clients and their helping professionals. New technology-leveraged methods of delivering services offer the opportunity for positive psychology to broaden its reach and build intervention effectiveness.

Therapeutic alliance is considered to be one of the most important and stable predictors of intervention outcome and early reports from practitioners suggest that a "positive" and "strengths" approach early on in an intervention may help establish a positive alliance. Positive psychology practitioners are becoming accustomed to hearing remarks such as "No one has ever been interested in what's right with me. They are always looking for what's wrong." Starting the helping process by looking at client strengths and resources may be strengthening the alliance and instilling hope. Recent research by Fluckiger and Holtforth has supported the alliance-building potential of a strengths-based approach which in turn resulted in improved outcomes. In this study of psychotherapy with general outpatients presenting with anxiety and depression disorders, therapists were primed for 10 min prior to the first five sessions. The priming focused therapists on the client's strengths. Results after 20 therapy sessions showed improved therapeutic alliance and outcomes compared to a control group.

Further, the short "communication bursts" that characterize email and text messaging allow for a density of interaction that can help strengthen the alliance. Simple supportive emails or text messages coming with appropriate frequency can go a long way in helping a client feel connected to their therapist or coach and imbue the client with a sense of therapist-caring. More importantly, though, new communication technology can be used as the *primary* modality for delivering services, not just as an adjunctive modality. Pioneering work at Hummingbird Coaching Services has found that intensity and term of engagement can be improved compared to face-to-face or telephonic delivery, and that the cost of services can be reduced significantly by making the helping process more time efficient from both the client and therapist/coach perspectives. Experimental studies have shown that online delivery of coaching services can be equally or more effective than face-to-face and telephonic delivery modalities.

The key seems to be *asynchronous communication*. While synchronous communication requires that two people communicate at the same time, asynchronous communication renders time and place irrelevant. Email is the most ubiquitous form of asynchronous communication, where the sender can communicate his/her message at a time of convenience for him/her, and the other party can then read and respond at a different time of their convenience. It seems that optimized convenience in helping relationships encourages better engagement than synchronous methods of delivery such as face-to-face or telephonic methods which require that the parties set aside time in, what for many are, busy and hectic life schedules. Further, asynchronous communication has grown in a culture of brevity while synchronous communication has evolved in a culture of expansiveness. While emails or text messages might take only seconds or a few minutes to compose or to read, phone calls and in-person communication typically takes much more time. It appears that 2 min at the right time may be as or more valuable than 20 min at a pre-appointed time. Such pre-appointed times are not designed to take advantage of "teachable moments," whereby asynchronous communication is perfectly designed to capture moments of heightened interest, motivation, and receptivity. As the saying goes, "timing can be everything."

Finally, the remarkable study by Seligman and colleagues (2005) showed that simple instructions delivered via the Internet *outside* the context of a relationship with a coach/therapist can produce significant increases in happiness and decreases in depression that last through 6-month follow-up assessment. This study shows the possibility that might lie in automated interventions delivered through the Internet or smart phones. Regarding the latter, smart phones are now being used to gather real-time self-observation data and brief survey data as well as to push messages that support, remind, and guide people in their efforts to change a variety of behaviors. This technology holds much promise due to its ability to keep change goals top-of-mind and its potential for informing clients and coaches with real-time, treatment-relevant data that are less biased than data collected retrospectively. Exploratory efforts also offer automated, self-guided happiness programs that people can download onto their cell phones. And, Internet-based social networks and blogs are commonplace venues now in which people share information and personal support with one another that can help in their pursuit of wellness.

In summary, early efforts to marry positive psychology with advanced communication technologies have shown promise in terms of improving engagement rates and bringing down cost of service. Broadening the accessibility of psychotherapy and coaching services by making them more convenient and cost effective will help positive psychology achieve its promise of helping people build good lives for themselves and tilt the world toward greater levels of virtuous behavior.

Finally, I received a commentary for this afterword from Ruut Veenhoven. Ruut is among the most well-respected happiness researchers in the world and, as a sociologist, has been concerned with happiness policy and social change for decades. His commentary speaks directly about the link between the individual and the collective:

Ruut Veenhoven: We live now longer than ever in human history. Life expectancy at birth is now about 80 years in western nations, while 100 years ago it was only some 50 years. This remarkable extension of our lifetime is largely due to the development of knowledge that allowed both better cure of the sick and better prevention of disease. This begs the question whether happiness can be furthered in a similar way. Can better knowledge about happiness help to make the next generations happier than we are now?

My answer to that question is "yes". Like in curative health care we can develop evidence-based interventions to "cure" unhappiness. Like in preventive health care we can also identify conditions for happiness and develop policies on that basis. Positive psychology is developing that kind of knowledge right now. I gather the fruits of that research in my World Database of Happiness (http://worlddatabaseofhappiness.eur.nl).

Will this create a heaven on earth? I think not. Perfect happiness is impossible, as is eternal life. Still we gain a lot. Average happiness in the world is now about 6 on scale 0–10. An average of 8.5 is possible, as the case of Denmark demonstrates. Will happier people make a better society? Probably "yes." Happiness enhances active involvement, creativity, and sociability. For that reason happy people tend to be better citizens and societies with responsible citizens are in a better position to deal with the future of mankind.

I respect Veenhoven's tempered answer. It is balanced and realistic, even as it is evidence based and hopeful. We must intervene at both the individual and group levels to promote positive emotion which, in turn, is a vital curative mechanism for relationships and psychological health. Fortunately, the information contained in the chapters of this book provides a number of practical ways of achieving the goal of positive social change. We will not all agree on which changes should take place, or on the pace at which they should be enacted. But consensus need not be a prerequisite for action. Instead, I would hope that this volume serves as a flashpoint for positive psychology, which is – after all – the science of a better world.

Coventry, UK   Robert Biswas-Diener

Index

Lightning Source UK Ltd.
Milton Keynes UK
17 January 2011

165847UK00005B/14/P

9 789048 199372